Handbook of Pediatric Retinal OCT and the Eye-Brain Connection

FIRST EDITION

Handbook of Pediatric Retinal OCT and the Eye-Brain Connection

Editor
CYNTHIA A. TOTH, MD
Joseph AC Wadsworth Professor of Ophthalmology and
Professor of Biomedical Engineering
Duke University
Durham, NC

Associate Editor
SALLY S. ONG, MD
Vitreoretinal Surgery Fellow
Ophthalmology
Johns Hopkins University
Baltimore, MD

ELSEVIER

Handbook of Pediatric Retinal OCT and the Eye-Brain Connection   ISBN: 978-0-323-60984-5

Notices

Practitioners and researchers must always rely on their own experience and knowledge in evaluating and using any information, methods, compounds or experiments described herein. Because of rapid advances in the medical sciences, in particular, independent verification of diagnoses and drug dosages should be made. To the fullest extent of the law, no responsibility is assumed by Elsevier, authors, editors or contributors for any injury and/or damage to persons or property as a matter of products liability, negligence or otherwise, or from any use or operation of any methods, products, instructions, or ideas contained in the material herein.

Library of Congress Control Number: 2019937966

Content Strategist: Kayla Wolfe
Content Development Manager: Katie De Francesco
Content Development Specialist: Angie Breckon
Publishing Services Manager: Deepthi Unni
Project Manager: Janish Ashwin Paul
Design Direction: Ryan Cook

Printed in China
Last digit is the print number: 9 8 7 6 5 4 3 2 1

1600 John F. Kennedy Blvd.
Ste 1800
Philadelphia, PA 19103-899

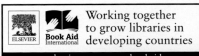

Working together
to grow libraries in
developing countries

www.elsevier.com • www.bookaid.org

To my husband, David F. Katz, for his understanding and support; to The Rockefeller Foundation, for providing me with a nurturing space to develop this book; to the children and their families, who have inspired, participated in research, and advanced our understanding of pediatric eye and brain development; and to Sally Ong, who was a remarkable powerhouse in the organization and editing of this book.

— Cynthia Toth

To my husband, Luke, for his unwavering encouragement and love. To my parents, Henry and Julie, and brothers Colin, Jeremy and Joshua, who have always supported my dreams through the years. To my mentor, Dr. Toth, a trailblazer for women and men in retina who has inspired me and many others with her countless contributions to our profession.

— Sally Ong

FOREWORD

The textbook, *Handbook of Pediatric Retinal OCT and the Eye-Brain Connection,* edited by Cynthia A. Toth and Sally S. Ong provides an invaluable and easy-to-use resource for pediatric retina specialists, pediatric ophthalmologists and many other clinicians who care for infants and children. There are practical tips for hands-on use of OCT in infants and children and ways to set up programs in the clinic, operating room or neonatal nursery. In addition, there is information on structural features of the retina in developmental, acquired or inherited conditions that affect the retina, optic nerve and visual pathways in children.

OCT imaging has improved our abilities to diagnose causes of reduced vision acuity in infants or children by providing structural information of the macula in association with visual acuity. In addition, our understanding of the development of visual acuity and function in children is optimized through longitudinal evaluations that identify changes in macular structure over time with development of visual acuity. Besides alerting the clinician to seek a diagnosis to align with macular abnormalities, OCT structural features can encourage physicians early on to emphasize the importance of enriched environments to maximize visual development and quality of life of the child. The structural changes identified by OCT and OCTA enable us to formulate new ideas on the pathophysiology of vision loss and have steered us to alternative hypotheses in some conditions, enabling us to rethink experimental approaches to better understand pathophysiology and develop better managements. Several conditions connect the retinal structure and brain pathways, among these incontinentia pigmenti, albinism, and effects of prematurity, and sometimes alert us of possible brain abnormalities by detecting findings on retinal OCT.

The straight-forward ability to click figure links within the text to the actual figures allows easy reading and comprehension. There is easy access to sections within the chapter through the comprehensive Table of Contents and through the keyword search functionality in the interactive eBook. This textbook is a one-in-a kind and important resource for those caring for or studying conditions affecting the retina and vision in infants and children.

Mary Elizabeth Hartnett, MD, FACS, FARVO
Calvin S. and JeNeal N. Hatch
Presidential Endowed Chair in Ophthalmology and Visual Sciences
Vitreoretinal Medical and Surgical Service
Director of Pediatric Retina,
Adjunct Professor of Pediatrics,
Adjunct Professor of Neurobiology and Anatomy
Principal Investigator Retinal Angiogenesis Laboratory
John A. Moran Eye Center
Salt Lake City, UT

As many ophthalmic researchers have noted, the eye is an approachable part of the brain,[1] the retina is the entry to the visual pathway,[2] and the stratified retinal structures develop throughout early life.[3] Optical coherence tomography (OCT) imaging of the retina and optic nerve head, although still not offering the capacity to assess molecular structures or function, has transformed the diagnosis and management of retinal, optic nerve, and even central nervous system diseases. In general, however, OCT textbooks have been written with a focus on the mature retina, with inclusion of pediatric diseases primarily through images from children old enough to cooperate with the imaging procedure. The retina, the optic nerve head, and the choroidal layers are immature at birth and differ from those of adults, and their appearances on OCT imaging change with growth of the individual. These differences are more profound with preterm birth and with developmental abnormalities, diseases, and injuries that are unique to infants and children. This book was inspired by the research described previously, by the adult OCT handbook by Duker et al.,[4] and by our discovery that with the aid of OCT, we can visualize and monitor developing retinal structures at birth and throughout childhood.

In this handbook on pediatric OCT imaging, we address the differences between OCT imaging of the infant or young child's retina and that of the adult and how the OCT image may reveal associations between brain injury or disease and delayed neurodevelopment in the infant. Furthermore, we describe methods of imaging and ways to avoid pitfalls in the imaging of children and infants. Experts in pediatric OCT analysis provide guidance in identifying OCT layers and abnormalities and techniques to distinguish these from artifacts in pediatric diseases. Finally, our contributors provide relevant examples of OCT images of pediatric retinal and optic nerve diseases in clinical care, as well as suggestions for use of such images in pediatric research.

Our intent is that the compact format, the high-quality images, and the clear explanations provided in this book will be useful to ophthalmologists, neuroscientists, and other researchers working with children, technicians and photographers who work to capture these important images in young children, students, and multidisciplinary teams working to improve children's health and potential. We are indebted to many subspecialists who care for the eye and brain health of children and infants, and we are especially grateful to the children we have studied, as well as their families, who have taught us so much about caring for the whole child.

References

1. Dowling John E. *The Retina, An Approachable Part of the Brain.* Cambridge, MA: Harvard University Press; 1987.
2. Benjamin E. Reese. Development of the Retina and Optic Pathway. *Vision Res.* 2011 Apr 13;51(7):613–632.
3. Mann Ida C. *The Development of the Human Eye.* London: Cambridge University Press; 1928.
4. Duker Jay S, Waheed Nadia K, Goldman Darin R. *Handbook of Retinal OCT.* Philadelphia: Elsevier; 2014.

CONTRIBUTORS

Mohsin H. Ali, MD
Fellow in Vitreoretinal Surgery
Duke University Department of
 Ophthalmology
Durham, NC

Isaac Bleicher, BS
Medical Student
Duke University School of Medicine
Durham, NC

Xi Chen, MD, PhD
Assistant Professor of Ophthalmology
Duke University Department of
 Ophthalmology
Durham, NC

Alexandria Dandridge
Research Analyst
Duke University Department of
 Ophthalmology
Durham, NC

Mays El-Dairi, MD
Associate Professor of Ophthalmology
Duke University Department of
 Ophthalmology
Durham, NC

Amanda Ely, MD
Assistant Professor of Ophthalmology
Penn State Health Milton S. Hershey Medical
 Center Department of Ophthalmology
Hershey, PA

Avni P. Finn, MD, MBA
Fellow in Vitreoretinal Surgery
Duke University Department of
 Ophthalmology
Durham, NC

Sharon F. Freedman, MD
Professor of Ophthalmology
 Professor of Pediatrics
Duke University Department of
 Ophthalmology
Durham, NC

Hesham Gabr, MD, MSc
Research Fellow
Duke University Department of
 Ophthalmology
Durham, NC

Dilraj S. Grewal, MD
Associate Professor of Ophthalmology
Duke University Department of
 Ophthalmology
Durham, NC

Robert J. House, MD
Research Fellow
Duke University Department of
 Ophthalmology
Durham, NC

S. Tammy Hsu, BA
Medical Student
Duke University School of Medicine
Durham, NC

Michael P. Kelly, FOPS
Director of Duke Eye Imaging
Duke University Department of
 Ophthalmology
Durham, NC

Shwetha Mangalesh, MBBS
Research Fellow
Duke University Department of
 Ophthalmology
Durham, NC

Prithvi Mruthyunjaya, MD, MHS
Associate Professor of Ophthalmology
Stanford University Department of
 Ophthalmology
Palo Alto, CA

Sally S. Ong, MD
Research Fellow
Duke University Department of
 Ophthalmology
Durham, NC

Adam L. Rothman, MD
Resident in Ophthalmology
Duke University Department of
  Ophthalmology
Durham, NC

Neeru Sarin, MBBS
Research Analyst
Duke University Department of
  Ophthalmology
Durham, NC

Adrienne W. Scott, MD
Associate Professor of Ophthalmology
Johns Hopkins University Department of
  Ophthalmology
Baltimore, MD

Vincent Tai, MS
Research Analyst
Duke University Department of
  Ophthalmology
Durham, NC

Akshay Thomas, MD, MS
Fellow in Vitreoretinal Surgery
Duke University Department of
  Ophthalmology
Durham, NC

James Tian, BS
Medical Student
Duke University School of Medicine
Durham, NC

Cynthia A. Toth, MD
Joseph AC Wadsworth Professor of
  Ophthalmology
Professor of Biomedical Engineering
Duke University Department of
  Ophthalmology and Biomedical
  Engineering
Durham, NC

Du Tran-Viet, BS
Research Analyst
Duke University Department of
  Ophthalmology
Durham, NC

Lejla Vajzovic, MD
Assistant Professor of Ophthalmology
Duke University Department of
  Ophthalmology
Durham, NC

Christian Viehland, PhD
Graduate Student
Duke University Department of Biomedical
  Engineering
Durham, NC

Katrina Postell Winter, BS
Research Analyst
Duke University Department of
  Ophthalmology
Durham, NC

Glenn Yiu, MD, PhD
Associate Professor of Ophthalmology
  University of California, Davis Department
  of Ophthalmology
Sacramento, CA

Steven Yoon, BS
Medical Student
Duke University School of Medicine
Durham, NC

Wenlan Zhang, MD
Fellow in Vitreoretinal Surgery
Duke University Department of
  Ophthalmology
Durham, NC

Aniruddha Agarwal, MD
Advanced Eye Center, PGIMER
Chandigarh, India
Stanley M. Truhlsen Eye Institute
University of Nebraska Medical Center
Ocular Imaging Research and Reading Center
    (OIRRC)
Menlo Park, CA, United States

Isaac Bleicher, BS
Medical Student
Duke University School of Medicine
Durham, NC, United States

Nathan Cheung, OD
Medical Instructor
Duke University Department of
    Ophthalmology
Durham, NC, United States

Laura Enyedi, MD
Associate Professor of Ophthalmology
Duke University Department of
    Ophthalmology
Durham, NC, United States

Sharon Fekrat, MD
Professor of Ophthalmology
Duke University Department of
    Ophthalmology
Durham, NC, United States

Alessandro Iannaccone, MD, MS
Professor of Ophthalmology
Duke University Department of
    Ophthalmology
Durham, NC, United States

Miguel Materin, MD
Professor of Ophthalmology
Duke University Department of
    Ophthalmology
Durham, NC, United States

Hoan T. Ngo, PhD
Postdoctoral Scholar
Duke University Department of
    Ophthalmology
Durham, NC, United States

Mark Pennesi, MD, PhD
Associate Professor of Ophthalmology
Casey Eye Institute
Oregon Health and Science University
Portland, OR, United States

Camila Ventura, MD, PhD
Retina and Vitreous Specialist
Head of the Department of Clinical Research
Altino Ventura Foundation and HOPE Eye
    Hospital
Department of Ophthalmology
Altino Ventura Foundation
Recife, Brazil

Steven Yoon, BS
Medical Student
Duke University School of Medicine
Durham, NC, United States

Imaging the retina of infants and young children by using optical coherence tomography (OCT) would not be possible without the individual efforts of dedicated biomedical engineers, technicians, and clinician researchers or without funding from donors and research grants. Joseph Izatt, PhD, biomedical engineer at Duke, and his graduate students have innovated and translated their imaging discoveries into systems that are useful in the health care of children. Stephanie Chiu, PhD and Sina Farsiu, PhD developed pediatric-specific OCT image analytics. Dr. Sharon Freedman partnered with me from the start in advancing the care of children's eyes and in research. Dr. Michael Cotten, neonatologist, along with our nurses and the coordinators of the Intensive Care Nursery (ICN), believed in infant eye imaging and welcomed our research in the nursery. Dr. Lejla Vajzovic, Dr. Mays El-Dairi, our student researchers—notably Dr. Ramiro Maldonado, Dr. Adam Rothman and Dr. Shwetha Mangalesh—and the members of the Duke Advanced Research in SD/SS OCT Imaging (DARSI) Laboratory, Du Tran-Viet, Dr. Neeru Sarin, Michelle McCall, Vincent Tai, Alexandria Dandridge, and Katrina Winter, have performed translational research with dedication and with respect for the children and their families. James Andrew and the Andrew Family Charitable Foundation, The Hartwell Foundation, Research to Prevent Blindness, the Retina Research Foundation and additional donors each provided essential support, personal interest, and valuable guidance through the early development of OCT imaging for young children. Support was also provided by the National Institutes of Health (NIH) through competitive research grants.

CONTENTS

Introduction to Pediatric Retinal OCT Imaging

CHAPTER 1

Introduction to OCT Imaging in Infants and Children

Cynthia A. Toth

It has been over 25 years since the development of optical coherence tomography (OCT) and its rapid introduction for ophthalmic use. The first OCT imaging in a young child or in infants was with tabletop time domain OCT systems (Stratus; Carl Zeiss Meditec, Jena, Germany), with children/infants placed under general anesthesia and positioned either prone on an anti-Trendelenburg tilted table, with the neck extended to position on the chin rest,[1,2] or on the side.[3] We recognized the need for OCT systems that would enable imaging in the supine infant or child. We thus modified a portable nonhuman spectral domain (SD) OCT system by Bioptigen (now Leica) for investigational human use. In 2009, we published several reports of supine imaging of infants and children: bedside imaging in an awake infant to visualize preretinal neovascularization in aggressive posterior retinopathy of prematurity (ROP)[4] and imaging of retinal detachment in ROP, macular hole, retinal folds, and epiretinal membrane in infants with nonaccidental trauma, and in a young child with Hermansky-Pudlak syndrome to visualize persisting inner retinal layers in the fovea.[5,6] In each of these cases, the higher speed of SD-OCT has enabled us to capture a volume scan across the macula, ensuring that information about the fovea accurately represents the foveal center. These reports were soon followed by our reports of novel findings in infants based on more widespread use of handheld SD-OCT in awake infants at the bedside. We characterized the stages of preterm infant foveal development, discovered macular cystoid spaces in preterm infants,[7,8] and identified subfoveal fluid in some healthy newborn infants.[9] At the same time, in India, investigators modified a tabletop SD-OCT system (Spectralis; Heidelberg Engineering, Heidelberg, Germany) for research and also imaged macular cystoid spaces in awake supine preterm infants.[10] By 2012, the U.S. Food and Drug Administration (FDA) cleared the first handheld SD-OCT system for use in neonates (Envisu; Bioptigen/Leica, Morrisville, NC).

From the first applications of OCT in children, OCT images and data have brought new insight into retinal and optic nerve diseases of older children who can cooperate for tabletop imaging. Many eye researchers and specialists have contributed to improving our understanding of the pediatric retina and optic nerve head from birth and throughout childhood through OCT imaging.[11] As in adult disease, in pediatric cases, OCT imaging of the optic nerve head and retina captures microanatomic information on tissues that are an extension of the diencephalon. This opens the door for access to information on pathology related to brain injury and brain maldevelopment. In young children, eyes and the brain grow rapidly, and thus the microstructures undergo large developmental changes with growth. Retinal and optic nerve head abnormalities in infants and young children may thus reflect injuries, inherited or acquired diseases, tumors, or even abnormalities in brain development. These are very important considerations in infants and children who, unlike adults, may not be capable of reporting symptoms of disease or injury. The relevant retinal and optic nerve findings relative to the brain are thus highlighted in each chapter in this text.

This text takes a structured look at the advancing field of pediatric OCT imaging. We recognize the unique aspects of retinal and optic nerve head imaging in infants and children and its

2

relationship to brain development and disease. We also address working with children and their families to capture and share images. We have described methods for optimizing scan quality and imaging areas of interest and new modalities, such as swept-source OCT imaging and OCT angiography, and the relevance of OCT imaging across a range of pediatric diseases.

This is an exciting era where every day new imaging discoveries are changing our prior understanding of infant disease—for example, the impact of hypoxic ischemic encephalopathy on the retina, which had not previously been studied because of the difficulty in approaching infants with such diseases for conventional examination. We have been able to perform OCT imaging of the retina in the intensive care nursery, without the need for pharmacologic pupil dilation.[12] Such advances point toward a future of expanded applications for OCT imaging in children. This handbook provides a summary and a roadmap for those working in this field.

References

1. Patel CK, Chen SD, Farmery AD. Optical coherence tomography under general anesthesia in a child with nystagmus. *Am J Ophthalmol.* 2004;137(6):1127–1129.
2. Patel CK. Optical coherence tomography in the management of acute retinopathy of prematurity. *Am J Ophthalmol.* 2006;141(3):582–584.
3. Joshi MM, Trese MT, Capone Jr A. Optical coherence tomography findings in stage 4A retinopathy of prematurity: a theory for visual variability. *Ophthalmology.* 2006;113(4):657–660.
4. Chavala SH, Farsiu S, Maldonado R, Wallace DK, Freedman SF, Toth CA. Insights into advanced retinopathy of prematurity using handheld spectral domain optical coherence tomography imaging. *Ophthalmology.* 2009;116(12):2448–2456.
5. Chong GT, Farsiu S, Freedman SF, et al. Abnormal foveal morphology in ocular albinism imaged with spectral-domain optical coherence tomography. *Arch Ophthalmol.* 2009;127(1):37–44.
6. Scott AW, Farsiu S, Enyedi LB, Wallace DK, Toth CA. Imaging the infant retina with a hand-held spectral-domain optical coherence tomography device. *Am J Ophthalmol.* 2009;147(2):364–373.
7. Maldonado RS, Izatt JA, Sarin N, et al. Optimizing hand-held spectral domain optical coherence tomography imaging for neonates, infants and children. *Invest Ophthalmol Vis Sci.* 2010;51(5):2678–2685.
8. Lee AC, Maldonado RS, Sarin N, et al. Macular features from spectral-domain optical coherence tomography as an adjunct to indirect ophthalmoscopy in retinopathy of prematurity. *Retina.* 2011;31 (8):1470–1482.
9. Cabrera MT, Maldonado RS, Toth CA, et al. Subfoveal fluid in healthy full-term newborns observed by handheld spectral-domain optical coherence tomography. *Am J Ophthalmol.* 2012;153(1):167–175.
10. Vinekar A, Avadhani K, Sivakumar M, et al. Understanding clinically undetected macular changes in early retinopathy of prematurity on spectral domain optical coherence tomography. *Invest Ophthalmol Vis Sci.* 2011;52:5183–5188.
11. Lee H, Proudlock FA, Gottlob I. Pediatric optical coherence tomography in clinical practice-recent progress. *Invest Ophthalmol Vis Sci.* July 1, 2016;57(9). OCT69-79.
12. Tran-Viet D, Wong BM, Mangalesh S, Maldonado R, Cotten CM, Toth CA. Handheld spectral domain optical coherence tomography imaging through the undilated pupil in infants born preterm or with hypoxic injury or hydrocephalus. *Retina.* 2018;38(8):1588–1594.

CHAPTER 2

Basic Principles of OCT and OCTA Imaging of Infants and Children

Christian Viehland

Principles of OCT

Optical coherence tomography (OCT) is a cross-sectional imaging modality that uses infrared light to provide micron-scale resolution of in vivo tissue.[1] OCT can be viewed as the optical analogue of ultrasonography. However, the use of light instead of sound leads to micron-scale resolution instead of millimeter-scale resolution. OCT systems generate images by splitting light into sample and reference arms. Light back-scattered from the sample is compared with light from the reference arm to reconstruct sample reflectivity as a function of depth. Cross-sectional images (B-scans) and volumes are generated by scanning the OCT beam across the retina.

Most commercial OCT systems use an approach to OCT called *spectral-domain optical coherence tomography* (SD-OCT). Typical SD-OCT systems use 850-nm centered light, have a lateral resolution of approximately 12 μm, an axial resolution of approximately 4 μm, and can acquire individual depth scans (A-scans) between 20,000 and 80,000 times per second. Some of the newest commercial systems are swept-source optical coherence tomography (SS-OCT) systems. SS-OCT uses a different 1050-nm centered light source that is generally faster (>100 kHz A-scans), has better penetration in tissue, and has better depth of imaging. However, the longer wavelength results in lower resolutions (~20 μm lateral and ~8 μm axial).[2]

PORTABLE SYSTEMS FOR SUPINE IMAGING

Most OCT systems are tabletop systems that require a compliant, seated subject. Two commercial armature-based OCT systems are currently marketed—the Ivue/Istand from Optovue and the Heidelberg Flex. Both suspend full-sized OCT systems over the subject and can be used with cooperative subjects in the supine position or subjects under anesthesia. However, these systems are difficult to use in awake infants and cannot be used in an incubator. Most OCT imaging of infants is performed with handheld OCT systems. Handheld OCT systems provide the portability and flexibility needed for bedside imaging of noncompliant subjects. There is one commercially available handheld OCT probe designed for supine retinal imaging, the Bioptigen/Leica Envisu c2300. This system has been in use since 2009[3] for infant OCT imaging and has been utilized to image a wide range of pediatric pathologies.

Adjustments to Optimize Imaging of the Small Infant Eye

Retinal OCT scans are formed by scanning unfocused light into the eye. The OCT beam pivots in the pupil, and the light is focused by the eye's optics onto the retina. The width of the scan on the retina is a function of both the angle of the scan at the pupil and the subject's eye length. In infants, eye length changes from 15.1 mm at 30 weeks postmenstrual age (PMA) to 21.8 mm at 2 years of age. This causes a 10 × 10 mm scan in adults to shrink to 9.1 × 9.1 mm in a 2-year-old and 6.3 × 6.3 mm in an infant at 30 weeks PMA. The short length of the infant eye also causes the pivot of the scan to move anterior to the pupil. This results in significant vignetting (clipping of the OCT beam) and poor imaging quality. To account for this, the OCT reference arm must be shortened such that the scan pivots in the pupil plane. Careful system calibration is needed to generate accurate scan lengths and reference arm positions given a patient's age and eye length.[4]

Principles of OCTA

OCT angiography (OCTA) is a functional extension of OCT that allows for imaging of the retinal microvasculature.[5] OCTA is an active area of research in adult ophthalmology and has started to enter pediatric ophthalmology. OCTA generates contrast by analyzing the differences between regions of flow, where blood flow causes fluctuations in the OCT signal, and regions of static tissue, where the OCT signal remains relatively constant. OCTA scans consist of volumes where each B-scan is repeated multiple times. Taking a measure of variance or decorrelation across the repeated B-scans creates the OCTA B-scans, which contain depth-resolved flow information. Typically, enface projections of the OCTA volumes are created by using segmentation to separate the different layers of retinal vasculature.

Because OCTA volumes require multiple B-scans and are typically more densely sampled compared with regular OCT volumes, OCTA volumes require long acquisition times. Even with the fastest OCT systems, acquisition time is often greater than 3 seconds. This makes OCTA images particularly sensitive to saccades and other sources of motion that become bright streaks on OCTA images. There are two common approaches for removing motion artifacts.[6] The first is to acquire multiple OCTA images at the same location and use software to remove the motion artifacts and register the volumes together. The second is to use a scanning laser ophthalmoscope to detect eye motion and rescan corrupted parts of the image.

References

1. Huang D, Swanson EA, Lin CP, et al. Optical coherence tomography. *Science.* 1991;254(5035):1178–1181.
2. Choma M, Izatt J. Theory of optical coherence tomography. In: Drexler W, Fujimoto JG, eds. *Optical Coherence Tomography.* Springer, Berlin, Heidelberg; 2008:47–72.
3. Scott AW, Farsiu S, Enyedi LB, Wallace DK, Toth CA. Imaging the infant retina with a hand-held spectral-domain optical coherence tomography device. *Am J Ophthalmol.* 2009;147(2):364–373. e362.
4. Maldonado RS, Izatt JA, Sarin N, et al. Optimizing hand-held spectral domain optical coherence tomography imaging for neonates, infants, and children. *Invest Ophthalmol Vis Sci.* 2010;51(5):2678–2685.
5. Zhang A, Zhang Q, Chen CL, Wang RK. Methods and algorithms for optical coherence tomography-based angiography: a review and comparison. *J Biomed Opt.* 2015;20(10):100901.
6. Camino A, Zhang M, Gao SS, et al. Evaluation of artifact reduction in optical coherence tomography angiography with real-time tracking and motion correction technology. *Biomed Opt Express.* 2016; 7(10):3905–3915.

CHAPTER 3

Optimizing Systems and Setup for OCT and OCTA Imaging of Children and Infants in the Nursery, Clinic, and Operating Room

Du Tran-Viet ■ Michael Kelly ■ Sally S. Ong

CHAPTER OUTLINE

The introduction of portable systems has greatly increased access to OCT imaging in the pediatric population. Because tabletop OCT imaging requires the use of a chin rest, patient cooperation, and adequate fixation, infants and young children were traditionally excluded from OCT imaging when only tabletop systems were available. With the commercial availability of both portable and tabletop systems, OCT imaging is now possible in diverse clinical settings (nursery, clinic, and operating room) and in children of all ages (neonates to teenagers).

OCT imaging in the pediatric population requires special considerations. The portable system, in particular, has been optimized for the unique biometric properties of the small infant eye (as briefly discussed in Chapter 2, and further discussed below). In both portable and tabletop systems, there are also setup considerations to optimize imaging in infants and children. This is important because most OCT systems were built with the adult patient in mind. Infants and prepubertal children have smaller body habitus and often lack the ability to comprehend and follow instructions.

OCT angiography (OCTA) is relatively new to the field of ophthalmology, and consequently, only a few imaging studies use this modality in the pediatric population. Also, as discussed in Chapter 2, OCTA requires long acquisition times and is exquisitely sensitive to saccades and other motion artifacts. For this reason, it is currently not possible to perform OCTA in awake infants and young children who are unable to comply with the instruction to be still. Tabletop OCTA images may be obtained in older, compliant children in the clinic. Currently, an investigational OCTA armature system allows for the imaging of children under anesthesia. Because of the long duration of the scanning procedure, adequate pupillary dilation and lubrication are especially important when acquiring OCTA images.

Optimization of Handheld OCT System for the Pediatric Eye

Axial length, refractive error, corneal curvature, and astigmatism are all properties that affect optical imaging, and these values change with age:

Axial length: Changes rapidly in the neonatal period at 0.16 mm per week. This change slows with age, and after age 15 years, the growth is no longer significant.[1,2]

Refractive error: At 30 to 35 weeks postmenstrual age (PMA), mean refractive errors are reportedly −1.00 +/− 0.90 diopter (D) (range −3.00 to + 1.00 D) with a shift to hyperopia (mean + 0.50 +/− 0.2 D) from age 36 weeks to 6 years.[1,2]

Corneal curvature: The newborn cornea is typically steeper compared with the adult cornea (mean central corneal power 48.00–58.50 D) and after 3 months decreases to adult values.[1,3-7]

Astigmatism: The newborn eye also has greater astigmatism compared with that of the adult and decreases by half after approximately 6 months.[4]

These characteristics result in a model infant/young child eye that is different from that of an adult (Fig. 3.1). The commercially available handheld OCT system (Bioptigen/Leica Envisu C2300), which was developed with neonates and children in mind, can and should be optimized to adjust for these biometric differences across ages.[8]

Reference arm: The default reference arm setting provided by the manufacturer is designed for a standard adult eye and therefore will cause clipping/vignetting at the side of the images, if not properly adjusted for infants and children (see Chapter 6 for an example of this artifact). To adjust the reference arm according to age, it is useful to refer to an age-corrected standard reference table (Table 3.1). On the basis of the adjusted values, the imager can turn the handle of the reference arm to minimize loss of quality at the edge of the scan. If adjustments have been made but the imager is still experiencing clipping and vignetting, the pupil may not be the optimal size for alignment.[8]

Refractive error: The autofocus feature is not available on the handheld system, so diopter correction must be made manually to get high-quality images. To do so, the imager must adjust the diopter by twisting the bore on the handheld probe in a clockwise/counterclockwise manner until the label indicating the desired refractive value is reached. The reference table (Table 3.1) provides calibrated refractive errors according to age and can be used as a starting point to set the focus. Additional adjustments to the focus may be necessary to optimize image quality. Because changes less than 2.00 D do not produce a noticeable improvement in image quality, we most often adjust in 2.00 D jumps.[8]

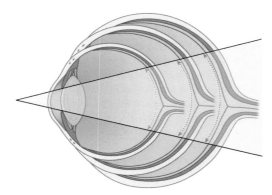

Fig. 3.1 Axial length growth in eye of an infant *(red arrowed line),* young child *(green arrowed line),* and adult *(blue arrowed line);* it can affect optical imaging of the retina.

TABLE 3.1 ■ **Age-Corrected Scan Length and Reference Arm Settings for the Bioptigen/Leica Envisu C2300**

Group Age	Refractive Error (D)	Axial Length (mm)	Reference Arm Change	Relative Scan Length on the Retina Relative to That of an Emmetropic Adult (%)
30–35 wk	−1.00	15.1	−48	63
35–39 wk	0.30	16.1	−43	67
39–41 wk	0.40	16.8	−39	70
0–1 mo	0.90	17.4	−36	73
1–2 mo	0.30	18.6	−29	78
2–6 mo	0.50	18.9	−28	79
6–12 mo	0.60	19.2	−26	80
12–18 mo	0.70	20.1	−21	84
18 mo – 2 yr	0.90	21.3	−15	89
2–3 yr	1.00	21.8	−12	91
3–4 yr	0.60	22.2	−10	93
4–5 yr	−0.80	22.3	−9	93
5–9 yr	−0.60	22.7	−7	95
10 yr – adult	−0.50	24.0	0	100
Axial myopia		26.0	+11	

Adapted from Maldonado RS, Izatt JA, Sarin N, et al. Optimizing hand-held spectral domain optical coherence tomography imaging for neonates, infants and children. *Invest Ophthalmol Vis Sci.* 2010;51(5):2678-2685. doi:10.1167/iovs.09-4403.

Scan length: In infants, the very short eye length will result in a scan that spans a much smaller area than in an adult eye. It is thus important to adjust the scan length according to age (see Table 3.1).[8]

Scan density (number of A-scans and B-scans per millimeter of retina): This is also impacted by the smaller eyes of infants. For example, a 35-degree spectral-domain OCT (SD-OCT) scan for an adult retina spans 10 mm in the adult and only 6.3 mm of retina of an infant 32 weeks of PMA (see Table 3.1). Therefore if the same A-scans per the B-scan parameters for an adult are used, then the density of the A-scans and B-scans would be higher in the infant retina. Because of the interest in rapid scanning in moving infants, the oversampling wastes scanning time. An imager can avoid this by reducing the number of scans.[8]

Optimization of OCT Setup in the Pediatric Population

In general, the child's pupil should be pharmacologically dilated to optimize imaging. This is important, even though the infrared OCT light does not constrict the pupil and imaging of a physiologically dilated pupil can be achieved under low ambient lighting.[9] Good quality imaging is also possible through a 1 mm pupil, though the alignment and distance from the eye are within a tight range.[9] Pharmacologic dilation (e.g., to a 6 mm pupil) lessens capture challenge, which reduces artifacts (see Chapter 6), especially for a novice imager. In addition, imagers should know in advance the areas of interest for imaging and, if possible, the fixation capability of each eye (e.g., fixation would be poor in an amblyopic eye or an eye with a macular lesion).

Besides these general tips to optimize OCT imaging in children, it is important to consider the individual setting (nursery, clinic, or operating room) and the age of the child (varying body habitus and degree of cooperation). Different strategies can be employed to image those without the ability to cooperate (infants, toddlers, and children with intellectual disability), those who can be coaxed to cooperate (young children), and those who can easily follow instructions (older children and teenagers).

INTENSIVE CARE NURSERY

Neonates in the intensive care nursery (ICN) often must be imaged at the bedside because they need continuous systemic monitoring. The handheld SD-OCT is the system of choice as a result of its portability. Before imaging, scan protocols should be prepared and loaded, and the imager should be positioned such that the infant's head is aligned with the imager's chest. The imager can then align himself or herself with the viewing screen and can image with the handheld probe over the infant's head (Fig. 3.2). When imaging within an incubator is necessary, this imaging setup ensures adequate space for the SD-OCT hand piece. Infants with continuous positive airway pressure (CPAP) masks can also be imaged without removing the mask. During imaging, small lateral movements are critical to aligning the scanner toward the area of interest. If images have poor signal quality, artificial tears (usually single-use, preservative-free tears in the nursery) can be used to help lubricate the cornea. As previously mentioned, adjusting the focus to correct for refractive error could also improve the signal quality.[8,9]

When possible, there should be a second person to help the primary imager. This second person can assist with operating the computer software while the imager performs the scanning. When an infant is restless, the second person can also help with soothing the infant by swaddling the infant while the imager is setting up the OCT system. The second person can also wrap his or her hands

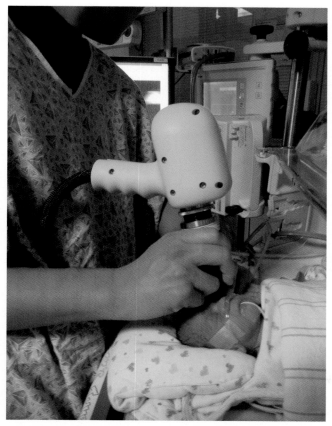

Fig. 3.2 Imaging an infant over the head in the intensive care nursery with a handheld portable system (Bioptigen/Leica Envisu C2300).

around the infant's head or body to apply warmth and pressure for comfort before, during, and after imaging. With caregiver approval, pacifiers and oral sucrose can also be used to calm the infant.[9]

CLINIC

Infants and toddlers who are too young to sit upright or stand to reach a tabletop chinrest can be imaged with a portable OCT system in the clinic. The techniques used in clinic are similar to those used in the ICN. If small enough, the infant can be laid flat across the parent's or imager's legs, with the head positioned toward the imager's chest (Fig. 3.3). When the infant is restless, a pacifier or oral sucrose can be used for soothing. The infant can also be imaged while bottle feeding. Toys and videos can be used to further distract and relax the infant. Some older infants can be imaged while sitting upright on the parent's lap.[10] A portable armature OCT system is under investigational use and may become commercially available in the future. However, the system generally does not shift fast enough for an awake and mobile infant or toddler.

If a child can stand or sit to reach the chinrest, he or she can be imaged on the tabletop OCT system. However, it is important to keep the imaging session short, with quick breaks, if necessary, because a young patient's attention span is short, and fatigue and disinterest can set in quickly. Depending on the height and size of the child, a chair or a stepstool, which should be readily available in the room, can be used (Fig. 3.4). The monitor of the OCT system should be out of the child's view to avoid distraction, and the scan protocols should be loaded and prepared before the child enters the room. The imager should warmly greet the parents and children by name and bring them

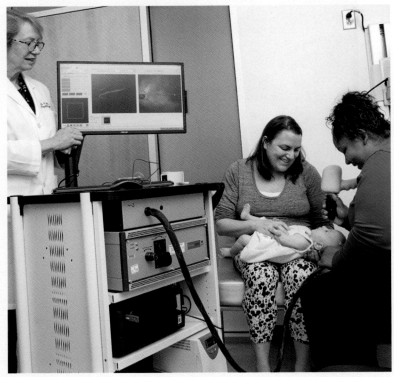

Fig. 3.3 Imaging an infant in the clinic with a handheld portable system (Bioptigen/Leica Envisu C2300).

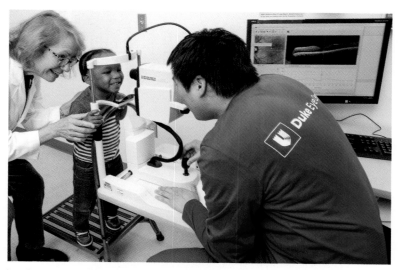

Fig. 3.4 Imaging a young child in the clinic with a tabletop system (Heidelberg Spectralis) and use of a footstool.

into the well-lit OCT room and a brief description of the imaging process should be provided to build trust. During this time, the device can be adjusted to the height of the child while engaging with the child to help keep him or her in place at the device. Smaller children can sit in the parent's lap or can kneel on the seat, with the parent holding the head in place at the chinrest. Older children may be able to stand to reach the chinrest with or without using a step stool. If the child is tall enough, he or she may sit as adults do. If standing, ensure that the child's feet are flat on the floor to reduce body movement during scanning.

Regardless of the methods chosen, ensure that the child can easily keep the forehead against the headrest and the chinrest. Adjust the headrest and the chinrest to place the lateral canthus in the middle range of the up–down movement of the imaging head. The use of a foot pedal to capture images frees the imager's hands to manage the device and the child. If the child refuses to sit and is restless during image capture, offer to image the parent or an older sibling first to reduce anxiety and provide reassurance. During imaging, determine immediately whether the system's internal or external fixation device is effective. If not effective, affix a Post-it note on the wall facing the child or use verbal instructions to direct the patient's gaze. A smartphone, tablet, or toy can be held by another person to provide a fixation target as well.[10]

OPERATING ROOM

Infants and children undergoing surgery or an examination under anesthesia in the operating room can be imaged with a handheld, armature stand, or surgical microscope–integrated OCT system. The imager should be positioned behind the infant such that the infant's head is positioned toward the imager's chest and the handheld probe/armature is situated across the infant's forehead and not over the infant's body (Fig. 3.5).[9] Use artificial tears to constantly lubricate the infant's eye to obtain good images. The imager must also be aware that the child's eye may drift as a result of the Bell's reflex. Communication with the anesthesia team may be useful and the use of a scleral depressor may assist with ocular alignment.

Below is a list of a few commercially available OCT systems. All of these systems are SD-OCT except the Topcon Triton, which is swept-source OCT (SS-OCT).

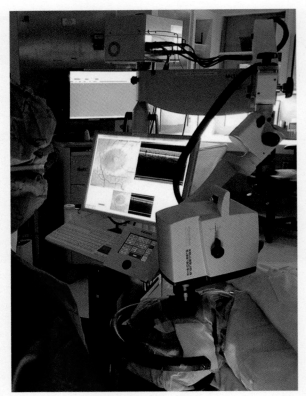

Fig. 3.5 Imaging a young child in the operating room with the Heidelberg Spectralis with Flex Module system, an investigational armature system.

Handheld

Bioptigen/Leica Envisu C2300 (Fig. 3.6)

Tabletop

Heidelberg Engineering Spectralis (Fig. 3.7)*
Zeiss Cirrus (Fig. 3.8) with OCT angiography (AngioPlex)
Optovue iVue 2 (Fig. 3.9) with OCT angiography (Angiovue)
Topcon Triton (Fig. 3.10)[†]

Armature

Heidelberg Engineering has an investigational SD-OCT and OCTA system that has yet to receive FDA approval; this research system is called *Spectralis with Flex Module* (Fig. 3.11).

---

*Heidelberg Engineering Spectralis has an investigational tabletop OCTA system, which has yet to receive approval from the U.S. Food and Drug Administration (FDA).

[†]Topcon has an investigational SS-OCTA system, which is used in Europe and Japan but is not yet FDA approved in the United States.

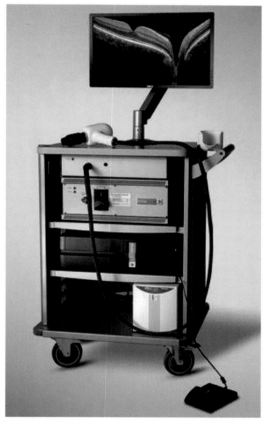

Fig. 3.6 Image of Bioptigen/Leica Envisu C2300 handheld optical coherence tomography (OCT) system. (With permission of Leica Microsystems.)

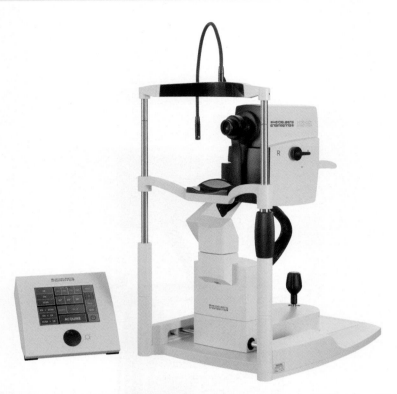

Fig. 3.7 Image of Heidelberg Spectralis tabletop optical coherence tomography (OCT) system. (Printed with permission of Heidelberg Engineering).

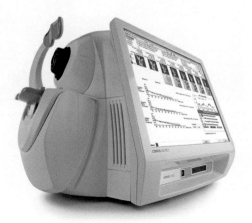

Fig. 3.8 Image of Zeiss Cirrus tabletop optical coherence tomography (OCT) system. (With permission of Carl Zeiss Meditec, AG.)

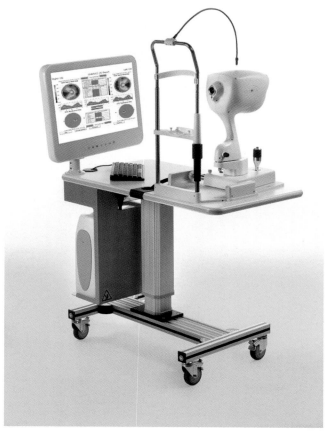

Fig. 3.9   Image of Optovue iVue2 tabletop optical coherence tomography (OCT) system. (With permission of Optovue.)

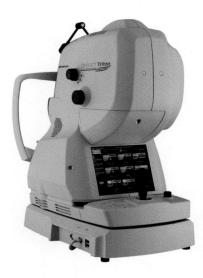

Fig. 3.10   Image of DRI OCT Triton tabletop optical coherence tomography (OCT) system. (Used by permission of Topcon (Great Britain) Medical Ltd.)

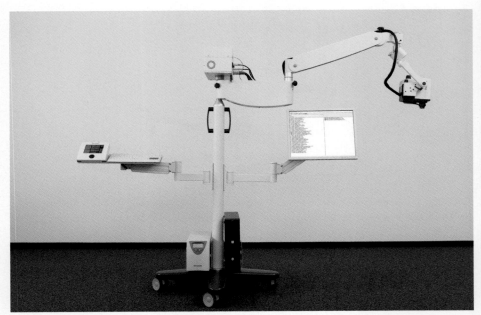

Fig. 3.11   Image of armature Heidelberg Spectralis with Flex Module optical coherence tomography (OCT) system, which is an investigational device. (Printed with permission of Heidelberg Engineering).

References

1. Gordon RA, Donzis PB. Refractive development of the human eye. *Arch Ophthalmol.* 1985;103(6):785–789.
2. Cook A, White S, Batterbury M, Clark D. Ocular growth and refractive error development in premature infants without retinopathy of prematurity. *Invest Ophthalmol Vis Sci.* 2008;49(12):5199–5207.
3. Friling R, Weinberger D, Kremer I, Avisar R, Sirota L, Snir M. Keratometry measurements in preterm and full term newborn infants. *Br J Ophthalmol.* 2004;88:8–10.
4. Isenberg SJ, Del Signore M, Chen A, Wei J, Christenson PD. Corneal topography of neonates and infants. *Arch Ophthalmol.* 2004;122:1767–1771.
5. Inagaki Y. The rapid change of corneal curvature in the neonatal period and infancy. *Arch Ophthalmol.* 1986;104:1026–1027.
6. Mohindra I, Held R, Gwiazda J, Brill S. Astigmatism in infants. *Science.* 1978;202:329.
7. Howland HC, Atkinson J, Braddick O, French J. Infant astigmatism measured by photorefraction. *Science.* 1978;202:331–333.
8. Maldonado RS, Izatt JA, Sarin N, et al. Optimizing hand-held spectral domain optical coherence tomography imaging for neonates, infants and children. *Invest Ophthalmol Vis Sci.* 2010;51(5):2678–2685.
9. Tran-Viet D, Wong BM, Mangalesh S, Maldonado R, Cotten CM, Toth CA. Handheld spectral domain optical coherence tomography imaging through the undilated pupil in infants born preterm or with hypoxic injury or hydrocephalus. *Retina.* 2018;38(8):1588–1594.
10. Lee H, Proudlock FA, Gottlob I. Pediatric optical coherence tomography in clinical practice-recent progress. *Invest Ophthalmol Vis Sci.* 2016;57(9):OCT69–79. https://doi.org/10.1167/iovs.15-18825.

CHAPTER 4

OCT and OCTA Image Capture in the Nursery, Clinic, and Operating Room

Du Tran-Viet ■ Michael P. Kelly ■ Mays El-Dairi ■
Sally S. Ong ■ Cynthia A. Toth

It is generally helpful to know which scan protocols to acquire before commencing optical coherence tomography (OCT) in patients of any age. This is especially important in infants and children because the amount of time available to capture images in this population is limited. Loss of interest and ability to cooperate as time passes is an important concern in examining and imaging the eyes of young children. Neonates in the nursery may be ill or premature; lengthy imaging sessions are undesirable, especially in these patients, and additional stimulation should be kept to a minimum.

Listed in the following sections are OCT scan acquisition protocols and their strengths and weaknesses with regard to pediatric scanning of the retina and optic nerve head. The names of scan modalities may vary, and some modalities are system specific (e.g., enhanced depth imaging [EDI] on selected spectral domain OCT [SD-OCT] systems), but they are available on most commercial OCT systems. Further details on glaucoma specific scans can be found in Chapter 70.

Aligning OCT Images

When planning imaging and orienting scans, it is important to note that OCT images in children may not be aligned as traditionally viewed in the adult eye. This may occur for many reasons: children may tilt their heads during tabletop imaging, a portable handpiece or armature may not be aligned along the sagittal or transverse planes, infants do often not fixate on a target, or the imaging system display may not invert the images captured from over the top of the head in a supine infant rather than from an upright position. Because of these effects, especially in handheld imaging of infants, such structures as the papillomacular bundle may be oriented and measured relative to the fovea to optic nerve head organizing axis.[1]

OCT Scan Acquisition Protocols

VOLUMETRIC, THREE-DIMENSIONAL (3D), CUBE SCANS

Volumetric scans (also known as 3D or cube scans) obtain multiple-raster B-scans aligned horizontally (transverse) or vertically (sagittal) across the retina. This is the most common scan protocol utilized by the retina specialist for imaging of children. These scans are especially useful for imaging of infants and children across all settings (nursery, clinic, and operating room) because these scans can capture an adequate area of OCT images of the retina and/or optic nerve even in the absence of fixation. By reviewing the entire volume in multiple views, one can determine and extract the correct location of the center of the optic nerve or foveal center.[2,3]

An OCT volume scan can be viewed (1) in 3D as a volume or cube (Fig. 4.1A), or (2) by scrolling through the successive B-scans to identify foveal or other structures (see Fig. 4.1B), (3) in an en face retinal view that sums the layers producing a retinal map in which retinal vascular structures stand out because of their shadowing (see Fig. 4.1C) and (4) by scrolling through successive C-scans (along a coronal [frontal] plane), which may be confusing because of the curvature of the posterior globe (see Fig. 4.1D). It is important to note that adequate C-scan views requires high-density scans, and because this has required more acquisition time, it has not been routinely performed in the pediatric population. Combining multiple viewpoint options (1–3 listed earlier in this section), it is much easier to determine where the foveal depression or optic nerve head is located in a volume scan of a nonfixating child.

With a handheld OCT system, volumetric scans are usually the scan protocol of choice for infants who are awake, moving their eyes, and cannot fixate. On either portable or tabletop systems, volumetric scans are also a great way to obtain high-quality scans in children with nystagmus.[4]

The imager must prioritize to ensure that the optic nerve head or foveal center is within the volumes captured.[5–7] The imager can also consider capturing a wider field so that both the macula and the optic nerve are captured in the same volume scan to allow for subsequent analysis of structures organized by the fovea to optic nerve head axis (see Fig. 4.1E). If the infant is restless, crying, looking away, or moving excessively, scan parameters like the number of A-scans and B-scans can be lowered to achieve faster acquisition speed (albeit with lower resolution as a trade-off). We recommend obtaining approximately 35 degree (10 × 10 mm adult emmetropic eye setting) scans that are centered on the macula, centered on the optic nerve, and aimed toward the temporal periphery of the retina, and then covering other areas of the periphery. These will vary, depending on the condition.

For children undergoing examination under anesthesia or older children/teenagers who can fixate, excessive movement is not as much of a concern. In these populations, higher-resolution volumetric scans can be captured. The higher-resolution scans may be viewed in the conventional modes or as C-scans (see Fig. 4.1D).

On the tabletop SD-OCT system, volumetric scans are focused over the macula, optic nerve, or area of interest, and this is easiest by using internal or external fixation targets to align the eyes. On Spectralis, for example, the typical protocol is a 30 × 25 degree (9.0 × 7.5 mm), 61-line B-scan volume with automatic real-time tracking (ART) set at 9 linear scans per B-scan. Reducing scan density will improve scan acquisition speed in children who are less cooperative.

As discussed in Chapter 3, imagers should be aware that an approximately 35-degree volume scan that crosses approximately 10 × 10 mm in an adult emmetropic eye will cross a shorter span (in millimeters) in the shorter infant eye; the actual scan length will vary with the size of the eye (and thus with patient age or axial myopia).[8] Adjusting the number of A-scans and B-scans will prevent oversampling in the infant because this causes too much time per image. For those with high myopia (if it is caused by greater axial length), smaller scans should be considered because the OCT scan will cross a greater span of retina (per the discussion in Chapter 3). In those with high myopia, often vertical (sagittal) line scanning provides better scan alignment and image and therefore more accurate autosegmentation compared with horizontal (transverse) scanning.

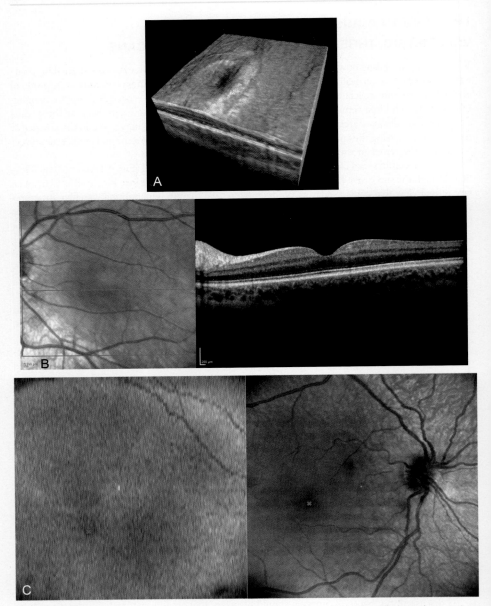

Fig. 4.1   (A) Volumetric scan at the fovea on handheld system (Leica) reconstructed in a 3D view using a custom software program in a 7-year-old child. The foveal depression and the vessels can be appreciated from this perspective. (B) Infrared orienting image *(left)* and single cross-sectional horizontal B-scan (selected from the volume) centered at the fovea, from a tabletop system in a cooperative 15-year-old (Spectralis). (C) Two examples of the en face retinal view from volumetric scans across the fovea *(red cross)* on handheld system (Leica). Note that in both cases, the fovea is not in the center of the image. The pixels in the volume have been summed to produce the retinal view in a 35-week postmenstrual-age premature infant *(left)* and a 15-month-old infant *(right)*. The visibility of the vessels is more limited in the image on the left, which is from a faster low-resolution scan, whereas the view on the right is from a higher-resolution, wider-field scan in which the retinal vessel are quite useful for orientation.

Continued

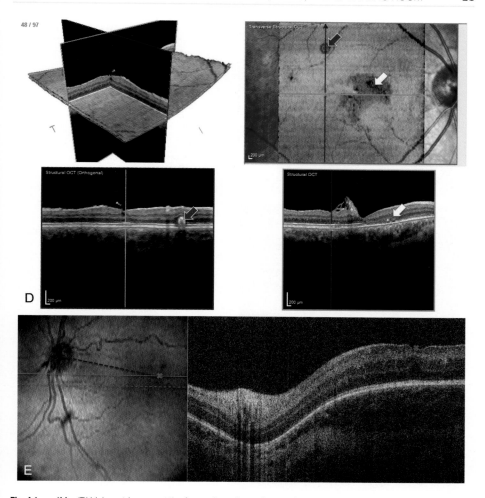

Fig. 4.1, cont'd (D) Volumetric scan at the fovea viewed as a C-scan (*red border,* between the red lines on the B-scan) on tabletop system in a cooperative 17-year-old (Spectralis). Retinal pigment epithelium (RPE) defects from trauma can be visualized as a dark hyporeflective area *(white arrow),* and a subretinal lesion *(purple arrow)* casts a shadow producing a hyporeflective circle in the C-scan view. (E) An en face view of the fovea and optic nerve head *(left)* and cross-sectional horizontal B-scan across the foveal center *(right,* extracted from this same SD-OCT volume at the location of the *solid green line*) in a 1-month-old infant on handheld SD-OCT system (Leica). Note that the B-scans were used to help determine the location of the displaced fovea *(red cross on both views).* Because the eye of the supine infant or the position of the handheld scanner was rotated, analysis should be organized around the optic nerve-foveal axis *(dotted blue line).* The *dotted green line* is approximately where one would guess the fovea was located based on clinical view.

Continued

Many commercially available tabletop systems offer an eye-tracking feature that is used to actively track the eye during scanning to reduce motion artifact. This feature also allows for repeat scanning in the exact retinal location, and this is useful for follow-up evaluation. This eye-tracking feature is useful even in children who have a difficult time fixating because it pauses the scanning during interruption of scan acquisition. For example, when the child looks away, the scanning will

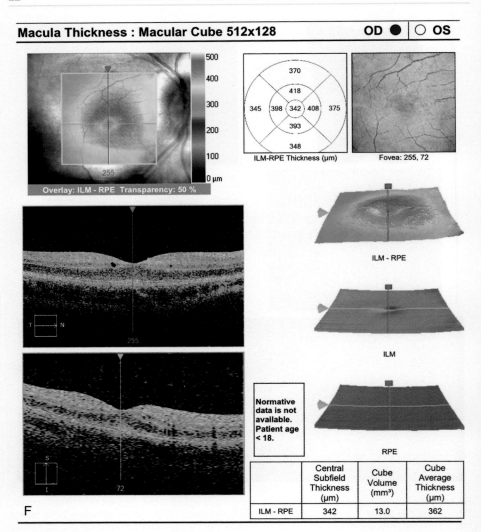

Fig. 4.1, cont'd (F) Macular thickness map generated from a volumetric scan of a cooperative 8-year-old (Zeiss Cirrus). The fovea is reasonably centered, and although normative data was not available on the system, the thickness maps are of good quality.

pause. When the child fixates again on the tabletop, the eye-tracking feature will resume the scanning. If necessary, this eye-tracking feature can be turned off to decrease the scan acquisition time.

Many commercially available OCT systems can produce macular maps by using volumetric scans as well. The integration of the multiple lines generates a topographic map centered on the foveal center (see Fig. 4.1F) and provides the total retinal thickness in three concentric rings (at 1, 3, and 6 mm, centered on the fovea) or even segment different layers of the retina for individual retinal thicknesses.[9]

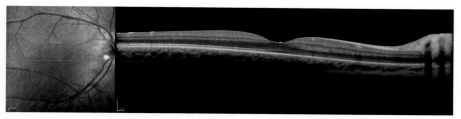

Fig. 4.2 Infrared orienting image *(left)* and high-resolution summed single-line scan *(right)* through the fovea in a cooperative 15-year-old (Spectralis).

HIGH-RESOLUTION LINEAR SCANS

High-resolution linear scans may be single or multiple (typically 5–9 raster scans). These are high-quality scans that enable the detailed interpretation of the vitreo–retinal interface, optic nerve head, and retinal and subretinal layers (Fig. 4.2). Successively acquired B-scans across the same location are averaged to reduce speckle noise and enhance the ability to perceive details. The successive scans, however, take longer to acquire compared with a single nonaveraged B-scan, and thus these scans are less useful in infants and young children because these patients are usually restless and cannot maintain steady fixation for the duration of the repeat scanning. These scan patterns are a great option for children who can cooperate and fixate while being imaged on a tabletop system or when aligned with a structure of interest during examination under anesthesia. On Spectralis, for example, we recommend a 30-degree (9-mm) scan with up to 60 ART. On the Spectralis system, the infrared retinal image is used to register/align the successive OCT scans at the same location. The ART number signifies the number of B-scans that are successively imaged, and typically the higher the number averaged (e.g., 56 rather than 12), the better is the image quality but the greater is the risk for motion artifact.

One caution with linear or raster scans in infants and young children is that depending on the size of the interval between raster scans (or "off alignment" of a single-line scan), none of the linear scans may cross the foveal center. In such cases, an off-center scan may be misinterpreted as foveal and interpreted as disease (e.g., as foveal hypoplasia). Imaging the foveal center in such cases is optimally determined from a higher-density volume scan.[2,3]

RADIAL SCANS

Radial scans are volumetric scans that capture multiple B-scans centered on an area of interest in a star-shaped or cross pattern (Fig. 4.3). Good centration on the target of interest is essential for a good-quality and useful radial scan. A smaller but detailed scan length of 6 × 6 mm or even 3 × 3 mm is recommended for evaluation of infants and children with suspected macular hole. Radial patterns can be used in the clinic on a tabletop system or in the operating room with the handheld or armature systems. This scan pattern is not generally recommended for awake children who have difficulty fixating, but if needed, scan density, quality, and eye tracking can be modified and reduced for faster acquisition speed.

CIRCULAR/ANNULAR SCANS FOR PERIPAPILLARY RFNL MEASUREMENTS

Circular or annular scans capture multiple A-scans in a ring (circular) or in concentric rings (annulus) centered on an area of interest. The most common use of these patterns are to capture the peripapillary retina for retinal nerve fiber layer (RNFL) measurements (Fig. 4.4A) used in the analysis of glaucoma and optic atrophies, as well as severity of certain degenerative neuro-ophthalmic

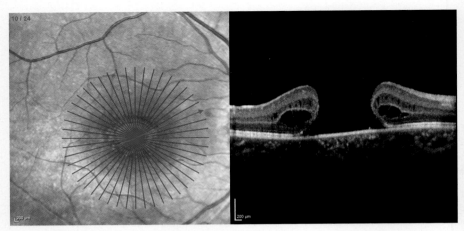

Fig. 4.3   Infrared orienting image *(left)* and B-scan image *(right)* selected from multiple radial scans (at the *green lines*) centered on a macular hole in a cooperative 6-year-old (Spectralis).

conditions. This imaging pattern is usually obtained in cooperative children on the tabletop system in clinic or with the handheld/armature system in the operating room. The diameter of the scan circle used in adults is usually approximately 12 degrees, which spans a 3.5- to 3.6-mm diameter.[1,3,5]

For infant eyes, alternate A-scans at the appropriate location for a circular scan may be extracted from volume scans across the optic nerve head. Because of the difference in axial length in the newborn eye, the RNFL thickness was evaluated for multiple diameters in infants, and a diameter of 3.0 mm was determined to be proportional to the standard location relative to the optic nerve and the fovea in adults (see Fig. 4.4B).[5]

Imaging the Choroid and EDI

Optimal imaging of the full thickness of the choroid, of lesions within the choroid, and of the lamina cribrosa and deep optic nerve structures may be challenging, caused by insufficient SD-OCT signal; this may occur in eyes with greater choroidal thickness or with loss of signal caused by overlying signal reflectance or absorption, which interfere in OCT signal from the deeper choroid or optic nerve head. EDI is an SD-OCT imaging mode that provides better visualization of the choroid because the zero delay line location is set so that SD-OCT image sensitivity is highest in the choroid (Fig. 4.5). It can be used to visualize the choroid and to determine choroidal thinning/thickening or if choroidal tumors are present. Other options that may improve choroidal imaging include summing low-signal scans or imaging with swept-source OCT (SS-OCT), which has a longer wavelength with greater depth of signal at the optic nerve and choroid. With adequate depth of imaging from either of these techniques, one can also determine the direction of bowing of the optic nerve in cases when high intracranial pressure is suspected and can measure Bruch membrane opening in cases when optic nerve hypoplasia is suspected. EDI can be used in conjunction with different SD-OCT scan patterns and can be obtained with the handheld system in the nursery or clinic, tabletop system in clinic, and handheld/armature system in the operating room.

OCT Angiography

As discussed in Chapters 2 and 3, OCT angiography (OCTA) acquisition times are longer than for standard OCT. This represents an additional challenge when working with children. The only

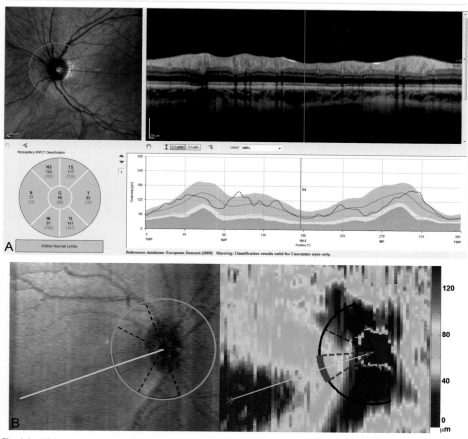

Fig. 4.4   (A) Infrared orienting image *(left)* and circular/annular scan *(right)* of the optic nerve for RNFL analysis (lower section of image) in a cooperative teenager (Spectralis). (B) Images of the optic nerve head in an infant (Leica). The en face retinal view with the optic nerve-foveal axis *(yellow line)* is obtained from volumetric scans across the optic nerve head (similar to Fig. 4.1C). Circular/annular location from which data were extracted for retinal nerve fiber layer (RNFL) analysis are shown over the en face image *(green circle, left)* and over a nerve fiber layer thickness map extracted from the segmented volume *(right)*. The color scale shows the thicknesses. The arc has a diameter of 3 mm and is centered on the optic nerve. The fovea is located at the red star. The papillomacular bundle analysis was performed within the thick solid pink arc, which extends 15 degrees above and below the axis.

commercially available OCTA systems are tabletop systems and require children who are able to cooperate and fixate in clinic. If the child is capable of cooperating for the full amount of capture time, high-quality images may be obtained. In the event the child has a short attention span, several steps can be taken to reduce the amount of capture time. These include (1) choosing a smaller scan size, (2) reducing the scan density (or increasing the distance between B scans), and (3) reducing the number of B-scans averaged across each location. Heidelberg Engineering has an investigational portable armature SD-OCTA system (Spectralis with Flex Module) that has been used in research protocols in children who are undergoing examination under anesthesia. Because the child is under anesthesia, movement and duration of scanning become less of a concern. Scan patterns have typically been a 10- or 20-degree square volume (Figs. 4.6A and 4.6B). There are other portable investigational SS-OCTA systems in research use in children, and these studies point to the future benefits of OCTA imaging in young children and infants.[10-13]

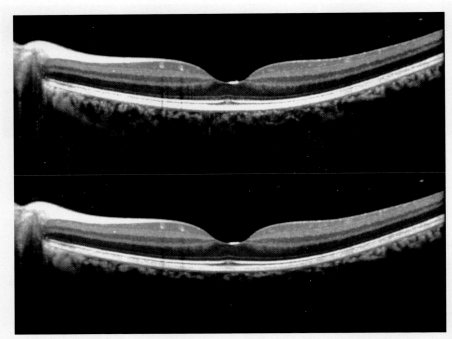

Fig. 4.5 Two images of the choroid beneath the fovea, one with *(top)* and one without *(bottom)* enhanced depth imaging (EDI) in a 13-year-old child (Spectralis). Note the difference in the outer border of the choroid and choroidal features with EDI.

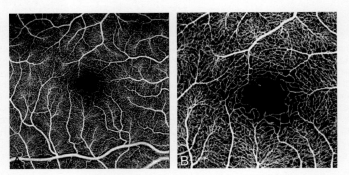

Fig. 4.6 An en face view of optical coherence tomography angiography (OCTA) of the macula extracted from an OCTA volume captured without injection of fluorescein dye in a 3-month-old child. The volume was captured across 20 × 20 degrees (5.7 × 5.7 mm) in image A and 10 × 10 degree (3.1 × 3.1 mm) in image B. Images obtained from an investigational device (Spectralis HRA + OCT with OCTA software and Flex module).

References

1. Rothman AL, Sevilla MB, Mangalesh S, et al. Thinner retinal nerve fiber layer in very preterm versus term infants and relationship to brain anatomy and neurodevelopment. *Am J Ophthalmol.* 2015;160(6): 1296–1308.
2. Chong GT, Farsiu S, Freedman SF, et al. Abnormal foveal morphology in ocular albinism imaged with spectral-domain optical coherence tomography. *Arch Ophthalmol.* 2009;127(1):37–44.

3. Avery RA, Rajjoub RD, Trimboli-Heidler C, Waldman AT. Applications of optical coherence tomography in pediatric clinical neuroscience. *Neuropediatrics.* 2015;46(2):88–97. https://doi.org/10.1055/s-0035-1549098.

4. Lee H, Sheth V, Bibi M, et al. Potential of handheld optical coherence tomography to determine cause of infantile nystagmus in children by using foveal morphology. *Ophthalmology.* 2013;120(12):2714–2724. https://doi.org/10.1016/j.ophtha.2013.07.018.

5. Rothman AL, Sevilla MB, Freedman SF, et al. Assessment of retinal nerve fiber layer thickness in healthy, full-term neonates. *Am J Ophthalmol.* 2015;159(4):803–811.

6. Tran-Viet D, Wong BM, Mangalesh S, Maldonado R, Cotten CM, Toth CA. Handheld spectral domain optical coherence tomography imaging through the undilated pupil in infants born preterm or with hypoxic injury or hydrocephalus. *Retina.* 2018;38(8):1588–1594.

7. Rajjoub RD, Trimboli-Heidler C, Packer RJ, Avery RA. Reproducibility of retinal nerve fiber layer thickness measures using eye tracking in children with nonglaucomatous optic neuropathy. *Am J Ophthalmol.* 2015;159(1):71–77.

8. Maldonado RS, Izatt JA, Sarin N, et al. Optimizing hand-held spectral domain optical coherence tomography imaging for neonates, infants and children. *Invest Ophthalmol Vis Sci.* 2010;51(5):2678–2685.

9. FF1 Ghasia, Freedman SF, Rajani A, Holgado S, Asrani S, El-Dairi M. Optical coherence tomography in paediatric glaucoma: time domain versus spectral domain. *Br J Ophthalmol.* 2013 Jul;97(7):837–842.

10. Campbell JP, Nudleman E, Yang J, et al. Handheld optical coherence tomography angiography and ultrawide-field optical coherence tomography in retinopathy of prematurity. *JAMA Ophthalmol.* 2017;135 (9):977–981.

11. Viehland C, LaRocca F, Tran-Viet D, et al. In: *Imaging of pediatric pathology in the intensive care nursery using a custom handheld, ultra-compact, swept-source OCT probe*: Proc. SPIE 10474, *Ophthalmic Technologies XXVIII, 1047416*; March 14, 2018. https://doi.org/10.1117/12.2290627. Published in SPIE Proceedings Vol. 10474: Ophthalmic Technologies XXVIII.

12. Chen X, Viehland C, Carrasco-Zevallos OM, et al. Microscope-integrated optical coherence tomography angiography in the operating room in young children with retinal vascular disease. *JAMA Ophthalmol.* 2017;135(5):483–486.

13. Vinekar A, Chidambara L, Jayadev C, Sivakumar M, Webers CA, Shetty B. Monitoring neovascularization in aggressive posterior retinopathy of prematurity using optical coherence tomography angiography. *J AAPOS.* 2016 Jun;20(3):271–274.

CHAPTER 5

Analyzing Structural Optical Coherence Tomography Images

Katrina Postell Winter

Optical coherence tomography (OCT) has greatly evolved from its conception as a time-domain (TD) imaging system to the now widely used spectral-domain (SD) imaging systems. More recently, swept-source (SS) imaging systems have also become available. As OCT evolves, the number of axial scans per second has increased from 400 scans per second with TD-OCT to upward of 70,000 with SD-OCT. Axial resolution has remained at 2 to 10 µm with resolution based on wavelength. This increased acquisition speed have resulted in better image quality by enabling averaging of multiple scans, increasing layer resolution, minimizing image artifacts, and even allowing for 3-D reconstruction or projection of retinal images. Many systems have also incorporated eye-tracking capabilities and image registration, which help minimize motion artifacts.

Many systems also have high-definition fundus cameras or scanning laser ophthalmoscopes (SLOs), which allow the scan location to be projected onto the fundus image (Fig. 5.1) and inform the examiner of the scan orientation. The fundus and SLO images are also used for registration of images obtained from one visit to the next to show changes in the map thickness of segmented retina over time. The ability to identify scan location and orientation is important in identifying retinal structures and determining the impact of certain pathologies on visual and anatomical outcomes. Furthermore, scan orientation and registration allows the examiner to determine proximity to the foveal center (of greatest visual significance) and identify retinal structure (e.g., to differentiate a vessel from an intraretinal plaque causing shadowing).

Qualitative Interpretation of OCT Images

Qualitative interpretation involves the examiner reviewing the individual B-scans or line scans within the area of interest (e.g., retina or optic nerve) and making a qualitative assessment concerning the presence or absence of pathology. Qualitative interpretation can also involve analyzing the development of the retina in neonates and infants. Layers may be displayed in gray scale or with false color, representing the reflectivity of the different layers or structures. Gray scale may be displayed with greater reflectivity as the white or the black end of the spectrum. Throughout this text, we depict gray scale with highest relative reflectivity as white.

Reflectivity is described as varying degrees of hyper- or hyporeflectivity compared with standard regions of the retina or of the vitreous body.

28

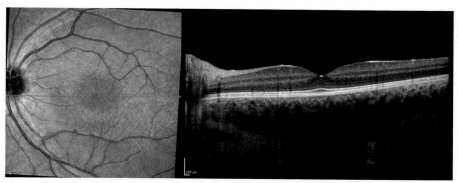

Fig. 5.1   In a 10-year-old boy, the image was acquired on the Heidelberg Spectralis, demonstrating the location of the B-scan projected onto the scanning laser ophthalmoscope (SLO) image. (With permission of Heidelberg Engineering)

- Hyperreflective bands of the retina are layers that appear whiter in varying degrees when viewed in gray scale in contrast to retinal nuclear layers. Examples of the more hyperreflective layers of the normal retina from vitreous outward include the retinal nerve fiber layer, inner and outer plexiform layers, external limiting membrane, ellipsoid zone, interdigitation zone, retinal pigment epithelium (RPE), and parts of the choroid.
- Relatively hyporeflective layers of the normal retina from vitreous outward include the ganglion cell (nuclear) layer, inner nuclear layer, Henle fiber layer (HFL), outer nuclear layer, and photoreceptor outer segments. Note that reflectivity of retinal structures, such as the HFL, can change with the alignment/entrance of the OCT beam relative to the visual axis of the eye (Fig. 5.2).[1]
- Hyperreflective abnormalities include hard exudates, epiretinal membranes, preretinal neovascular tufts, choroidal neovascular membranes, and intra- and subretinal tumors, which may also be hyperreflective.
- Hyporeflective abnormalities include areas of fluid, such as intraretinal cystoid spaces, subretinal fluid, and vessel lumens, which may appear as dark as or darker than the vitreous body.

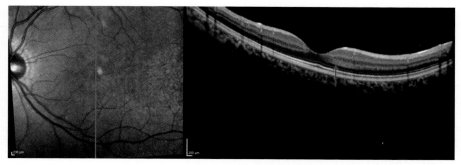

Fig. 5.2   Vertical displacement of the optical coherence tomography (OCT) entrance beam to the edge of a dilated pupil will cause the vertical scan to appear tilted. Similarly, horizontal translation of the OCT entrance beam relative to the center of the pupil will cause the horizontal scan to appear tilted. In a 13-year-old boy, the OCT entrance beam was displaced inferiorly to the edge of the pupil, and Henle fiber layer (HFL) on the same side of the fovea where the light was displaced (inferior) appeared hyporeflective, whereas the HFL on the opposite side of the fovea (superior) appeared hyperreflective *(red arrow)*.[1]

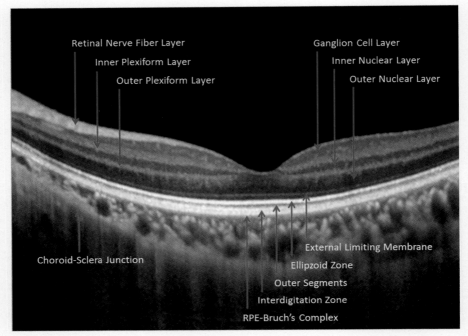

Fig. 5.3 Healthy retina of a 14-year-old boy imaged using Heidelberg Spectralis system. Nomenclature for normal anatomical landmarks seen on spectral-domain optical coherence tomography (SD-OCT) images, as proposed and adopted by the International Nomenclature for Optical Coherence Tomography Panel.[2]

- Shadowing occurs when there is an increased absorption of light in a given area compared with surrounding tissue or structures. Larger vessels, vitreous debris, exudates, blood, and highly pigmented structures often create optical shadowing, which results in decreased visualization of underlying structures.
- Hypertransmission (sometimes called *reverse shadowing*) occurs when there is increased light transmission to deeper tissue layers as a result of atrophy or loss of pigmented layers. Hypertransmission is most commonly seen with RPE and outer retinal atrophy, in which there is hypertransmission of light into the choroidal layer (choroidal hypertransmission) such that it becomes more hyperreflective compared with the adjacent areas of the choroid where the RPE layer is intact.

Proper identification of the retinal layers and ocular structures (anatomical and pathological) is essential for OCT analysis (Fig. 5.3)[2] (also discussed in greater detail in Chapter 10). The examiner should be aware of structural or anatomical differences associated with the disease, age, and even ethnicity of the subject (Fig. 5.4). There is currently a critical need for a normative database for neonates showing the range of normal as well as delayed development of the retina and optic nerve.

Quantitative Interpretation of OCT

Quantitative interpretation of OCT images relies on the ability of the OCT software to define individual retinal layers (segmentation) and provide depth information (thickness calculations) within tissue. This calculation of retinal layer thicknesses and/or retinal volume can then be compared with

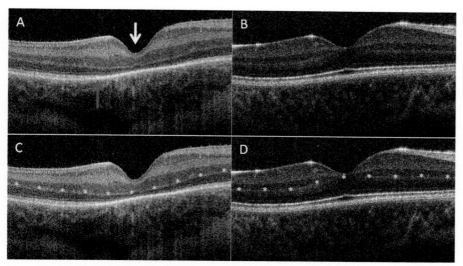

Fig. 5.4 Image A is a spectral-domain optical coherence tomography (SD-OCT) image of a neonate 35 weeks postmenstrual age (PMA) and image B is that of an 8-year-old child. Both patients were imaged on the Bioptigen commercial system. Note the persistent inner retinal layers at the foveal center *(white arrow)* and the absence of the external limiting membrane (ELM) and ellipsoid zone (EZ) at the foveal center (both the ELM and EZ are seen lateral to the foveal center as denoted by the red arrow) in the neonate in comparison with the older child. In images C and D, note the yellow asterisks along the outer plexiform layer (OPL) denoting the inner retina versus the outer retina in the neonate (C) and in the older child (D). Images A and C have been corrected for axial and lateral sizing in the neonate.

that in age-matched controls for assessment of normalcy or monitored over time to assess development of layers or progression/regression of disease (i.e., edema). It is important to be cognizant of the fact that the normative database included in commercial OCT systems was obtained from findings in adults. Thus quantitative measurements obtained in children should be compared with normative pediatric reference values published in the literature. Normative data for each retinal layer and the peripapillary retinal nerve fiber layer has been reported for children from birth to age 17 years.[3-11]

Image registration features on most commercial OCT systems allow for comparison of thickness maps captured over time. When comparing thickness maps, it is important to compare scans captured on the same commercial system, whenever possible, because different OCT systems may plot the outer retinal boundary at different layers (Fig. 5.5). It is also important to consider the age of the patient because the presence of retinal layers varies throughout early life (see Chapter 10). If it is necessary to compare images captured on different systems, the examiner can redraw to the desired outer boundary by using segmentation correction tools provided in most systems. Segmentation correction tools are often utilized also extremely helpful to correct segmentation errors caused by infant age, scanning artifacts, or severe pathology.

Third-party segmentation programs and algorithms are often most useful for research purposes because typically more options are available, for example, ability to mark an area en face by using a drawing function, ability to choose which layers you wish to segment, ability to segment a greater number of layers, ease of correction, ability to create thickness maps of desired boundaries, and ability to mark points of interest by using markings of foci. Fig. 5.6 is an example of a 10-layer segmentation of pediatric retina by using specialized algorithms (DOCTRAP V63.9) developed in MATLAB (Mathworks, Inc., Natick, MA).

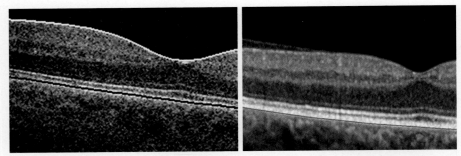

Fig. 5.5 Segmented adult image on the left was captured on a Zeiss Cirrus system, which plots the bottom boundary at the inner aspect of the retinal pigment epithelium (RPE) and the outer aspect of the interdigitation zone. (With permission of Carl Zeiss Meditec, AG.) The segmented image on the right was captured on the Heidelberg Spectralis system and shows the bottom boundary at the outer aspect of the RPE–Bruch membrane complex.

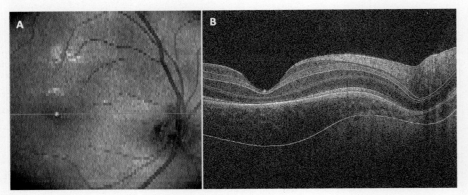

Fig. 5.6 The image on the left (A) is a created summed voxel projection (SVP) of the B-scans, with the green line indicating the location of the segmented B-scan and the yellow asterisk marking the foveal center. The image on the right (B) is a segmented pediatric image (41 weeks postmenstrual age [PMA]) showing segmentation of 10 layers. From top: internal limiting membrane (ILM), nerve fiber layer to ganglion cell layer (NFL-GCL), ganglion cell layer to inner plexiform layer (GCL-IPL), inner plexiform layer to inner nuclear layer (IPL-INL), inner nuclear layer to outer plexiform layer (INL-OPL), outer plexiform layer and outer nuclear layer (OPL-ONL), inner segment-outer segment junction (IS-OS) (also known as ellipsoid zone), outer segment and retinal pigment elipthelial layer (OS-RPE), Bruch membrane, and choroidal–scleral junction (CSJ). The *two red arrows* indicate age-appropriate underdevelopment of the ellipsoid zone (EZ) in the foveal region.

Measuring calipers are available on most commercial OCT systems. Measurements using calipers can be confounded by a variety of factors, including image quality, segmentation errors, scan tilt, corneal curvature, axial length, and lens status. Traditionally, OCT images have a higher axial resolution than lateral resolution, resulting in the image being stretched axially for better visualization of the retinal layers. This ratio of axial to lateral resolution is approximately 2:1 for Zeiss Cirrus and 3:1 for Heidelberg Spectralis scans acquired in the default high-speed mode. Uji et al.[12] reported that measuring perpendicular to the RPE in tilted images introduces greater error in true retinal thickness than simply measuring parallel to the A-scan. This difference in the ratio of axial to lateral aspect between systems is another vital reason for comparing map values captured on the same system, whenever possible.

References

1. Lujan BJ, Roorda A, Knighton RW, Carroll J. Revealing Henle's fiber layer using spectral domain optical coherence tomography. *Invest Ophthalmol Vis Sci*. 2011;52:1486–1492.
2. Staurenghi G, Sadda S, Chakravarthy U, Spaide RF. International Nomenclature for Optical Coherence Tomography (IN-OCT) Panel. Proposed lexicon for anatomic landmarks in normal posterior segmentation spectral-domain optical coherence tomography: the IN-OCT consensus. *Ophthalmology*. 2014;121(8):1572–1578.
3. Lee H, Purohit R, Patel A, et al. In vivo foveal development using optical coherence tomography. *Invest Ophthalmol Vis Sci*. 2015;56:4537–4545.
4. Huynh SC, Wang XY, Rochtchina E, Mitchell P. Distribution of macular thickness by optical coherence tomography: findings from a population-based study of 6-year-old children. *Invest Ophthalmol Vis Sci*. 2006;47:2351–2357.
5. Gupta G, Donahue JP, You T. Profile of the retina by optical coherence tomography in the pediatric age group. *Am J Ophthalmol*. 2007;144:309–310.
6. Yanni SE, Wang J, Cheng CS, et al. Normative reference ranges for the retinal nerve fiber layer, macula, and retinal layer thicknesses in children. *Am J Ophthalmol*. 2013;155:354–360. e1.
7. Turk A, Ceylan OM, Arici C, et al. Evaluation of the nerve fiber layer and macula in the eyes of healthy children using spectral-domain optical coherence tomography. *Am J Ophthalmol*. 2012;153:552–559. e1.
8. Allingham MJ, Cabrera MT, O'Connell RV, et al. Racial variation in optic nerve head parameters quantified in healthy newborns by handheld spectral domain optical coherence tomography. *J AAPOS*. 2013;17:501–506.
9. Rothman AL, Sevilla MB, Freedman SF, et al. Assessment of retinal nerve fiber layer thickness in healthy, full-term neonates. *Am J Ophthalmol*. 2015;159:803–811.
10. El-Dairi MA, Asrani SG, Enyedi LB, Freedman SF. Optical coherence tomography in the eyes of normal children. *Arch Ophthalmol*. 2009;127:50–58.
11. Lee H, Proudlock FA, Gottlob I. Pediatric optical coherence tomography in clinical practice—recent progress. *Invest Ophthalmol Vis Sci*. 2016;57:69–79.
12. Uji A, Abdelfattah NS, Boyer DS, Balasubramanian S, Lei J, Sadda SR. Variability of retinal thickness measurements in tilted or stretched optical coherence measurements. *Transl Vis Sci Technol*. 2017;6(2):1.

CHAPTER 6

Identifying Artifacts and Outliers in Structural Optical Coherence Tomography

Du Tran-Viet ■ Katrina Postell Winter ■ Xi Chen

Suboptimal scans and imaging artifacts, although often unavoidable, can affect the analysis of optical coherence tomography (OCT) images and lead to incorrect interpretation of data. Table 6.1[1-4] lists the common artifacts seen on OCT images. The table also provides suggestions on how to identify these artifacts and how to avoid the errors to improve the quality of the scans. Some examples of artifacts are shown below.

Artifact	How to Identify	How to Avoid
Vignetting	Scan clipping on the edges when OCT signal is blocked as a result of lack of pupil dilation or mismatching of eye length and reference arm length such that the OCT beam pivot is not axially aligned within the pupil.	Increase pupil size and/or adjust reference arm to the eye length.[1]
Out-of-range error	Image is too high or too low in scan window. It may occur if the scanner is too close or too far away from the eye or if the subject moves during imaging. It may also occur when there is ocular pathology (e.g., high myopia, severe edema, vitreous traction, or other pathology).	Adjust working distance accordingly to position area of interest in scan window.

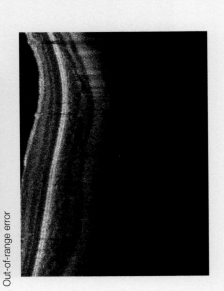

Continued on following page

TABLE 6.1 ■ Suboptimal Scans and Artifacts from SD-OCT Imaging (Continued)

Artifact		How to Identify	How to Avoid
Mirror artifact	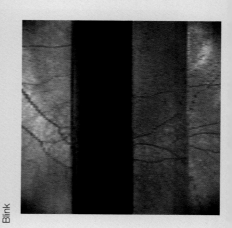	Image crosses zero delay line and results in an inverted image or vitreous pathology superimposed on top of retinal image. It occurs when the scanner is too close to the eye or when opacity is elevated within the vitreous (e.g., asteroid hyalosis).	Adjust working distance accordingly to obtain area of interest in scan window.
Blink		Child blinked resulting in dark or vignetted frames.	Try to reobtain image.

Images are tilted at an angle. This may affect reflectance of retinal layers, such as Henle fiber layer, which may further affect visualization, and qualitative and quantitative grading. Severely tilted scans may also affect accurate thickness measurements.[3]

Make lateral pivoting motions to correct the tilt and straighten the scan.

Area of interest (e.g., fovea or optic nerve) is not centered in the retinal view/volume.

Make sliding motion on same plane to center, and obtain image of area of interest.

Tilt

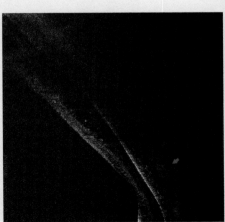

Misalignment

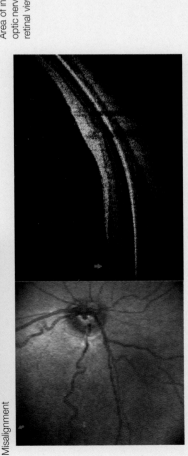

Continued on following page

TABLE 6.1 ■ Suboptimal Scans and Artifacts from SD-OCT Imaging (Continued)

Artifact	How to Identify	How to Avoid
Motion	Child moves during scanning (tracking, active sucking on pacifier, or axial motion with heartbeat when supine) or has saccades or nystagmus.[4]	Try to reobtain image with less motion. Increase scan speed by reducing number of A-scans and B-scans. Provide an external fixation object (telephone screen or toy).[4]
Out of focus	Image is less saturated and appears fainter as a result of uncorrected refractive error or misalignment of scan.	Correct imaging system for refractive error and realign.[1]

Before focus adjustment   After focus adjustment

Signal blocking

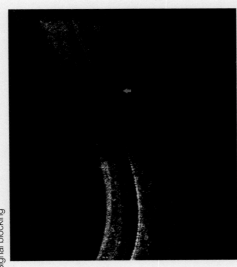

Media opacities including vitreous hemorrhage, cataract, or corneal opacity may block signal to retina. Inner retinal reflective structure (e.g., large retinal vessels or hemorrhage) may shadow deeper structures.

Recognize the blocking and image off axis, if needed.

Scanner artifact

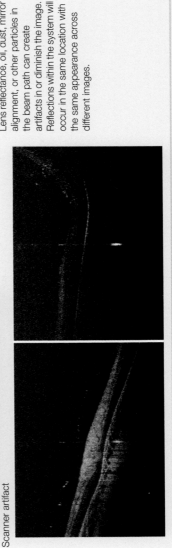

Lens reflectance, oil, dust, mirror alignment, or other particles in the beam path can create artifacts in or diminish the image. Reflections within the system will occur in the same location with the same appearance across different images.

Cannot avoid lens reflectance. For other artifacts, clean the optical pathway of the imaging system.

OCT, Optical coherence tomography; SD-OCT, spectral-domain OCT.

Reference

1. Maldonado RS, Izatt JA, Sarin N, Wallace DK, Freedman S, Cotten CM, Toth CA. Optimizing hand-held spectral domain optical coherence tomography imaging for neonates, infants and children. *Invest Ophthalmol Vis Sci.* 2010;51(5):2678–2685.
2. Lujan BJ, Roorda A, Knighton RW, Carroll J. Revealing Henle's fiber layer using spectral domain optical coherence tomography. *Invest Ophthalmol Vis Sci.* 2011;52(3):1486–1492.
3. Uji A, Abdelfattah NS, Boyer DS, Balasubramanian S, Lei J, Sadda SR. Variability of retinal thickness measurements in tilted or stretched optical coherence measurements. *Transl Vis Sci Tech.* 2017;6(2):1.
4. Lee H, Proudlock FA, Gottlob I. Is handheld optical coherence tomography reliable in infants and young children with and without nystagmus? *Invest Ophthalmol Vis Sci.* 2013;54(13):8152–8159.

CHAPTER 7

Analyzing Optical Coherence Tomography Angiography

S. Tammy Hsu ■ Lejla Vajzovic

Optical coherence tomography angiography (OCTA) provides information regarding blood flow and may aid in monitoring or identifying various pathologies. The principles of OCTA are covered in Chapter 2. The initial OCTA image contains vascular flow signaling from within both the retina and the choroid. The analysis of OCTA images begins with segmentation of the scans into retinal and choroidal vascular sublayers, as described in Table 7.1. This segmentation determines en face slab definition, which subsequently provides visualization of the detected blood flow segmented into various vascular layers. After segmentation, one can then perform qualitative and quantitative analyses of the vascular flow within the en face OCTA layers (Figs. 7.1 and 7.2, *lower rows*). Table 7.1 provides general guidelines for segmentation of commonly analyzed vascular layers, although the presence of some of these layers is dependent on the location relative to the optic disc and fovea.

Automated segmentation of the retinal layers may work well in healthy eyes without pathology. However, careful review of the segmentation of the retinal layers is needed for the retinal layers that may not conform to the standard retinal layers in a healthy adult retina, for example, in a premature infant (Fig. 7.3).

Qualitative analysis involves descriptive examination of vasculature.[2] For pathologies in which the retinal layers are unclear and therefore difficult to segment, potential misinterpretation of OCTA images (see Chapter 8 regarding segmentation artifacts) can be avoided by scrolling through the retinal vasculature as en face OCTA slices from the inner layer to the outer layer of the retina, rather than only reviewing the vasculature segmented into the OCTA vascular layers, such as the superficial vascular complex (SVC) and deep vascular complex (DVC). Additionally, reviewing the retinal vasculature by scrolling through the OCT/OCTA volume from the en face superficial layer to the deep retinal layer may be helpful in evaluating and tracing vessel flow, especially in eyes with complex pathology.

Quantitative analysis of OCTA images (Fig. 7.4) can be performed to measure the diameter and area of the foveal avascular zone, parafoveal and peripapillary vessel density, perfusion density, and flow voids.[2-5] Quantification of OCTA images remains challenging because of the difficulties in identifying and resolving artifacts that may affect these analyses (see Chapter 8). Further verification of the methods that have been developed for quantifying various measures is needed, and work in this area by numerous groups is in progress.

TABLE 7.1 ■ **Retinal Vascular Layers Commonly Used in Analysis of Optical Coherence Tomography Angiography (OCTA) Images[1]**

Retinal Vascular Layer	General Guidelines for Segmentation Boundaries[a]
Retina	Internal limiting membrane (ILM) to Bruch membrane
Superficial vascular complex (SVC)	SVC = RPCP + SVP
Radial peripapillary capillary plexus (RPCP)	Nerve fiber layer (NFL) (Note this is only surrounding the optic nerve head and is not found in the macula.)
Superficial vascular plexus (SVP)	Ganglion cell layer through 80% of the inner plexiform layer (IPL)
Deep vascular complex (DVC)	DVC = ICP + DCP
Intermediate capillary plexus (ICP)	Posterior 20% of IPL through the inner 50% of the inner nuclear layer (INL)
Deep capillary plexus (DCP)	Inner 50% of the INL through the outer plexiform layer (OPL)
Avascular complex	Posterior boundary of OPL to Bruch membrane
Choriocapillaris	0–20 μm posterior to Bruch membrane
Choroid	After choriocapillaris to choroidal–scleral junction (CSJ)

[a]The segmentation boundaries may vary, depending on the commercial software used.
[1]Adapted from Campbell JP, Zhang M, Hwang TS, et al. Detailed vascular anatomy of the human retina by projection-resolved optical coherence tomography angiography. *Sci Rep.* 2017;7:42201.

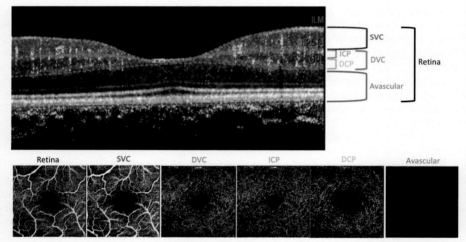

Fig. 7.1 Example foveal optical coherence tomography/optical coherence tomography angiography (OCT/OCTA) B-scan of a 13-year-old patient. The image is segmented into en face OCTA layers. Layer definitions are provided in Table 7.1. Images obtained from an investigational device (Heidelberg Spectralis HRA + OCT with OCTA Module). (Image courtesy of Nathan Cheung, MD.)

Fig. 7.2 Example foveal optical coherence tomography/optical coherence tomography angiography (OCT/OCTA) B-scan of a 72-year-old. The image is segmented into en face OCTA layers. Images obtained from Zeiss AngioPlex. (Images courtesy of Stephen Yoon and Sharon Fekrat, MD.)

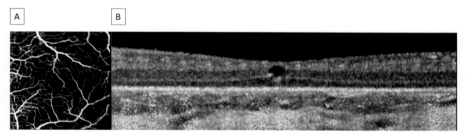

Fig. 7.3 En face optical coherence tomography angiography (OCTA) of (A) the retinal vasculature in a 3-month-old infant with retinopathy of prematurity, born at 23 weeks' gestational age. On the (B) OCT/OCTA B-scan, note the challenges of segmenting premature infant retinal layers compared with that of an older child (as shown in Fig. 7.1) or adult (as shown in Fig. 7.2). (Image courtesy of Cynthia A. Toth, MD.)

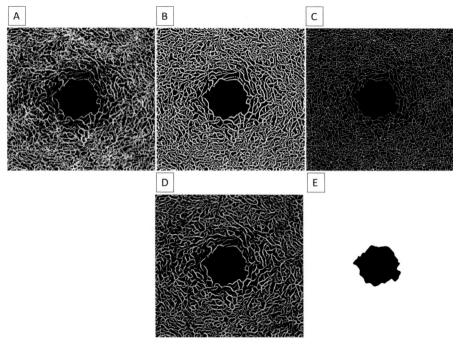

Fig. 7.4 Quantification of (A) the deep vascular complex (DVC) vessel density by (B) binarization to measure vessel area density, (C) skeletonization to measure vessel length density, and (D) foveal avascular zone (FAZ) boundaries with (E) the resulting FAZ area in a 4-month-old infant. (Quantification method and images courtesy of Hoan T. Ngo, PhD, and patient recruitment courtesy of Sharon Freedman, MD.)

References

1. Campbell JP, Zhang M, Hwang TS, et al. Detailed vascular anatomy of the human retina by projection-resolved optical coherence tomography angiography. *Sci Rep.* 2017;7:42201.
2. Lumbroso B, Huang D, Jia Y, Fujimoto J, Rispoli M. *Clinical Guide to Angio-OCT: Non Invasive, Dyeless OCT Angiography.* 1st ed. New Delhi, India: Jaypee Brothers Medical Pub; 2015.

3. Zhang Z, Huang X, Meng X, et al. In vivo assessment of macula in eyes of healthy children 8 to 16 years old using optical coherence tomography angiography. *Sci Rep.* 2017;7(1):8936.
4. Chu Z, Lin J, Gao C, et al. Quantitative assessment of the retinal microvasculature using optical coherence tomography angiography. *J Biomed Opt.* 2016;21(6):66008.
5. Liu L, Jia Y, Takusagawa HL, et al. Optical coherence tomography angiography of the peripapillary retina in glaucoma. *JAMA Ophthalmol.* 2015;133(9):1045–1052.

CHAPTER 8

Identifying Artifacts in OCT Angiography

S. Tammy Hsu ■ Lejla Vajzovic

TABLE 8.1 ■ **Artifacts on OCTA Images Can Lead to Misinterpretation of Data**
It is important to be able to identify and avoid these artifacts.

Artifact
Out of focus

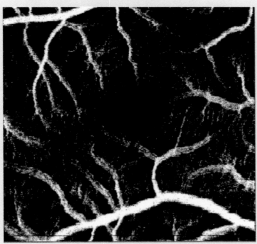

Out-of-focus camera causing blurring and doubling of vessels on en face optical coherence tomography angiography (OCTA) images of retinal vasculature in a 3-month-old patient.

Misinterpretation	How to Identify	How to Avoid
Increased vessel caliber of larger vessels and decreased density of finer vessels	While imaging, the confocal scanning laser ophthalmoscopy image appears out of focus. Images show blurring and doubling of vessels.	Adjust focus. Use the appropriate eye length settings. For high astigmatism, image the patient through their glasses.

Continued on following page

TABLE 8.1 ■ **Artifacts on OCTA Images Can Lead to Misinterpretation of Data** (Continued)

Artifact

Motion

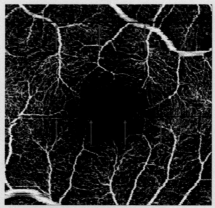

Optical coherence tomography angiography (OCTA) of retinal vasculature in a 6-year-old demonstrating motion artifact, indicated by the red arrows pointing to the sharp, linear changes.

Misinterpretation	How to Identify	How to Avoid
Flow void	During imaging, the child's head or eyes are moving (tracking, saccades); flipped B-scans from movement may result.	Reimage with stabilization of patient, if possible.

Continued on following page

ABLE 8.1 ■ **Artifacts on OCTA Images Can Lead to Misinterpretation of Data** (Continued)

Artifact

Dry eye and blinking

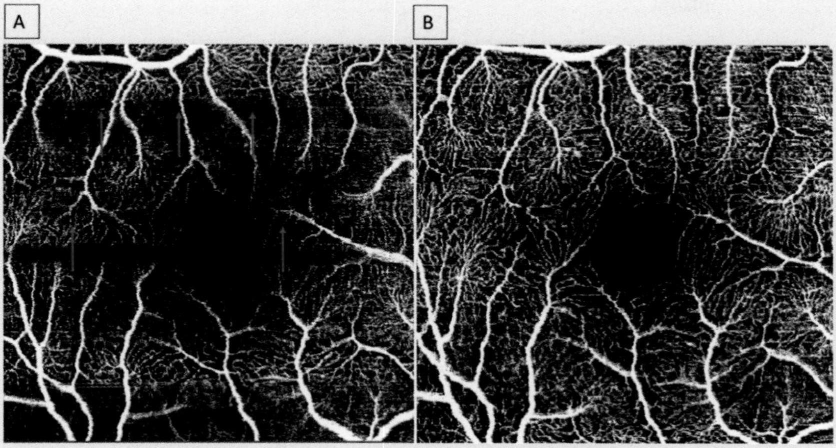

Optical coherence tomography angiography (OCTA) of the superficial venous complex (SVC) in a 14-year-old with (A) dry eyes and blinking artifacts indicated by the red arrows, and (B) reimaging after application of artificial tears. (Image courtesy of Dr. Nathan Cheung.)

Misinterpretation	How to Identify	How to Avoid
Flow void	Gradual fading in and out in a linear pattern across several consecutive B-scans; coincides with the scans being acquired before and after the patient blinks.	Reimage with artificial tears

Continued on following page

TABLE 8.1 ■ **Artifacts on OCTA Images Can Lead to Misinterpretation of Data** (Continued)

Artifact

Anterior opacity (cataract, vitreous floater)

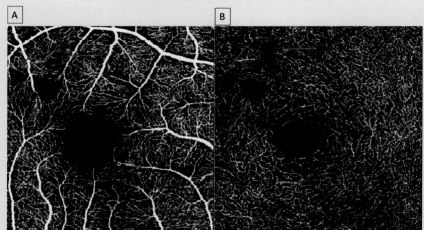

Vitreous floaters in a 17-year-old causing shadowing on the optical coherence tomography angiography (OCTA) images through all retinal layers, such as (A) superficial venous complex (SVC) and (B) deep venous complex (DVC).

Misinterpretation	How to Identify	How to Avoid
Flow void	When imaging, moving shadows caused by floaters may be visible. B-scans show shadowing and lack of flow through all layers; OCTA shows sharply demarcated spots. When reimaged, the areas with shadowing will typically change.	Reimage, and recognize the artifact.

Continued on following pa

TABLE 8.1 ■ **Artifacts on OCTA Images Can Lead to Misinterpretation of Data** (Continued)

Artifact
Shadowing

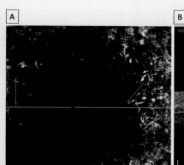
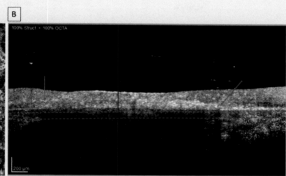

Shadowing artifact in a 14-year-old with old toxoplasma chorioretinitis scar seen on (A) en face optical coherence tomography angiography (OCTA) of the choroid layer and (B) the corresponding B-scan at the green and blue crosshairs indicated in the en face OCTA image; the yellow dots represent flow, and the red lines indicate the upper and lower boundaries used to generate the en face OCTA image in (A). Note the lack of flow seen under the hyperreflective scar in (B). Arrows point to the edges of the shadowing caused by the hyperreflective scar.

Misinterpretation	How to Identify	How to Avoid
Flow void	B-scan shows an opacity/obstruction causing an attenuation of signal in the deeper retinal layers underneath. Commonly seen in retinas with scarring or edema.	Recognize the artifact.

Continued on following page

TABLE 8.1 ■ Artifacts on OCTA Images Can Lead to Misinterpretation of Data (Continued)

Artifact
Hypertransmission

Hypertransmission of optical coherence tomography (OCT) signal in a 15-year-old with laser pointer injuries seen on (A) en face OCT angiography (OCTA of the choroid layer and (B) the corresponding B-scan at the green and blue crosshairs indicated in the en face OCTA image; the yellow dots represent flow, and the red lines indicate the upper and lower boundaries used to generate the en face OCTA image in (A). Note the increased flow caused by increased transmission through the retinal pigment epithelium (RPE) defects in (B).

Misinterpretation	How to Identify	How to Avoid
Increased flow in a nonvascular pattern	When there is increased OCT signal, such as in the choroid beneath defects in the RPE layer (choroidal hyperreflectance), or at sites of exudates, this can result in erroneous flow signal.	Recognize the artifact.

Continued on following page

TABLE 8.1 ■ **Artifacts on OCTA Images Can Lead to Misinterpretation of Data** (Continued)

Artifact
Suspended particles in motion

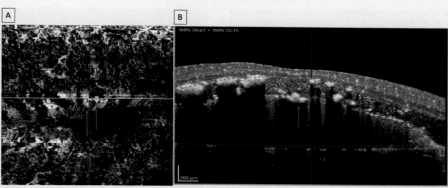

Hyperreflective particles *(red arrows)* in a patient with Coats disease appear as patches of flow on (A) the en face optical coherence tomography angiography (OCTA) image of the avascular complex layer shown in (B) the corresponding B-scan at the green and blue crosshairs indicated in the en face OCTA image; the yellow dots represent flow, and the red lines indicate the upper and lower boundaries used to generate the en face OCTA image in (A).

Misinterpretation	How to Identify	How to Avoid
Increased flow in a nonvascular pattern	Suspended hyperreflective particles moving in fluid[1]	Recognize the artifact.

Continued on following page

TABLE 8.1 ■ Artifacts on OCTA Images Can Lead to Misinterpretation of Data (Continued)

Artifact

Incorrect segmentation

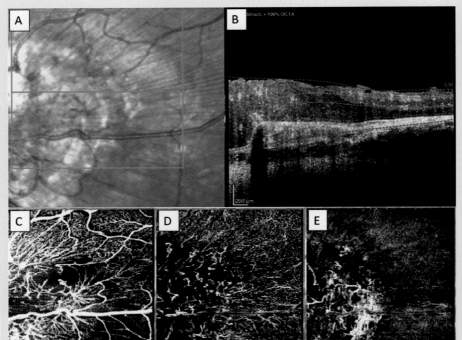

Abnormal retinal layers in a 3-year-old result in incorrect automatic segmentation (shown by the dotted lines) that results in an incorrect (A) superficial venous complex (SVC) and (B) deep venous complex (DVC).

Misinterpretation	How to Identify	How to Avoid
Blood vessels at the wrong retina layers	Review B-scans for segmentation, particularly in patients with abnormalities in retinal layers.	Correct the segmentation.

Continued on following page

BLE 8.1 ■ Artifacts on OCTA Images Can Lead to Misinterpretation of Data (Continued)

Artifact

Projection

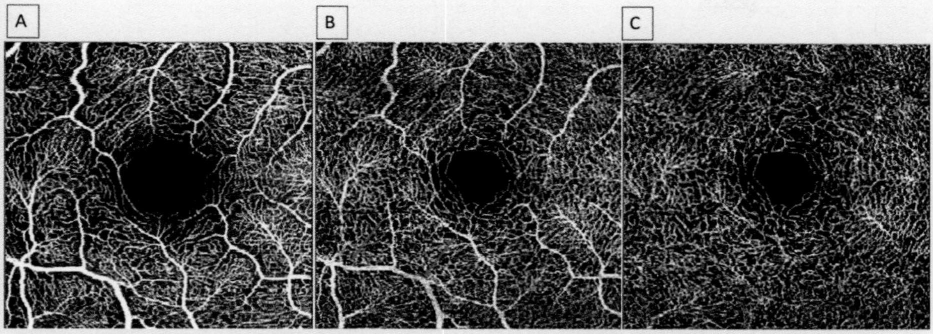

Optical coherence tomography angiography (OCTA) of a 14-year-old showing projection artifact of the larger vessels from the (A) superficial venous complex (SVC) to the (B) deep venous complex (DVC) (indicated by the red arrows). (C) DVC image after projection artifact removal. (Images obtained from an investigational device [Heidelberg Spectralis HRA+OCT with OCTA Module]. Image courtesy of Dr. Nathan Cheung.)

Misinterpretation	How to Identify	How to Avoid
ncorrect vessel density in he DVC	Vessels in the DVC appear to have the same pattern as those on the SVC. On the B-scan, look for flow coinciding with a vessel in the more superficial layers of the retina.	Remove projection artifact.

Continued on following page

TABLE 8.1 ■ **Artifacts on OCTA Images Can Lead to Misinterpretation of Data** (Continued)

Artifact
Projection removal

Optical coherence tomography angiography (OCTA) of (A) SVC and (B) DVC with projection artifact removal. Red arrows point to the area in which a superficial venous complex (SVC) large vessel projected onto the deep venous complex (DVC) was removed; however, the finer DVC vessels along that area may also have been removed.

Misinterpretation	How to Identify	How to Avoid
Decreased vessel density	Vessels in the DVC are blurred or obscured as a result of removal of the vessels projected from the SVC.	Recognize the artifact.

DVC, Deep vascular complex; OCT, optical coherence tomography; OCTA, OCT angiography; RPE, retinal pigment epithelium; SVC, superficial vascular complex.

Reference

1. Kashani AH, Green KM, Kwon J, et al. Suspended scattering particles in motion: a novel feature of OCT angiography in exudative maculopathies. *Ophthalmol Retina.* 2018;2(7):694–702.

SECTION 2

Evaluating Pediatric OCT Images: Age-Dependent Features and Common Abnormalities

CHAPTER 9

Introduction to Age-Dependent Features in Pediatric OCT Imaging

Akshay Thomas ■ Cynthia Toth

Optical coherence tomography (OCT) has revolutionized, and become an essential tool for, the diagnosis and management of retinal diseases in older children and adults. Handheld, microscope-integrated, and stand-based OCT imaging in supine patients and handheld OCT imaging in awake young children and infants have allowed us to better understand pediatric retinal and optic nerve morphology in normal and diseased states. Because of the rapid changes in eye development, especially early in life, the interpretation of pediatric OCT images can be a challenge. The effects of disease on eyes must be interpreted relative to the ongoing retinal and optic nerve development.

The subsequent chapters will discuss how OCT has revolutionized our understanding of the timeline of the complex processes of foveal development—the rate and period of centripetal movement of cone photoreceptors into the foveal center, distinct from the rate and period of centrifugal migration of inner retinal layers away from the foveal center, and the continued development through adolescence.[1] We will additionally address how certain disease states can perturb this process, resulting in morphological changes, such as persistence of foveal retinal inner layers and vasculature and reduced foveal pit depth (and increase in the central subfield thickness). Other disease processes that affect ganglion cells and their axons or that affect photoreceptors will be considered for their direct disease effects, their effects on retinal maturation, and their assessment compared with age-appropriate normative data.[2,3] Throughout this text, we will point out the strength and limitations of current pediatric normative data for OCT analyses.

The fovea and ganglion cells are not the only areas of development in the pediatric retina. In the chapters to follow, we address OCT analysis of the normal and diseased retinal and choroidal vascular development through OCT angiography (OCTA) and through imaging of the vascular/avascular junction. We will also provide insight into the unique impact of age and development on diseases of the fetal vasculature and those of the vitreoretinal interface. In each of these areas, we recognize the unique patterns of diseases of the vitreoretinal interface, retina, choroid, and optic nerve of pediatric patients and how they compare with those found in the adult eye.

With OCT imaging of the natural history of normal and perturbed retinal and optic nerve development, we have a better understanding of periods of plasticity in the microanatomy of the retina, choroid, and optic nerve in childhood. This points to the possibility that novel therapeutics may someday be developed and administered during this period of plasticity to optimize visual development and function in disease states. During these same periods, the brain (and the remainder of the visual pathway) is also undergoing rapid development, and thus OCT ocular findings may also reflect brain development and health. Noncontact OCT imaging is likely to provide useful monitoring of the microanatomy of eyes at risk and of response to novel treatments.

References

1. Vajzovic L, Hendrickson AE, O'Connell RV, et al. Maturation of the human fovea: correlation of spectral-domain optical coherence tomography findings with histology. *Am J Ophthalmol*. 2012;154(5):779–789. e2.
2. Tong AY, El-Dairi M, Maldonado RS, et al. Evaluation of optic nerve development in preterm and term infants using handheld spectral-domain optical coherence tomography. *Ophthalmology*. 2014;121(9): 1818–1826.
3. El-Dairi MA, Asrani SG, Enyedi LB, Freedman SF. Optical coherence tomography in the eyes of normal children. *Arch Ophthalmol*. 2009;127(1):50–58.

Foveal Development

Lejla Vajzovic

Introduction

The fovea is the most import part of human retina that enables fine visual acuity and color vision. Our understanding of foveal development is based primarily on histopathology studies of primates. The fovea begins to develop at 12 weeks' gestational age, and then the inner retinal layers begin to displace outward to form a foveal pit at midgestation, followed by an inward displacement of the photoreceptors and increased foveal cone density at term gestation.[1] By age 2 years, the foveal is fully developed and resembles that one of an adult (Fig. 10.1).

The Brain Connection

Neurosensory retina is central nervous system (CNS) tissue and therefore is likely to reflect ongoing brain development or maldevelopment. Although brain development cannot be readily visualized because of the complexity of repeat magnetic resonance imaging (MRI) in infants, optical coherence tomography (OCT), as described in the next section, has allowed for in vivo visualization of neurosensory retinal development.

Clinical Features

On clinical examination, the luteal pigment and foveal reflex are the visible hallmarks of the healthy macula and foveal pit.

OCT Features

Bedside spectral domain–optical coherence tomography (SD-OCT) imaging allows for in vivo visualization of the foveal developmental process.[2] SD-OCT images illustrate the persistence of the inner retinal layers at the fovea of immature neonates compared with that of adults, the centrifugal development of the inner layers, and a concurrent centripetal development of the outer layers (Fig. 10.2).[3] Retinal vascular development, including of the foveal avascular zone, starts to

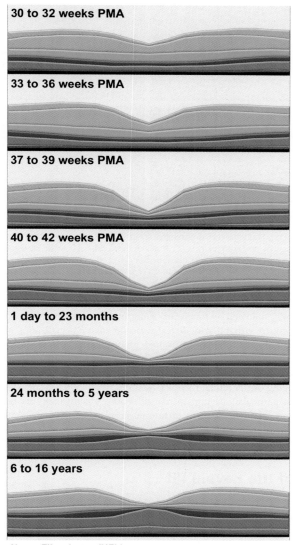

30 to 32 weeks PMA

33 to 36 weeks PMA

37 to 39 weeks PMA

40 to 42 weeks PMA

1 day to 23 months

24 months to 5 years

6 to 16 years

Nerve Fiber Layer (NFL)
Ganglion Cell Complex (GCL+IPL)
Inner Nuclear Layer (INL)
Outer Plexiform Layer or Photoreceptor Synapse Layer (OPL/PSL)
Outer Nuclear Layer and Henle's Fiber Layer (ONL+HFL)
Inner Segment Ellipsoids and Outer Segments (ISE+OS)
Retinal Pigment Epithelium (RPE)

Fig. 10.1   Diagram of foveal development from 30 weeks postmenstrual age (PMA) to 16 years, illustrated on the basis of spectral domain–optical coherence tomography (SD-OCT) volumes with centrifugal development of the inner layers and a concurrent centripetal development of the outer layers throughout age groups. Orange, nerve fiber layer (NFL); green, ganglion cell complex (GCL + IPL); light blue, inner nuclear layer (INL); dark blue, outer plexiform layer or photoreceptor synapse layer (OPL/PSL); lavender, outer nuclear layer and Henle fiber layer (ONL + HFL); red, inner segment ellipsoids and outer segments (ISE + OS); black, retinal pigment epithelium (RPE).

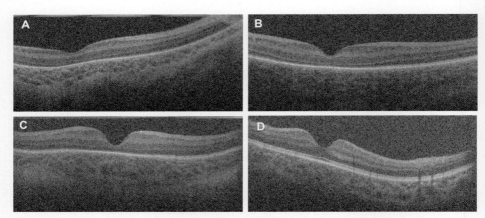

Fig. 10.2 Spectral domain–optical coherence tomography (SD-OCT) images of different stages of early foveal development: a 31-week-PMA (postmenstrual age) infant illustrating shallow foveal pit, persistence of inner retinal layers at the foveal pit, and immature outer retinal layers (A); a 37-week-PMA infant with migration of inner retinal layers out of foveal pit and immaturity of outer retinal layers (B); a 41-week-PMA infant with deeper foveal pit and developing peripheral photoreceptors (C); a 3-year-old child with fully developed inner and outer retinal layers with deep foveal pit and elongated inner and outer segments in the outer retina.

form at the optic disc, followed by formation along nasal and temporal meridians. At birth, the retina is fully vascularized with maturing foveal avascular zone.[4] Visualization of the human retinal vascular development, to date, has been limited to histopathologic studies.[4] Although current modes of imaging, such as fluorescein angiography, can provide retinal vascular information, the advent of OCT angiography (OCTA), particularly portable OCTA devices, has enabled in vivo depth-resolved imaging of the retinal microvasculature.[5-7] OCTA has the added benefit of being noninvasive and, in particular, having no risk of serious anaphylactic reaction while providing significant insight into the development of normal human foveal microvasculature and into the pathogenesis of many retinal vascular diseases.

Formation of the Foveal Pit

By using SD-OCT, one can visualize progressive increase in neurosensory retinal thickness from early gestation through late teenage years. The total neurosensory retinal thickness consistently is least in the fovea and greatest in the periphery. Initially, in early gestation, the pit is shallow and then deepens, with the pit shoulders increasing in height around full term, followed by overall increase in retinal thickness and relative shallowing of the foveal pit (see Fig. 10.2).[4]

Formation of the Foveal Avascular Zone

At 25 to 26 weeks' gestation, the developing retinal vascular network reaches the nasal foveal pit margin, whereas the temporal side vascularizes later. By 37 weeks' gestation, the foveal avascular zone (FAZ) has fully formed and continues to mature through birth and then even up to 15 months after birth.[4] In vivo imaging of FAZ by OCT-A technology illustrated that FAZ significantly varied with race, but not with age, gender, or axial length (Fig. 10.3).[6]

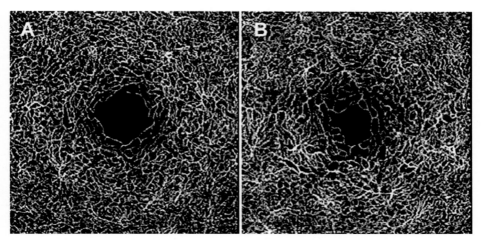

Fig. 10.3   Optical coherence tomography (OCT) angiography (OCTA) images of pediatric foveal avascular zone (FAZ) in term infant (A) and premature infant (B). Note variation in FAZ size on these deep vascular complex images. Larger FAZ correlates with wider foveal pit.

Photoreceptor Development

By using SD-OCT, one can visualize progressive thickening of the foveal outer nuclear layer after birth as cone packing and elongation of inner and outer segments (IS and OS). The inner segment ellipsoid zone (EZ) is an array of longitudinally oriented mitochondria that appears as a hyperreflective band on OCT. Initially, IS and OS are noted as hyperreflective retinal pigment epithelium (RPE) thickening approximately 33 to 36 weeks postmenstrual age (PMA) in the pericentral macula; subsequently, EZ is separated from similarly reflective RPE by the elongating hyporeflective OS approximately 37 to 39 weeks PMA in that annular region.[8] Over time, this process progresses into the central fovea. The final elongation of the photoreceptor outer segments occurs after birth (up to age 5 years), and at birth approximately one-third of term infants do not have the EZ present at the foveal center.[9] Disruptions in this process of photoreceptor development, particularly disruption of EZ development, may lead to poorer visual acuity.

Photoreceptor Maturation and Development of a Distinct Interdigitation Zone

Peripheral IS/OS are longer until well after birth, and it is not until 15 months that the foveal IS/OS length begins to overtake the peripheral length. At approximately 5 years of age, foveal IS and OS are at adult length, and the distinct interdigitation zone is visible on OCT.[8] The retinal pigment epithelium thickens through a similar age range.[10]

Ancillary Testing

Functional testing, such as electroretinography (ERG) and visual evoked potentials, although complex to perform in young infants and children, provides complementary information on the functional development of the retina. Visual acuity testing through preferential looking and later HOTV eye chart also provides functional information.

References

1. Hendrickson A, Possin D, Vajzovic L, Toth CA. Maturation of the human fovea. 1. Histological development from midgestation to maturity. *Am J Ophthalmol.* 2012;154:767–778.
2. Lee H, Purohit R, Patel A, et al. In vivo foveal development using optical coherence tomography. *Invest Ophthalmol Vis Sci.* 2015;56(8):4537–4545. https://doi.org/10.1167/iovs.15-16542.
3. Maldonado RS, O'Connell RV, Sarin N, et al. Dynamics of human foveal development after premature birth. *Ophthalmology.* 2011;118:2315–2325.
4. Provis JM, Hendrickson AE. The foveal avascular region of developing human retina. *Arch Ophthalmol.* 2008;126(4):507–511.
5. Chen X, Viehland C, Carrasco-Zevallos OM, et al. Microscope-integrated optical coherence tomography angiography in the operating room in young children with retinal vascular disease. *JAMA Ophthalmol.* 2017;135(5):483–486.
6. Hsu ST, Ngo H, House R, et al. Foveal vascular development in pediatric eyes assessed using optical coherence tomography angiography. In: *Paper presentation. ARVO Meeting.* Hawaii: Honolulu; 2018.
7. Campbell JP, Nudleman E, Yang J, et al. Handheld optical coherence tomography angiography and ultra-wide-field optical coherence tomography in retinopathy of prematurity. *JAMA Ophthalmol.* 2017;135(9):977–981.
8. Vajzovic L, Hendrickson A, O'Connell R, et al. Maturation of the human fovea. 2. Correlation of spectral domain optical coherence tomography findings with histology. *Am J Ophthalmol August.* 2012;13.
9. Vajzovic L, Rothman AL, Tran-Viet D, Cabrera MT, Freedman SF, Toth CA. Delay in retinal photoreceptor development in very preterm compared to term infants. *Invest Ophthalmol Vis Sci.* 2015;56 (2):908–913.
10. Lee H, Purohit R, Patel A, Papageorgiou E, Sheth V, Maconachie G, Pilat A, McLean RJ, Proudlock FA, Gottlob I. In Vivo Foveal Development Using Optical Coherence Tomography. *Invest Ophthalmol Vis Sci.* 2015;56(8):4537–4545. https://doi.org/10.1167/iovs.15-16542.

CHAPTER 11

Development of Retinal and Choroidal Vasculature and Peripheral Retina

Xi Chen

Our understanding of the development of retinal and choroidal vasculature and peripheral retina in humans largely relies on histopathological studies.[1-3] Optical coherence tomography (OCT) provides us with the opportunity to visualize the development of retinal structures in a noninvasive manner. Here, we briefly discuss our current knowledge and timeline of human vascular and peripheral retinal development. This information forms the basis of pediatric retinal structural and vascular imaging and contributes to our understanding of pathologic processes.

During embryonic development, closure of the eye cup fissure occurs at 5.5 weeks' gestation.[4] This is followed by development of the three vascular systems of the eye: the choroidal vasculature develops first, followed by the hyaloid vasculature and lastly the retinal vasculature.[4]

Choroidal vasculature: A single layer of choroid capillaries forms at 7 weeks' gestation. Larger choroidal vessels form and mature from 12 to 22 weeks' gestation.[2]

Hyaloid vasculature: Hyaloid artery forms by 7 weeks' gestation, the anterior portion of which supplies the developing lens, whereas the posterior portion supplies the inner retina till formation of the retinal vasculature.[2] The hyaloid vasculature starts to regress at around 13 weeks' gestation, in coordination with the formation and perfusion of the inner retina by the retinal vasculature. Failure of regression of the hyaloid vascular system causes persistent fetal vasculature (PFV) (Chapter 54).

Retinal vasculature: The retinal vasculature is the last to develop. Retinal vasculature, on *en face* view, is divided into the lobular system (perfusing the peripheral retina) and the macular system (perfusing the macula). The formation of the lobular system is largely accomplished by outward migration of endothelial cells from the optic disc to the retinal periphery, starting from 12 weeks' gestation and completed around term birth.[2] The endothelial cell migration follows the routes established by glial cells and retinal ganglion cells.[5] The macular vasculature, however, is less well understood because of the lack of fovea in common murine models. Formation of foveal avascular zone and foveal development, as visualized with OCT, are detailed in Chapter 10. In cross-sectional view, there are three layers of retinal vasculature, which are divided on OCT angiography (OCTA) into the superficial and deep vascular complexes (with the deep vascular complex subdivided into the intermediate and deep capillary plexuses), as previously discussed in detail in Chapter 7. The superficial capillary plexus forms first, followed by the intermediate and deep vascular plexuses.[1,2] Pathologic development of the retinal vasculature causes pediatric retinal vascular diseases, such as retinopathy of prematurity (ROP), familial exudative vitreoretinopathy (FEVR), incontinentia pigmenti (IP), and Norrie disease (see Section V).

Structural development of the peripheral retina is hypothesized to derive from regions in the eye cup distinct from the central retina in the eye cup[6] and is largely complete before retinal vascularization.[7] Indeed, no significant retinal structural changes between vascularized retina and avascular retina was observed across the vascular–avascular junction on OCT imaging in infants with no or stage 1 ROP (Chapter 28). Detailed human retinal vascular development and its interaction with the central and peripheral neural retina is still under active investigation. We look forward to new findings in this area, informed by structural OCT and OCT angiography in neonates, as an understanding of the developmental process will inform us of the pathologic process of the retinal and choroidal vascular system and the peripheral retina.

References

1. Hughes S, Yang H, Chan-Ling T. Vascularization of the human fetal retina: roles of vasculogenesis and angiogenesis. *Invest Ophthalmol Vis Sci.* 2000;41(5):1217–1228.
2. Lutty GA, McLeod DS. Development of the hyaloid, choroidal and retinal vasculatures in the fetal human eye. *Prog Retin Eye Res.* 2018;62:58–76.
3. Provis JM, Hendrickson AE. The foveal avascular region of developing human retina. *Arch Ophthalmol.* 2008;126(4):507–511.
4. Mann IC. *The Development of the Human Eye.* Cambridge: University Press; 1928.
5. Chan-Ling T, McLeod DS, Hughes S, et al. Astrocyte-endothelial cell relationships during human retinal vascular development. *Invest Ophthalmol Vis Sci.* 2004;45(6):2020–2032.
6. Venters SJ, Mikawa T, Hyer J. Central and peripheral retina arise through distinct developmental paths. *PLoS One.* 2013;8(4):e61422.
7. Hendrickson A. Development of Retinal Layers in Prenatal Human Retina. *Am J Ophthalmol.* 2016;161:29–35. e21.

CHAPTER 12

Vitreoretinal Abnormalities

Hesham Gabr ■ Alexandria Dandridge

Vitreoretinal Abnormalities

Optical coherence tomography (OCT) allows for visualization of a wide range of vitreoretinal abnormalities.

Vitreoretinal Interface Disorders

These include epiretinal membranes (ERMs) or vitreoretinal adhesions/traction (Fig. 12.1). In children, in contrast to adults, partial or complete vitreous separation from the retinal surface is less common, and idiopathic ERMs are thus less common.[1] Also, compared with adults, children are less likely to have any ERM separation from the macula (Fig. 12.2). This results in the different appearance of vitreoretinal traction and epiretinal membranes.

Differential diagnosis includes:
1. Familial exudative vitreoretinopathy (FEVR)
2. Retinopathy of prematurity (ROP)
3. Idiopathic ERM
4. Combined hamartoma of the retina and retinal pigment epithelium
5. Retinoschisis
6. Chronic retinal detachment (including with proliferative vitreoretinopathy)
7. Trauma
8. Posterior uveitis
9. Norrie disease
10. Incontinentia pigmenti (IP)

Macular Cystoid Spaces and/or Edema

These areas appear as hyporeflective spaces, usually involving all retinal layers but may be more noticeable in the inner nuclear layer, especially in infants with ROP. Fluorescein angiography

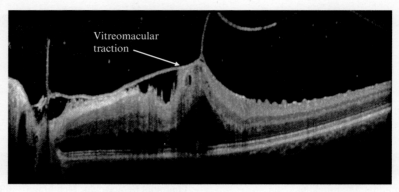

Fig. 12.1 Vitreomacular traction in a 16-year-old boy.

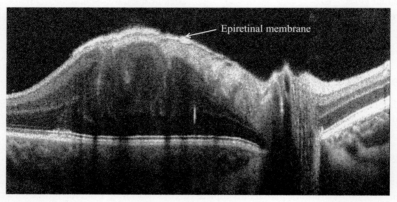

Fig. 12.2 Epiretinal membrane (ERM) in a 13-year-old girl; the ERM is within the condensed posterior hyaloid over the combined hamartoma of the retina and retinal pigment epithelium.

(FA) often reveals leakage from cystoid macular edema. In contrast, intraretinal cystoid spaces associated with juvenile X-linked retinoschisis and retinitis pigmentosa do not typically leak on FA.

Differential diagnosis includes:

A. Cystoid macular edema associated with:
1. ROP (Fig. 12.3)
2. Chronic retinal detachment
3. Trauma
4. Posterior uveitis
5. Posterior segment tumor
6. Coats disease
7. Optic pit maculopathy
8. Central serous chorioretinopathy

B. Macular cystoid changes are associated with:
1. Juvenile X-linked retinoschisis (Fig. 12.4)
2. Retinitis pigmentosa

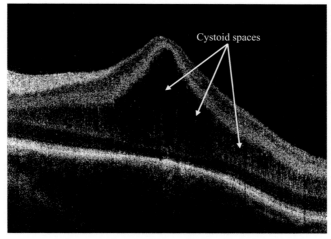

Fig. 12.3 Macular cystoid spaces in the inner nuclear layer in a 37 weeks' postmenstrual age infant with retinopathy of prematurity.

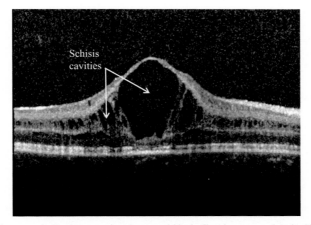

Fig. 12.4 Cystoid spaces in the inner nuclear layer and Henle fiber layer associated with juvenile X-linked retinoschisis in a 6-year-old boy.

Subretinal Fluid

See Fig. 12.5.

Accumulation of a clear (serous) or lipid-rich (exudative) fluid in the subretinal space appears hyporeflective/optically empty on OCT.

Differential diagnosis includes:

1. Coats disease
2. FEVR
3. Retinal detachment—serous, rhegmatogenous, or tractional
4. Trauma
5. Posterior uveitis

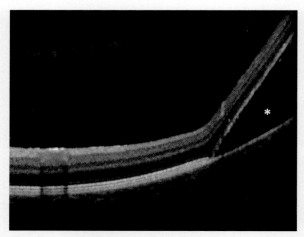

Fig. 12.5 Subretinal fluid (*) in an 11-year-old boy with retinal detachment.

6. Posterior segment tumor
7. Optic pit
8. Optic nerve and chorioretinal coloboma
9. Central serous chorioretinopathy

Intraretinal and Subretinal Deposits

See Fig. 12.6.

These appear as hyperreflective foci within or under the retina with shadowing of the underlying tissues. They may represent lipid exudation, old subretinal/intraretinal hemorrhage, pigmentation, or calcification.

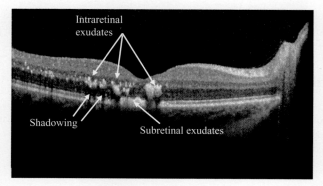

Fig. 12.6 Intraretinal and subretinal hyperreflective exudates with shadowing of the underlying tissues in a 10-year-old boy with Coats disease.

Differential diagnosis includes:
1. Coats disease
2. FEVR
3. ROP
4. Posterior uveitis
5. Posterior segment tumor (e.g., retinoblastoma)
6. Sickle cell retinopathy
7. Diabetic retinopathy

Choroidal Neovascular Membrane

See Fig. 12.7.

This is the growth of new blood vessels that originate from the choroid through a break in the Bruch membrane into the sub–retinal pigment epithelium (RPE) space or the subretinal space. On OCT, they appear as highly reflective tissue with margins that can be sharp or poorly defined. They may be associated with intraretinal, subretinal, or sub-RPE fluid. Over time, they may be associated with RPE atrophy and retinal disorganization and thinning. Subretinal neovascularization may also rarely occur from a retinal vascular source.

Differential diagnosis includes:
1. Optic nerve coloboma with peripapillary choroidal neovascular membrane (CNVM)
2. Optic nerve edema with peripapillary CNVM
3. Optic nerve drusen with peripapillary CNVM
4. Angioid streaks (pseudoxanthoma elasticum, Ehlers-Danlos syndrome, Paget disease, sickle cell disease, idiopathic) with peripapillary CNVM
5. Retinal dystrophies with CNVM
6. Myopia
7. Trauma with choroidal rupture
8. Presumed ocular histoplasmosis syndrome
9. Posterior uveitis
10. Posterior segment tumors, such as choroidal hemangioma or osteoma
11. Combined hamartoma of the retina and RPE
12. Idiopathic

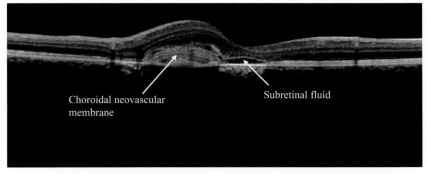

Fig. 12.7 Choroidal neovascular membrane (CNV) in a 12-year-old boy. Image shows also distorted retina and subretinal fluid resulting from leakage from the CNV.

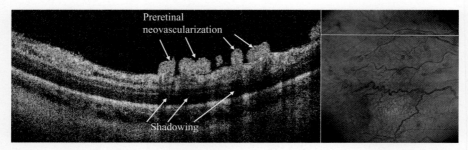

Fig. 12.8 Preretinal neovascularization with shadowing of the underlying tissues in a 44 weeks' postmenstrual age infant with retinopathy of prematurity.

Preretinal Neovascularization

See Fig. 12.8.

This appears as extraretinal tissue above the retina. The abnormal vasculature casts a shadow on OCT.[2]

Differential diagnosis includes:

1. ROP
2. FEVR
3. Norrie disease
4. IP
5. Hyperviscosity syndrome or retinal artery or vein occlusion
6. Sickle cell retinopathy
7. Proliferative diabetic retinopathy
8. Retinal detachment
9. Eales disease

Loss of Retinal Tissue

See Figs. 12.9 and 12.10.

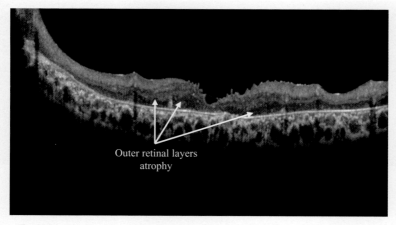

Fig. 12.9 Atrophy of the outer retinal layers in a 10-year-old boy with Coats disease.

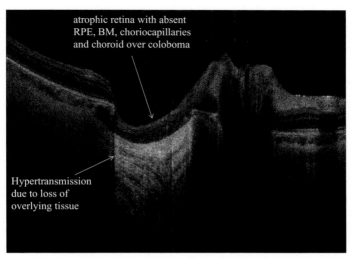

Fig. 12.10   Hypertransmission caused by loss of overlying tissue in a 2-year-old boy with bilateral chorioretinal colobomas and CHARGE (coloboma, heart anomaly, choanal atresia, retardation, genital and ear anomalies) syndrome. The lack of retinal pigment epithelium (RPE) and choroid at the site of the chorioretinal coloboma results in hypertransmission of optical coherence tomography (OCT) signal into the sclera producing the intense bright white reflected signal beneath the lesion.

This refers to the atrophy or decrease in size of the inner retinal layers (nerve fiber layer to inner nuclear layer) and/or outer retinal layers (outer plexiform layer to retinal pigment epithelium).
   Differential diagnosis includes:
   1. Retinal artery or vein occlusion
   2. Inflammatory or infectious retinitis or chorioretinitis
   3. Trauma
   4. Coats disease
   5. FEVR
   6. IP
   7. ROP
   8. Norrie disease
   9. Retinal degenerations and dystrophies
   10. Optic nerve and chorioretinal coloboma
   11. After retinal detachment

Loss of Retinal Vasculature

See Fig. 12.11.
   Differential diagnosis includes:
   1. Trauma
   2. Retinal artery or vein occlusion
   3. Inflammatory or infectious retinitis or chorioretinitis and residual scar
   4. Coats disease
   5. FEVR
   6. IP
   7. ROP
   8. Norrie disease

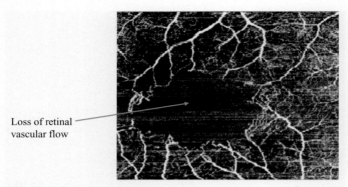

Loss of retinal vascular flow

Fig. 12.11 Loss of retinal vasculature caused by scarring in a 14-year-old boy.

References

1. Rothman AL, Folgar FA, Tong AY, Toth CA. Spectral domain optical coherence tomography characterization of pediatric epiretinal membranes. *Retina.* 2014;34(7):1323–1334.
2. Maldonado RS, Toth CA. Optical coherence tomography in retinopathy of prematurity: looking beyond the vessels. *Clin Perinatol.* 2013;40(2):271–296.

CHAPTER 13

Normal Optic Nerve Head: Anatomy and Development

Mays El-Dairi ■ Robert James House

Introduction

Understanding the normal anatomy of the optic nerve head allows clinicians to more effectively recognize pathology and abnormalities in patients of a similar developmental stage. The invention of optical coherence tomography (OCT), more specifically handheld OCT, has provided quantitative values of the normal pediatric optic nerve head and has allowed for measurement of the retinal nerve fiber layer (RNFL) and optic disc.

Eye–Brain Connection

The optic nerve is part of the central nervous system (CNS) and is composed of densely packed retinal ganglion cell (RGC) axons,[1] which send information from the retina to the brain. The optic nerve is mostly unmyelinated at birth, with myelination beginning posterior to the lamina cribrosa soon after and stabilizing at around age 4 years, and it remains there until late adulthood.[1]

Clinical Features

In pediatric patients, examinations of the optic nerve head are performed with a dilated fundus examination because children (especially those under age 5 years or those with developmental delay) can have problems cooperating and focusing for imaging. Other clinical examinations to evaluate functionality, such as visual acuity, color vision, visual field, grating acuity, and motility examinations, can give clinical clues to ocular abnormalities, including those associated with the optic nerve.

OCT Features

OCT is a relatively quick and noninvasive imaging modality that can enhance the pediatric clinical examination, when indicated. Different protocols can be used when OCT is required. In neuro-ophthalmology, in particular, the interpretation of OCT images frequently requires a macular map (Fig. 13.1), as well as scans of the peripapillary RNFL (Fig. 13.2), the retina, and the optic

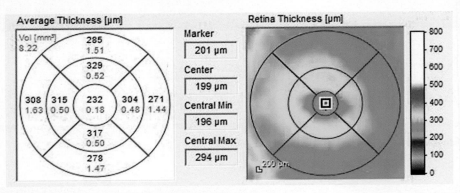

Fig. 13.1 Macular map of a healthy 6-year-old boy. Numbers on the map are the average volumes of each sector per the Early Treatment Diabetic Retinopathy Study (ETDRS) map.

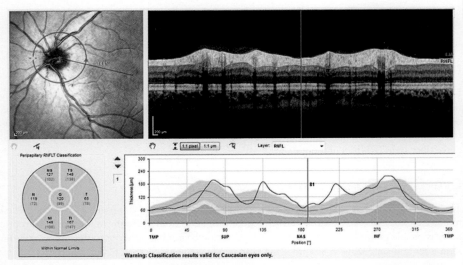

Fig. 13.2 Retinal nerve fiber layer (RNFL) scan from a healthy 6-year-old white boy. Average RNFL is 120 (average is 107 per published normative database). The cursor indicates the nerve fiber layer thickness in that position (81 μm in this example)

nerve (Figs. 13.3 and 13.4). When only a limited amount of scans can be obtained because of lack of patient cooperation, the authors recommend obtaining a central macular scan through the fovea and an RNFL scan.

OCT values are affected by several variables, including age, axial length, and race.[2-8] Optic disc diameter increases with age, as demonstrated by Patel et al.[3] who found that mean disc diameter increased from 1.14 mm at birth to 1.49 mm at age 13 years. Increasing disc size has a nonlinear growth pattern, being rapid in the first 3 to 4 years of life and eventually tapering off and reaching adult size by 12 years.[1,3] In the same cohort of patients, Patel et al.[3] also showed an increase in axial length from 16.8 mm at birth to 24 mm at age 13 years, as well as an increase in cup size (0.4 mm at birth to 0.56 mm at age 13 years.) Measurements of the cup[7] tend to correlate with axial length,[2]

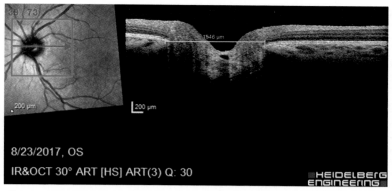

Fig. 13.3 Enhanced depth imaging (EDI) map through the Bruch membrane opening in a healthy 6-year-old white boy. The Bruch membrane is flat (no upward bowing). The maximal Bruch membrane opening distance is 1546 μm, which is normal.

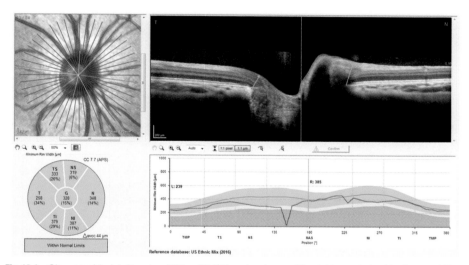

Fig. 13.4 Glaucoma Module Premium Edition (GMPE) protocol scan of the right eye of a healthy 8-year-old boy. The placement of the Bruch membrane opening is seen as red dots in the image. The sectors display the neuroretinal rim volume, and the disc area is noted in the bottom right corner of the infrared image (1.92 mm²).

and the cup-to-disc ratio often remains stable.[3] Longitudinal studies have also shown that global OCT measurements in children are reproducible over time despite changes in axial length.[4]

Racial differences have been described in analyses of the RNFL, the optic disc topography,[5,8] and the macula,[2] and these demographics can provide important information when there are differences between a physiologic nerve and a pathologic nerve.

RNFL thickness measurements do not seem to be dependent on age in children ages 3 to 18 years, with average thickness reported to be between 102 and 113 μm.[3] El-Dairi et al.[2] demonstrated that in children ages 3 to 17 years, mean RNFL ranges from 105.9 μm to 110.7 μm in white and black children, respectively. In preterm infants, a thinner RNFL has been associated with brain injury, as demonstrated on brain magnetic resonance imaging.[9]

Ancillary Testing

Additional testing outside of a funduscopic examination should be performed, as indicated, on the basis of clinical findings. If a patient with a normal ocular examination result fails to improve even after correcting for refractive error, other imaging modalities, such as OCT or visual field tests, may aid in the diagnosis if the child is capable of cooperating during the examination.

References

1. Dolman CL, McCormick AQ, Drance SM. Aging of the optic nerve. *Arch Ophthalmol.* 1980;98(11): 2053–2058.
2. El-Dairi MA, Asrani SG, Enyedi LB, Freedman SF. Optical coherence tomography in the eyes of normal children. *Arch Ophthalmol.* 2009;127(1):50–58.
3. Patel A, Purohit R, Lee H, et al. Optic nerve head development in healthy infants and children using hand-held spectral-domain optical coherence tomography. *Ophthalmology.* 2016;123(10):2147–2157.
4. Prakalapakorn SG, Freedman SF, Lokhnygina Y, et al. Longitudinal reproducibility of optical coherence tomography measurements in children. *J AAPOS.* 2012;16(6):523–528.
5. Tong AY, El-Dairi M, Maldonado RS, et al. Evaluation of optic nerve development in preterm and term infants using handheld spectral-domain optical coherence tomography. *Ophthalmology.* 2014;121(9): 1818–1826.
6. Allingham MJ, Cabrera MT, O'Connell RV, et al. Racial variation in optic nerve head parameters quantified in healthy newborns by handheld spectral domain optical coherence tomography. *J AAPOS.* 2013;17(5): 501–506.
7. Rothman AL, Sevilla MB, Freedman SF, et al. Assessment of retinal nerve fiber layer thickness in healthy, full-term neonates. *Am J Ophthalmol.* 2015;159(4):803–811.
8. Huynh SC, Wang XY, Rochtchina E, Mitchell P. Peripapillary retinal nerve fiber layer thickness in a population of 6-year-old children: findings by optical coherence tomography. *Ophthalmology.* 2006;113(9): 1583–1592.
9. Rothman AL, Sevilla MB, Mangalesh S, et al. Thinner retinal nerve fiber layer in very preterm versus term infants and relationship to brain anatomy and neurodevelopment. *Am J Ophthalmol.* 2015;160(6): 1296–1308.

CHAPTER 14

Optic Nerve Head Abnormalities

Mays Antoine El-Dairi ▪ Robert James House

Optical coherence tomography (OCT) can enhance clinical examination findings in the analysis of anomalous optic nerves because it adds quantification when describing optic nerve morphology, especially in the setting of optic nerve swelling or atrophy.[1]

Eye-Brain Connection

The ganglion cell axons that comprise the majority of the optic nerve extend to synapse within the brain. Thus optic nerve swelling or atrophy may signal one or more of many central nervous system events that are described in this chapter.

The Elevated Optic Nerve

See Fig. 14.1.

A clinically elevated optic nerve can appear on OCT as:

1. A thickened peripapillary retinal nerve fiber layer (pRNFL)
2. Thickened nasal segments of the macular map that correspond to the temporal peripapillary area
3. Possible upward bowing of the Bruch membrane.

Differential diagnosis includes:

1. Papilledema (Chapter 66) from increased intracranial pressure
2. Optic neuritis (acutely) (About 66% of pediatric optic neuritis patients have acutely swollen nerves as seen on clinical examination[2] and greater than 95% also have a thickened RNFL.[2])
3. Ischemic optic neuropathy (rare in children)
4. Pseudo–optic disc edema resulting from the acute phase of Leber hereditary optic neuropathy.
5. Optic nerve head drusen with segmentation errors (Chapter 69)
6. Pseudopapilledema with segmentation errors (Chapter 69)
7. High hyperopia
8. Neuroretinitis (Chapter 68)
9. Medication-induced toxic optic neuropathy—acute stage resulting from linezolid, ethambutol

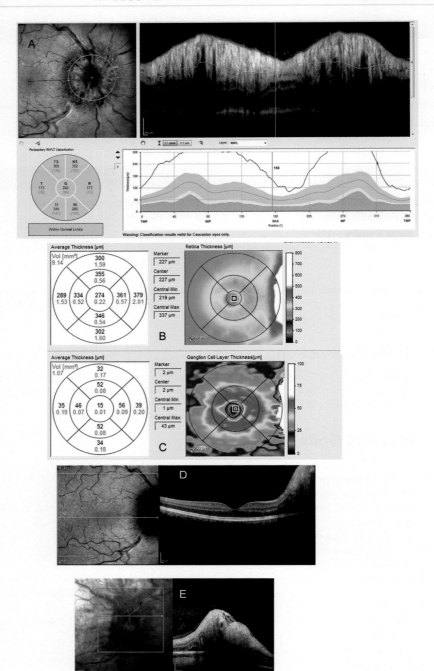

Fig. 14.1 Severe acute papilledema in a 14-year-old girl with aseptic meningitis. Optical coherence tomography (OCT) of the retinal nerve fiber layer (RNFL) (A) is thickened with an average of 242 microns. Total macular volume (B) shows thickened retina nasally, but the ganglion cell layer (C) is normal. Single-line OCT of the macula (D) shows elevated nasal macula. Enhanced depth imaging (EDI) scan through the optic nerve (E) shows upward bowing of the Bruch membrane, indicative of high intracranial pressure. When looking at optic disc edema, all protocols (RNFL, macular map, ganglion cell layer, and single-line macular scans and optic nerve head scan) need to be analyzed.

10. Infiltrative optic neuropathy—acute stage resulting from acute lymphocytic leukemia (ALL), lymphoma, optic nerve sheath meningioma
11. Traction to the optic nerve head from familial exudative vitreoretinopathy or other vitreoretinopathy (Chapter 29)

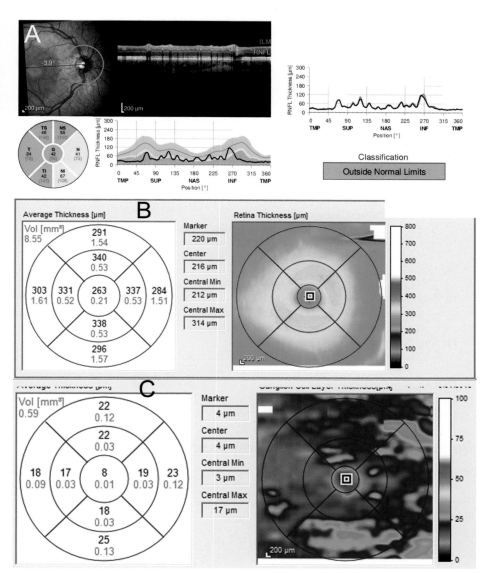

Fig. 14.2 Optic atrophy resulting from previous optic neuritis in a 6-year-old boy. Optical coherence tomography (OCT) scan of the retinal nerve fiber layer (RNFL) (A) demonstrated significant thinning, measured here at 42. Total macular volume (B) was normal at 8.55 mm³. Segmented ganglion cell layer map (C) shows abnormal thinning with total volume of 0.59 mm³. All protocol scans should be used to diagnose optic atrophy.

Optic Nerve Atrophy

See Fig. 14.2.

The RNFL is thin in optic atrophy, which is the end stage of optic neuropathy. It is seen in the period between 3 weeks and 3 months of the onset of the disease.[3]

On OCT, an atrophic optic nerve will manifest as:

1. Thin RNFL
2. Thin NFL, ganglion cell layer, and inner plexiform layer on the macular map
3. Possible inner cysts in the inner nuclear layer

Differential diagnosis includes:

1. Compressive lesions (brain tumor involving the anterior visual pathway, brain cysts, or orbital masses)
2. End-stage papilledema (Chapter 66)
3. End-stage optic neuritis
4. Genetic optic neuropathies, such as dominant optic atrophy or Wolfram (diabetes insipidus, diabetes mellitus, optic atrophy, and deafness [DIDMOAD]) syndrome
5. Vitamin B (riboflavin, folate, B^{12}) deficiencies
6. Medication-induced toxicity, such as from linezolid, ethambutol, methanol, and chloramphenicol; heavy metal toxicity; carbon monoxide poisoning
7. Traumatic
8. Infectious
   a. Neuroretinitis (Chapter 68)
   b. Direct invasion of the nerve from an infectious cause (often including meningitis)
      i. Herpetic (cytomegalovirus [CMV], herpes simplex virus [HSV]), syphilis, Lyme disease, influenza, *Cryptococcus* infection, brucellosis, and other rare causes
9. Infiltrative—end stage
   a. ALL, lymphoma, and optic nerve sheath meningioma
10. Glaucoma (Chapter 70)
    a. Glaucoma causes thinning of the RNFL and of the inner macula, but the nerve appears cupped as opposed to pale on clinical examination
11. Optic nerve hypoplasia (Chapter 62)
    a. This causes thinning of the RNFL and of the inner macula. The Bruch membrane will appear small, and there may be a "double ring" sign, but there should not be any pallor.
12. Optic atrophy (Chapter 64)
13. Hydrocephalus (see Fig. 14.1)
14. Ischemic from macro or microvascular disease or injury.

Optic Nerve Swelling Superimposed on Optic Atrophy

See Fig. 14.3.

In the early stages of optic neuropathy, a situation that can potentially cause confusion is optic nerve swelling superimposed on optic atrophy. In these cases, the RNFL may appear normal, and the ganglion cell layer will be thin.

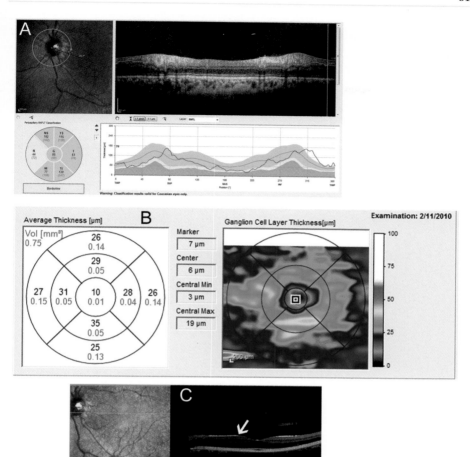

Fig. 14.3 Retinal nerve fiber layer (RNFL) thinning and ganglion cell layer atrophy resulting from chronic hydrocephalus in a 15-year-old girl. RNFL scan (A) looks almost normal with an average RNFL of 85. Macular ganglion cell layer map (B) shows diffuse thinning. Single-line optical coherence tomography (OCT) image of the macula (C) shows severely atrophic ganglion cell layer *(arrow)*. The RNFL protocol, used in isolation, would not have shown the pathology of vision loss in this case because the swelling of the nerve was masking the atrophy, making the RNFL look normal.

References

1. Kupersmith MJ. Optical imaging of the optic nerve: beyond demonstration of retinal nerve fiber layer loss. *J Neuroophthalmol.* 2015;35(2):210–219.
2. Walia S, Fishman GA. Retinal nerve fiber layer analysis in RP patients using Fourier-domain OCT. *Invest Ophthalmol Vis Sci.* 2008;49(8):3525–3528. https://doi.org/10.1167/iovs.08-1842.
3. El-Dairi MA, Ghasia F, Bhatti MT. Pediatric optic neuritis. *Int Ophthalmol Clin.* 2012;52(3):29–49. xii.

Research Considerations for OCT Studies in Children

CHAPTER 15

Introduction to Research in Pediatric OCT Imaging

Xi Chen ■ Katrina Postell Winter

Tabletop and handheld optical coherence tomography (OCT) systems have provided researchers and clinicians with valuable research tools to evaluate retinal development and pathology, offering the ability to assess qualitative changes (e.g., changes in retinal layers, cystoid macular edema, and photoreceptor maturation) with high-resolution and measure and record longitudinal quantitative changes in retinal layer thickness.[1-3]

The major benefit of using OCT for eye research is its noninvasive nature—it can be performed with or without pharmacologic dilation, it avoids contact, and it can be performed with minimal risk to infants and children at the bedside (handheld), during examination under anesthesia (handheld and armature-fixated), and in the clinic (handheld and tabletop). Prior investigations have established normative databases of optic nerve and retinal development in infants and children from term to age 16 years.[2,4,5] OCT has been shown to be effective in demonstrating pathologies that were less well appreciated by the human eye on direct fundus examination[1] and to help identify potential biomarkers of brain development.[6]

Research in pediatric OCT imaging should follow the same rigor and reproducibility that are exercised in studies of adult vitreoretinal diseases by using OCT as a primary or secondary outcome. As we have previously discussed, features of the growing pediatric eyes and their evolving retinal morphology necessitate methods for pediatric-specific image acquisition, segmentation, interpretation, and analysis.[7] Research in infants and children (those under 18 to 21 years of age, the age varies by jurisdiction), who are a vulnerable population, comes with its own rules and regulations. Indeed, any human research protocol involving the pediatric population requires additional review through the institutional review board (IRB), which will consider the child's health status, age, and ability to understand what is involved in the research. The IRB must also make a determination of the risks and the potential benefit(s) of the research to the subject, to other children with the same condition or disease, or to society as a whole (Office of Human Research Protections, Special protections for children as research subjects).

In this chapter, we discuss the special considerations in research involving children who are a vulnerable population, the benefits of nondilated imaging, quality assessment, reproducibility of imaging and interpretation, and secure OCT data storage and networking.

References

1. Maldonado RS, Toth CA. Optical coherence tomography in retinopathy of prematurity: looking beyond the vessels. *Clin Perinatol.* 2013;40(2):271–296.
2. Turk A, Ceylan OM, Arici C, et al. Evaluation of the nerve fiber layer and macula in the eyes of healthy children using spectral-domain optical coherence tomography. *Am J Ophthalmol.* 2012;153(3):552–559. e551.

3. Vajzovic L, Rothman AL, Tran-Viet D, Cabrera MT, Freedman SF, Toth CA. Delay in retinal photoreceptor development in very preterm compared to term infants. *Invest Ophthalmol Vis Sci.* 2015;56(2): 908–913.
4. Patel A, Purohit R, Lee H, et al. Optic Nerve head development in healthy infants and children using handheld spectral-domain optical coherence tomography. *Ophthalmology.* 2016;123(10):2147–2157.
5. Yanni SE, Wang J, Cheng CS, et al. Normative reference ranges for the retinal nerve fiber layer, macula, and retinal layer thicknesses in children. *Am J Ophthalmol.* 2013;155(2):354–360. e351.
6. Rothman AL, Sevilla MB, Mangalesh S, et al. Thinner retinal nerve fiber layer in very preterm versus term infants and relationship to brain anatomy and neurodevelopment. *Am J Ophthalmol.* 2015;160(6): 1296–1308. e1292.
7. Maldonado RS, Izatt JA, Sarin N, et al. Optimizing hand-held spectral domain optical coherence tomography imaging for neonates, infants, and children. *Invest Ophthalmol Vis Sci.* 2010;51(5):2678–2685.

CHAPTER 16

Considerations for Neonates and Children as a Vulnerable Research Population

Neeru Sarin

In human research, neonates and children are considered a vulnerable population for multiple reasons. First, they lack autonomy and the capacity to ethically and legally consent to participating in research. Neonates and children do not typically have the ability to assume and understand the risks involved in research. Furthermore, inequality in power exists between children and adults, leading to the risk of exploitation of children. Premature babies, in particular, are considered a highly vulnerable population because of their many systemic health issues, and this should be kept in mind when enrolling them into clinical studies. There has been lack of sufficient research in pediatric populations, and pediatric research has been encouraged through national and multinational policies.

Pediatric research must follow proper ethical standards that are designed to provide additional safeguards to protect children. This has been stated both in the Declaration of Helsinki (1964, with subsequent amendments) and in the U.S. Federal Policy for the Protection of Human Subjects (1991, with subsequent updates). U.S. regulations from the Department of Health and Human Services (DHHS), 45 CFR Part 46 (2009) include subparts that address additional protections for neonates and children.[1] In that document, research is described on the basis of the risk involved, the level of risk to the child, and the child directly benefiting from participation in research. When children are involved in a research study, it is important to obtain their assent (if they are capable) and the permission of their parents/legal guardians. Assent is described as a child's affirmative agreement to participate in research (45 CFR 46.402 [b]).[2]

Research guidelines and regulations may vary by country and, in some countries, may be institution specific.[3] For multinational pediatric trials, there is a wide variation in consent requirements, so standardization is needed. Local research oversight is typically provided by an institutional review board (IRB), also known as *ethical review board* or *research ethics board*.

In pediatric research studies, optical coherence tomography (OCT) is a noncontact method of imaging ocular pathology with near infrared light. OCT can be performed without pharmacologic pupil dilation; thus no exposure to mydriatic drops is needed to view the retina, which may decrease the potential risk of pediatric research imaging.

In studies governed by DHHS regulations, data pertaining to the conduct of the research study must be retained by the institution for at least 3 years after completion of the research. In addition, other regulations may apply, requiring retention of pediatric records for a longer period of time, and requirements vary by jurisdiction. This is an important aspect to consider when planning an OCT-based research study in children.

References

1. U.S. Department of Health & Human Services Office for Human Research. *45 CFR 46*. Available at https://www.hhs.gov/ohrp/regulations-and-policy/regulations/45-cfr-46/index.html; 2009. Accessed May 22, 2018.
2. Wendler DS. Assent in pediatric research: theoretical and practical considerations. *J Med Ethics*. 2006;32 (4):229–234.
3. Lepola P, Needham A, Mendum J, Sallabank P, Neubauer D, de Wildt S. Informed consent for paediatric clinical trials in Europe. *Arch Dis Child*. 2016;101(11):1017–1025.

CHAPTER 17

Benefit of Nondilated Imaging

Shwetha Mangalesh

The advent of spectral domain–optical coherence tomography (SD-OCT) imaging in infants has reminded us that the retina is an extension of the diencephalon, pointing to the potential for OCT imaging to revolutionize the diagnosis and monitoring of retinal, optic nerve, and neurologic diseases in infants. Traditionally, retinal and optic nerve evaluations have required pharmacologic dilation because the pupil constricts briskly to the visible light emitted by ophthalmoscopes and fundus cameras. However, the use of pharmacologic agents may not always be advisable, for example, in sick infants, given the risk of systemic side effects, and in patients with profound brain injury, given the need for continuous pupillary monitoring.[1] Optical coherence tomography (OCT), with its infrared light source, offers the advantage of imaging the retina and the optic nerve without need for pharmacologic dilation. Because infrared light from the OCT, does not constrict the pupil, by placing a patient in dim lighting, it is possible to image through a physiologically dilated pupil.

Furthermore, even when pupils are constricted, for example, as a result of the use of opiates or other parasympathomimetic agents, successful imaging of the macula and the optic nerve is possible with use of OCT. Because it avoids the need for daily dilation, this method is beneficial for repeat assessments to monitor changes in response to treatment (Fig. 17.1). Non-dilated OCT imaging of the structure and vascular flow in neurovascular tissue of the retina has potential value as a reflection of injury, disease and even development of the brain.

Techniques to obtain high-quality images in small pupils are similar to those that ensure the comfort and ergonomics of the child and imager during OCT imaging, as discussed in Chapter 3.[2] Alignment of the OCT probe with the visual axis of the eye is very important when pupils are small because small movement will shift the region of interest in the retina out of the pupil. It is also important to control the ambient illumination, adjust the positioning of the imager relative to that of the child, and stabilize the OCT probe. Thus having a second person to assist with the imaging is very useful.[2]

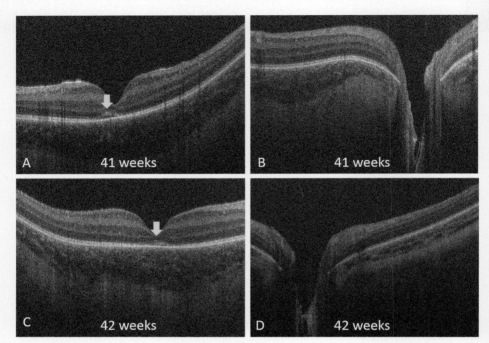

Fig. 17.1 Spectral domain–optical tomography (SD-OCT) images captured without pharmacologic dilation in a neonate with hypoxic ischemic encephalopathy (HIE). The pupil diameter was 2 mm at the first examination (A, B) and 3.5 mm 1 week later (C, D). The subfoveal fluid that was present at birth (A) decreased 1 week later (C). The optic nerve head was also imaged at both visits (B, D, different sections shown for each week) and demonstrated absence of swelling and presence of a deep cup.

References

1. Chen JW, Vakil-Gilani K, Williamson KL, Cecil S. Infrared pupillometry, the Neurological Pupil index and unilateral pupillary dilation after traumatic brain injury: implications for treatment paradigms. *Springerplus.* 2014;3:548.
2. Tran-Viet D, Wong BM, Mangalesh S, Maldonado R, Cotten CM, Toth CA. Handheld spectral domain optical coherence tomography imaging through the undilated pupil in infants born preterm or with hypoxic injury or hydrocephalus. *Retina.* 2017;38:1588–1594.

CHAPTER 18

Quality Assessment

Katrina Postell Winter ▨ Xi Chen

Quality assessment of optical coherence tomography (OCT) images involves the evaluation of factors that may impact the interpretation of the image. Poor image quality, as detailed below, may interfere in the ability of the clinician or researcher to identify and distinguish normal or abnormal structures and to measure relevant structures such as retinal thickness. Poor image quality contributes to greater confusion and disagreement in findings based on review of an OCT image, and therefore also contributes to a higher degree of inter-grader or intra-grader disagreement. The goals of clinical and research imaging are to produce useful images, and assessment of image quality is one measure of this product. Poor scan quality often results in a higher degree of inter-grader or intra-grader disagreement.

Assessing Image Quality

Image quality assessment parameters are usually established before the start of imaging or of the study to outline minimum quality standards to reliably perform image analysis for clinical evaluation or research criteria.

Image quality assessment is generally based on a few criteria:

1. *Is the area of interest included in the scanned area?* The area of interest should be of adequate lateral placement (centration) in the scan and of proper axial placement such that the image is not clipped or cropped.
2. *Is the signal/resolution sufficient to determine ocular structures and pathologies?* Signal strength with greater image resolution is, by far, the most critical factor for optimal imaging. Signal strength based on a 10-point scale for the Zeiss Cirrus system (displayed on the screen and in the scan name) and for the Heidelberg Spectralis system (displayed in the information tab). Not all commercial or research systems display signal strength.
3. *Does the acquired image(s) comply with the required scan protocol (research imaging)?* Scan protocols are often determined at the beginning of the study. This includes scan density (number of B-scans per volume), scan length, high speed versus high resolution (number of A-scans per B-scan), volume scan versus radial scan, and so on.
4. *Are there imaging artifacts that prevent or impair diagnosis or image analysis?* Imaging artifacts may distort or hinder evaluation of an examiner's interpretation of an image. For example, clipping of the scan within an area of interest and poor scan resolution may prevent proper identification of anatomic or pathologic features. Imaging artifacts are discussed in greater detail with example images in Chapters 6 and 8.

Patient-related factors may also confound image quality or hinder the imager from acquiring images of good quality. This includes media opacity (caused by vitreous hemorrhage, cloudy cornea, lens opacities, etc.), tear film quality, surface disease or injury, and small or undilated pupils. Patient cooperation factors, such as inability to focus (including tremors or nystagmus) and inability to obey commands (blinking, scan tracking, etc.), can frustrate even a seasoned operator and are unavoidable obstacles in most cases. These factors are discussed in more detail in Chapter 3.

Grading Scan Quality

When evaluating the quality of the scans obtained, the observer should establish a systematic approach with detailed criteria for assessing scan quality, and the minimum standards for useful images should be predetermined. An example of a data acceptance scoring system is shown below:

1. *Excellent:* Scan is of excellent resolution, saturation, and overall quality. Features and pathologies are easily discerned, layers are distinctly visible and can be segmented properly, and there is good centration such that the area of interest is represented.
2. *Acceptable:* Scan is of acceptable resolution and overall quality. Features and pathologies are discernable, layers are visible but not clearly distinct, segmentation may be possible on most if not all layers, and adequate centration of area of interest is represented.
3. *Poor:* Scan is of poor resolution and/or overall quality. Features and pathologies may not be readily discernable but may be interpreted by overall retinal structures. Layer boundaries may not be visible for some or all layers.
4. *Unusable:* Scan is of such poor quality that features, pathologies, and layers cannot be determined.

If multiple scans are obtained of the same area(s), the best scans are selected for a particular area of interest (e.g., fovea or optic nerve) for further analysis, such as stage of development, pathology assessment, or quantitative measurements.

CHAPTER 19

Reproducibility of Imaging and Interpretation

Xi Chen ■ Katrina Postell Winter

For any research imaging system, reproducibility of imaging and interpretation are essential for studies of optical coherence tomography (OCT) findings. Before initiation of studies using a research imaging system, the repeatability and reproducibility of imaging and interpretation should be rigorously tested, often in comparison with a standard system.[1] Outcome measures and milestones of repeatability and reproducibility should be defined before testing. Research imaging systems may be investigational devices and their use in human research should follow national regulatory guidelines, such as from the United States Food and Drug Administration (Title 21 of the Code of Federal Regulations Part 812), as well as local regulations.

Repeatability

Repeatability is the consistency of measurements when the same person measures the same item with the same procedure by using the same instrument multiple times. *Imager repeatability* refers to the same imager conducting repeated measures using the same instrument, and *grader repeatability* refers to the consistency of the same grader repeatedly grade the same scan.

Reproducibility

Reproducibility is the consistency of measurements by different appraisers using the same measuring equipment. Reproducibility to be tested may include *imager reproducibility* (multiple imagers using the same instrument) and *intragrader reproducibility* of interpretation (multiple graders grading the same scan). Agreement among the variables being assessed or between two different observers is often scored by using the correlation coefficient with a 95% confidence limit of agreement.[2] With variables at less than 95% agreement, there may be an issue of bias (judgment calls), a problem with the quality of the data being assessed, or an error in methods. For example, assessment of an OCT image for the presence of intraretinal fluid (cysts) is dependent on the quality of the scan and the determination of the observer if the scan appearance meets the perceived level of determination (bias) to conclude that intraretinal fluid is present and is not an imaging artifact.[3]

References

1. Folgar FA, Yuan EL, Farsiu S, Toth CA. Lateral and axial measurement differences between spectral-domain optical coherence tomography systems. *J Biomed Opt.* 2014;19(1):16014.
2. Bland JM, Altman DG. Statistical methods for assessing agreement between two methods of clinical measurement. *Lancet.* 1986;1(8476):307–310.
3. Folgar FA, Jaffe GJ, Ying GS, Maguire MG, Toth CA. Comparison of Age-Related Macular Degeneration Treatments Trials Research G. Comparison of optical coherence tomography assessments in the comparison of age-related macular degeneration treatments trials. *Ophthalmology.* 2014;121(10):1956–1965.

CHAPTER 20

Secure OCT Data Storage and Networking

Vincent Tai

Optical coherence tomography (OCT) provides high-resolution two- or three-dimensional images, which may contain labels that are considered protected health information (PHI). Therefore it is very important to maintain security and privacy when managing OCT image databases.

OCT Data Storage

OCT images are large digital files that follow the Digital Imaging and Communications in Medicine (DICOM) standard with regard to nonproprietary data interchange protocol, digital image format, and file structure for biomedical images and image-related information.[1] To meet the DICOM standard, images acquired from the OCT imaging device for clinical or research purposes should be transferred to a picture archiving and communication system (PACS).

Because OCT files may contain labels that are PHI,[2,3] the OCT imaging device and the PACS should meet pertinent regulatory security standards, such as the Health Insurance Portability and Accountability Act[4] (HIPAA) in the United States or the General Data Protection Regulation[5] (GDPR) in the European Union countries.

Access to OCT Data

Users who access OCT databases should be authorized by their respective institutions, completed the necessary training, and enrolled in a research protocol (if applicable when using images in the research setting). Access to the OCT databases should follow the DICOM standards and require encrypted connection, including secure authorization, secure shell, remote desktop protocol, or virtual private network[6] (VPN).

References

1. Bidgood Jr WD, Horii SC, Prior FW, Van Syckle DE. Understanding and using DICOM, the data interchange standard for biomedical imaging. *J Am Med Inform Assoc.* 1997;4(3):199–212.
2. Jannetti MC. Safeguarding patient information in electronic health records. *AORN J.* 2014;100(3):C7–C8.

3. Lemke J. Storage and security of personal health information. *OOHNA J.* 2013;32(1):25–26.
4. The Health Insurance Portability and Accountability Act of 1996 (HIPAA) P.L. No. 104-191, 110 Stat. 1938 (1996).
5. Regulation (EU) 2016/679 of the European Parliament and of the Council of 27 April 2016 on the protection of natural persons with regard to the processing of personal data and on the free movement of such data, and repealing Directive 95/46/EC (General Data Protection Regulation) Official Journal L. 2016;119(1).
6. Kruse CS, Smith B, Vanderlinden H, Nealand A. Security techniques for the electronic health records. *J Med Syst.* 2017;41(8):127.

Inherited Retinal Diseases

Best Disease

Avni P. Finn ■ Lejla Vajzovic

Introduction

Best vitelliform dystrophy is an inherited retinal disease involving the retinal pigment epithelium (RPE), leading to a characteristic bilateral yellow "egg yolk" appearance in the macula. The causative gene (*BEST 1/VMD2*) encodes the transmembrane protein bestrophin 1, causing abnormal chloride channel conductance, disrupting fluid transport across the RPE, and affecting RPE metabolism.[1]

Clinical Features

Best disease is classically a bilateral process but may be asymmetric. Abnormal chloride channel function in the RPE leads to the eventual buildup of lipofuscin between the outer retina and the RPE, causing a yellow vitelliform lesion in the macula[2] (Fig. 21.1). The disease evolves over five clinical stages. In the previtelliform stage, there are subtle RPE changes and minimal changes in vision. The vitelliform stage is marked by the classic "egg yolk" appearance and is followed by the pseudohypopyon stage with layering of the lipofuscin. Then the vitellidisruptive or "scrambled egg" stage occurs and is followed by atrophy and focal scar in the final stage. Often, visual acuity is minimally affected, especially in the early stages of the disease. Patients may note gradual vision loss or metamorphopsia as the disease progresses. Rarely, the disease can be complicated by secondary choroidal neovascularization (CNV), which can cause rapid significant vision loss.[3]

The Brain Connection

Bestrophin 1 is a multifunctional protein known to be expressed in a variety of tissues, including the brain.[4,5] In the brain, much like in the RPE, the protein functions as an anion channel. It is also a key regulator of various important brain functions, including the permeation and release of glutamate and gamma aminobutyric acid (GABA), which are important transmitters in the brain.[5]

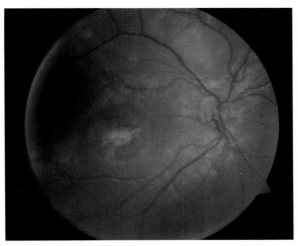

Fig. 21.1 Fundus photo of the right eye of a 6-year-old girl shows a yellow vitelliform lesion in the macula. There is also a temporal pigmented lesion in this eye, indicating possible choroidal neovascularization (CNV).

OCT Features

OCT demonstrates varying findings as the disease progresses. In the preclinical or previtelliform stage, OCT demonstrates thickening and increased hyperrflectivity at the level of the photoreceptor outer segments. In the vitelliform stage, OCT reveals hyperreflective dome-shaped material in the subretinal space, as well as persistent thickening of the photoreceptor outer segments (Fig. 21.2). This particular OCT image also shows subretinal fluid associated CNV temporal to the fovea. In the pseudohypopyon stage, the retina is elevated, with a clear space between the neurosensory retina and the RPE. There may be thinning of the outer nuclear layer and a variable degree of increased hyperreflectivity of the photoreceptor outer segments. In the vitellidisruptive stage, there may be hyperreflective subretinal mounds at the level of the RPE, with either underlying shadowing or increased hyperreflectivity of the underlying choroid and associated thinning of the outer retinal layers. In the atrophic stage, OCT shows overall thinning of the neurosensory retina and absent or thin ellipsoid zone or photoreceptor complex.[6,7]

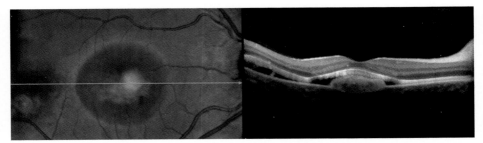

Fig. 21.2 Optical coherence tomography (OCT) image of the right eye of a 6-year-old girl shows subretinal hyperreflective material consistent with the vitelliform lesion, increased thickening and hyperreflectivity of the outer segments, and subretinal fluid from the nearby choroidal neovascularization (CNV).

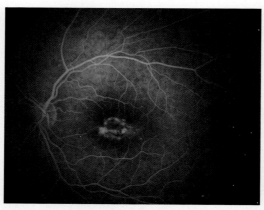

Fig. 21.3 Fluorescein angiogram of the left eye of a 10-year-old girl with a Best vitelliform lesion and choroidal neovascularization (CNV) confirms leakage in the area of suspected CNV.

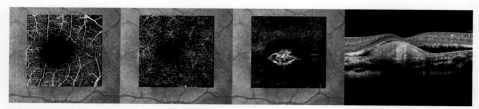

Fig. 21.4 Optical coherence tomography angiography (OCTA) image of the left eye of a 10-year-old girl reveals a choroidal neovascular membrane (CNVM) in the avascular layer (C). The superficial vascular plexus (A) and deep vascular plexus (B) appear normal. Segmentation of the three layers (D) is seen. Images obtained from an investigational device (Heidelberg Spectralis HRA + OCT with OCTA software).

Ancillary Testing

Electroretinography (ERG) results are typically normal, whereas electrooculography (EOG) results are abnormal, with an Arden ratio (light-to-dark) of 1.5 or less. Fluorescein angiography is helpful in demonstrating leakage in an area of suspected active CNV (Fig. 21.3). OCT angiography (OCTA) similarly may be helpful to determine whether choroidal neovascular membrane (CNVM) is present (Fig. 21.4).

Treatment

Currently, there is no treatment for Best disease. CNV may be treated with anti–vascular endothelial growth factor (VEGF) injections, alone or in conjunction with photodynamic therapy (PDT).

References

1. Boon CJ, Theelen T, Hoefsloot EH, et al. Clinical and molecular genetic analaysis of best vitelliform macular dystrophy. *Retina.* 2009;29(6):835–847.
2. O'Gorman S, Flaherty WA, Fishman GA, Berson EL. Histopathologic findings in Best's vitelliform macular dystrophy. *Arch Ophthalmol.* 1988;106(9):1261–1268.
3. Booij JC, Boon CJF, van Schooneveld MJ, et al. Course of visual decline in relation to the best1 genotype in vitelliform macular dystrophy. *Ophthalmology.* 2010;117(7):1415–1422.

4. Johnson AA, Guziewicz KE, Lee CJ, et al. Bestrophin 1 and retinal disease. *Prog Retin Eye Res.* 2017;58:45–69.

5. Oh SJ, Lee CJ. Distribution and function of the bestrophin-1 (Best1) channel in the brain. *Exp Neurobiol.* 2017;26(3):113.

6. Ferrara DC, Costa RA, Tsang S, Calucci D, Jorge R, Freund KB. Multimodal fundus imaging in Best vitelliform macular dystrophy. *Graefes Arch Clin Exp Ophthalmol.* 2010;248(10):1377–1386.

7. Querques G, Zerbib J, Georges A, et al. Multimodal analysis of the progression of Best vitelliform macular dystrophy. *Mol Vis.* 2014;20:575–592.

CHAPTER 22

Stargardt Disease (and Fundus Flavimaculatus)

Mohsin H. Ali ■ Lejla Vajzovic

Introduction

Stargardt disease, or fundus flavimaculatus, is a disease characterized by abnormal accumulation of liposfuscin within the retinal pigment epithelium (RPE). It is typically inherited in an autosomal recessive pattern with involvement of the *ABCA4* gene. Affected individuals often develop decreased central visual acuity in childhood or young adulthood and may reach a final visual acuity nadir of 20/200.

The Brain Connection

Neuroimaging (magnetic resonance imaging [MRI]) has demonstrated microstructural alterations in the brains of patients with Stargardt disease, and these alterations may, at least partially, correlate with the degree of retinal damage and visual impairment.[1] These changes include gray matter loss in the bilateral occipital cortex and frontobasal regions.[1]

Clinical Features

Stargardt disease has variable clinical features.[2] The classic features, although not present in every patient, include the following: (1) vermillion fundus—in which excessive pigmentation of the RPE leads to a darkly colored fundus with indistinct underlying choroidal details; (2) "dark" or "silent" choroid on fluorescein angiography—in which the normal choroidal fluorescence is masked by the diffuse lipofuscin accumulation in the RPE (Fig. 22.2C); (3) pisciform flecks—in which fishtail-shaped, light-colored or yellowish, lipofuscin deposits are seen in the posterior pole or periphery (Figs. 22.1 through 22.3); and (4) macular atrophy with peripapillary sparing (see Fig. 22.1), which may manifest as a "bull's eye" pattern, geographic atrophy, a "beaten bronze" appearance, or a metallic sheen.[2,3]

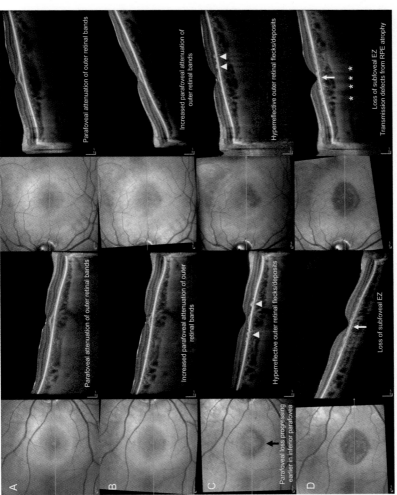

Fig. 22.1 Optical coherence tomography (OCT) findings in a 9-year-old male child with Stargardt disease, with a compound heterozygous mutation in the *ABCA4* gene. OCT was performed at the following time points: (A) initial presentation (visual acuity = 20/40 OD, 20/30 OS); (B) 6 months after initial presentation (visual acuity = 20/40 OD, 20/32 OS); (C) 11 months after initial presentation (visual acuity = 20/50 OD, 20/40 OS); (D) 18 months after initial presentation (visual acuity = 20/125 OD, 20/100 OS). Progressive macular atrophy is seen on both the en face and horizontal cross-sectional B-scan OCT images OU, beginning with parafoveal outer retinal loss (A, B) that progressed most rapidly in the inferior parafovea (C, *black arrow*), followed by the development of hyperreflective outer retinal deposits (C, *white arrowheads*), loss of the subfoveal outer retina (D, *white arrows*), and areas of enhanced light transmission suggestive of retinal pigment epithelium (RPE) atrophy (D, *white asterisks*). Abbreviations: EZ (ellipsoid zone).

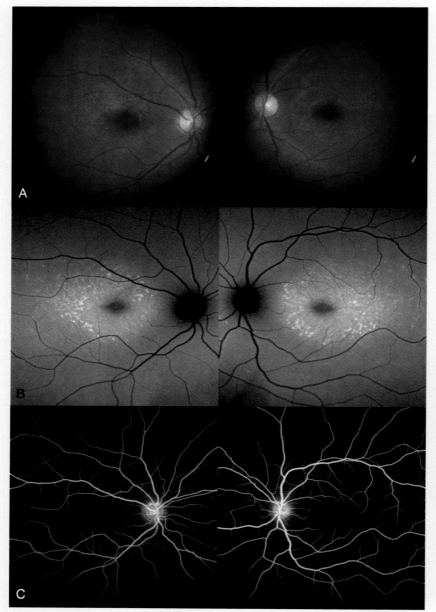

Fig. 22.2   Multimodal imaging in an 11-year-old male Stargardt disease patient with two mutations in the *ABCA4* gene reveals characteristic pisciform flecks in the posterior pole (A), which exhibit hyperautofluorescence on fundus autofluorescence (B) along with the classic "dark choroid" on fluorescein angiography (C).

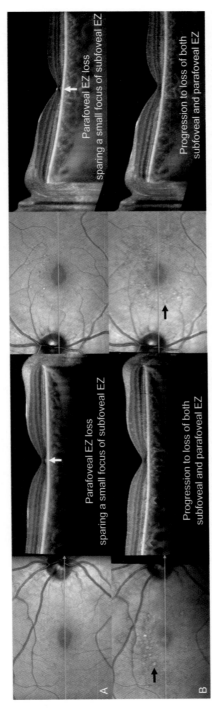

Fig. 22.3 Optical coherence tomography (OCT) images separated by 1 year from the same patient depicted in Fig. 22.2. (A) initial; (B) final. The en face infrared images reveal a significant increase in the number of flecks in both eyes (black arrows) from the initial (A) to the final (B) OCT images. The horizontal cross-sectional B-scan images show small, dome-shaped elevations at the level of the retinal pigment epithelium (RPE) with focal disruption of the overlying ellipsoid—these are the characteristic hyperreflective flecks (red arrowheads). Additionally, there is parafoveal loss of the ellipsoid zone (EZ) with a small focus of intact subfoveal EZ remaining (white arrows) in the initial OCT (A), which is ultimately lost on the final OCT image (B). The patient's vision remained stable in the range of 20/126 to 20/200 in both eyes.

OCT Features

OCT findings in Stargardt disease can be variable, given the range of phenotypic manifestations.[2-4] In general, OCT is helpful in identifying pisciform flecks and determining the degree and progression of macular atrophy (see Fig. 22.1). Flecks are seen as hyperreflective outer retinal deposits that interrupt one or more of the following hyperreflective outer retinal bands: external limiting membrane, ellipsoid zone, and interdigitation zone (see Fig. 22.1). There may also be subtle outer nuclear layer thinning overlying the flecks. Macular atrophy (see Fig. 22.1) can be detected as loss of the RPE (loss of the hyperreflective RPE–Bruch membrane complex band with corresponding increased light transmission to the choroid) and/or atrophy of the outer retinal bands (loss of the outer nuclear layer, external limiting membrane, ellipsoid zone, and interdigitation zone).[3,4] Outer retinal tubulations may also be seen in some patients. Thickening and hyperreflectivity of the external limiting membrane or the base of the outer nuclear layer may also commonly be seen.[5,6] Both en face and B-scan cross-sectional OCT images may be helpful in monitoring disease progression.

Ancillary Testing

Patients with suspected or confirmed Stargardt disease may benefit from additional testing to identify important findings on fluorescein angiography (e.g., "dark" or "silent" choroid), fundus autofluorescence (e.g., pisciform flecks and macular atrophy), perimetry (e.g., varying degrees of visual field constriction), and electroretinography (e.g., reduced amplitudes and delayed implicit times).

Genetic testing will often reveal a mutation in the *ABCA4* gene (and much less frequently in the *ELOVL4, PRPH2,* and *BEST1* genes). Family pedigree analysis will frequently demonstrate an autosomal recessive inheritance pattern.

Treatment

There are currently no established treatments for Stargardt disease, although gene replacement therapy, stem cell therapy, and drug-based therapy trials are ongoing.

References

1. Olivo G, Gaia O, Melillo P, et al. Cerebral involvement in Stargardt's disease: a VBM and TBSS Study. *Invest Ophthalmol Vis Sci.* 2015;56(12):7388–7397.
2. Tanna P, Strauss RW, Fujinami K, Michaelides M. Stargardt disease: clinical features, molecular genetics, animal models and therapeutic options. *Br J Ophthalmol.* 2017;101(1):25–30.
3. Cai CX, Light JG, Handa JT. Quantifying the rate of ellipsoid zone loss in Stargardt disease. *Am J Ophthalmol.* 2018;186:1–9.
4. Park JC, Collison FT, Fishman GA, et al. Objective analysis of hyperreflective outer retinal bands imaged by optical coherence tomography in patients with Stargardt disease. *Invest Ophthalmol Vis Sci.* 2015;56 (8):4662–4667.
5. Khan KN, Kasilian M, Mahroo OAR, Tanna P, Kalitzeos A, Robson AG, et al. Early Patterns of Macular Degeneration in ABCA4-Associated Retinopathy. *Ophthalmology.* May 2018;125(5):735–746.
6. Lee W, Nõupuu K, Oll M, Duncker T, Burke T, Zernant J, et al. The external limiting membrane in early-onset Stargardt disease. *Invest Ophthalmol Vis Sci.* Aug 2014;55(10):6139–6149.

CHAPTER 23

Retinitis Pigmentosa

Mohsin H. Ali ■ Alessandro Iannaccone ■ Lejla Vajzovic

Introduction

Retinitis pigmentosa (RP) is a term used to describe a heterogeneous group of disorders characterized by progressive retinal degeneration.[1] RP may be an isolated condition affecting the eyes or part of a broader systemic syndrome. The mode of inheritance may be autosomal recessive, autosomal dominant, X-linked, or so-called simplex (in which the mode of inheritance is unknown). The disease may manifest very early in childhood or in adulthood.

The Brain Connection

This section focuses on nonsyndromic RP, which typically is not associated with neurologic or systemic abnormalities. Patients with RP, however, may have secondary visual field remapping in the primary visual cortex without structural changes, as evidenced by functional magnetic resonance imaging (MRI) studies. The degree of visual field remapping may increase with more constricted visual fields.[2]

Patients with visual impairment secondary to inherited retinal dystrophies may exhibit alterations in multisensory processing – such that the impaired vision may result in compensatory neural processing leading to enhanced responsiveness to non-visual sensory stimuli.[3] This enhanced or more sensitized auditory processing has been demonstrated in patients with visual loss secondary retinitis pigmentosa, Bardet-Biedl syndrome (see Chapter 24), and cone-rod dystrophy.

Clinical Features

Affected individuals typically develop night blindness, progressive loss of peripheral vision, light aversion, and, ultimately, reduced central visual acuity. Anterior segment findings may include posterior subcapsular cataract formation and fine-pigmented vitreous cells or vitreous opacities. The fundus findings can be highly variable but classically consist of progressive, bilateral, fairly symmetric waxy pallor of the optic nerve, attenuated vessels, midperipheral granularity or mottling of the retinal pigment epithelium, and bone spicules (Figs. 23.1 and 23.3). Additionally, cystoid macular edema and epiretinal membrane may be present (see Fig. 23.1 and Fig. 23.2).

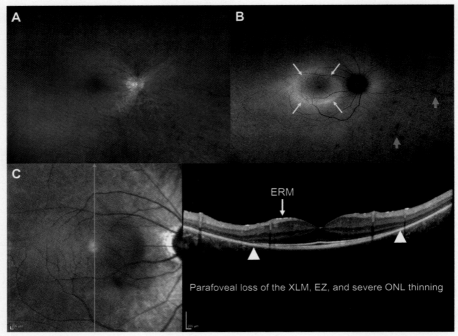

Fig. 23.1 Imaging findings in a 16-year-old male with autosomal dominant RP (*PRPF31* gene mutation). (A) Wide-field fundus image reveals moderate attenuation of the retinal vasculature, scattered bone spicule pigmentation, and moth-eaten peripheral RPE loss. (B) Fundus autofluorescence better highlights the hypoautofluorescent bone spicule changes and nummular RPE loss *(red arrows)* as well as a hyperautofluorescent parafoveal ring *(yellow arrows)* identifying the leading edge of the disease and the area of best preserved visual function, largely corresponding with the transition zone at the OCT level. (C) OCT imaging reveals severe parafoveal attenuation of the outer nuclear layer, loss of the external limiting membrane***, and marked thinning of the outer retinal bands,*** including the ellipsoid zone (beginning near the *white arrowheads*). Additionally, there is a trace epiretinal membrane *(white arrow)*. The fovea appears completely intact and visual acuity was 20/20 OU. Abbreviations: ONL (outer nuclear layer), XLM (external limiting membrane), EZ (ellipsoid zone). (Image courtesy of Alessandro Iannaccone, MD.)

OCT Features

Optical coherence tomography (OCT) findings in RP[4-8] typically reveal attenuation of the outer nuclear layer thickness, loss of the external limiting membrane, and loss of the ellipsoid zone that occurs centripetally toward the foveal center (see Figs. 23.1 and 23.2). OCT is particularly helpful in delineating a transition zone between severely diseased retinal regions exhibiting OCT structural changes (namely, attenuation of retinal layers) and relatively healthy retinal regions near the foveal center, without apparent morphologic changes on OCT. In the transition zone, following the retinal morphology on OCT from the foveal center to the midperiphery will typically reveal progressive thinning of the outer segment of the photoreceptors, progressive thinning of both the outer segment and outer nuclear layer, loss of the ellipsoid zone and outer segment, complete loss of the outer nuclear layer, and finally disruption and loss of the retinal pigment epithelium. In some forms of RP, measurements of various OCT parameters, in particular ellipsoid zone width and outer nuclear layer thickness, have been used to determine rates of progression and serve as structural biomarkers of disease severity. Therefore as treatment options continue to evolve, these and other OCT parameters will likely be increasingly used to assess the efficacy of various interventions.

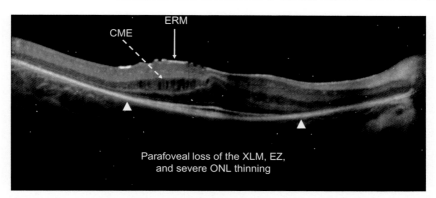

Fig. 23.2 Optical coherence tomography (OCT) imaging of the 18-year-old older brother of the patient in Fig. 23.1, with the same genetically confirmed form of autosomal dominant RP, reveals mild cystoid macular edema (*white dashed arrow*) and epiretinal membrane (*white arrow*) in addition to parafoveal loss of outer retinal layers (beginning near the *white arrowheads*). The foveal area is largely spared by both the cystoid changes and the epiretinal membrane, and the ellipsoid zone, external limiting membrane, and outer nuclear layer are intact, supporting a visual acuity of 20/20 OU. (Image courtesy of Alessandro Iannaccone, MD.)

Cystoid intraretinal spaces may also be seen on OCT (see Fig. 23.2). Bone spicule pigmentation manifests as discrete intraretinal hyperreflective foci in various retinal layers on OCT. Hyperreflective epiretinal membranes may also be seen (see Figs. 23.1 and 23.2).

Ancillary Testing

Visual field testing and electroretinography are essential in diagnosing RP and monitoring disease progression. Multiple visual field loss patterns can occur. More typically, field loss begins in the midperiphery and progressively enlarges in a pattern termed *ring scotoma*. In other cases, there can either be a slowly progressive generalized constriction or selective losses in certain quadrants only, more often the superior and/or the temporal ones. Fundus autofluorescence may accentuate the findings of bone spicules (see Fig. 23.1) and atrophy of the retinal pigment epithelium (RPE), both of which will present as hypoautofluorescence. Fluorescein angiography may also reveal retinal pigment epithelial atrophy and often may show angiographic leakage and petaloid pooling in the macula in the presence of cystoid intraretinal spaces on OCT and occasionally elsewhere. Genetic testing is essential to determine the causative genetic mutation(s) for diagnostic, prognostic, reproductive risk assessment, and – nowadays, in the era of molecular ophthalmology – also for therapeutic purposes.

Treatment

Dietary supplementation with vitamin A, lutein, and zeaxanthin have been investigated and shown, on average, to slow down the progression of RP, and docosahexaenoic acid (DHA) has been shown to slow down X-linked RP.[9] Topical and/or oral carbonic anhydrase inhibitors, as well as subtenon and intravitreal steroids, may be beneficial for concurrent cystoid macular edema.[9] FDA-approved artificial retinal implants are also available for end-stage cases (Fig. 23.4). Gene therapy, stem cell therapy, editing antisense oligonucleotide therapy, and drug-based therapy trials are ongoing.

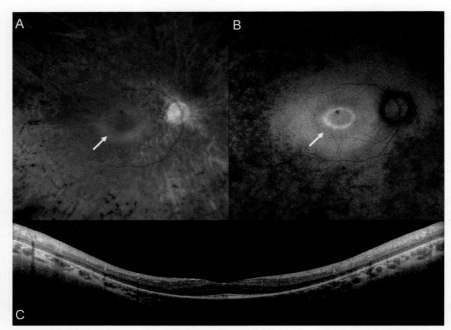

Fig. 23.3 Imaging findings in of a 17-year-old female with autosomal recessive early-onset RP (*PDE6B* gene mutations) with a history of night blindness since childhood, and progressive peripheral vision loss. (A) Wide-field fundus image demonstrates the classic findings of widespread bone spicules, vascular attenuation, a mild form of bull's eye maculopathy (*white arrow*), and waxy pallor of the optic nerve. (B) Wide-field fundus autofluorescence shows diffuse speckled hypo-autofluorescence corresponding to both bone spicule pigment deposits and moth-eaten RPE loss, and a bright ring of perifoveal hyper-autofluorescence surrounded by a halo of faint hypo-autofluorescence configuring a bull's eye pattern (*white arrow*). (C) OCT reveals moderate loss of the outer retinal bands including the external limiting membrane and ellipsoid zone outside of the foveal region, and good foveal preservation. Visual acuity was 20/32 OD and 20/60 OS. Visual field testing showed severe constriction to the central 10–15 degrees of vision with large U-shaped far peripheral temporal, inferior and nasal islands in both eyes. (Image courtesy of Alessandro Iannaccone, MD.)

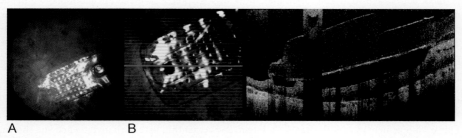

Fig. 23.4 (A) Fundus image of an ARGUS II Retinal Prosthesis System (ARGUS II, Second Sight Medical Products, Sylmar, CA) in a patient with retinitis pigmentosa (RP). This device consists of an electrode array containing 60 platinum electrodes and is secured in an epiretinal position overlying the macula with a retinal tack. This electrode array generates electrical pulses that stimulate retinal neurons in response to visual information processed from a camera affixed to custom glasses worn by the patient. (B) Optical coherence tomography (OCT) with the same ARGUS II device depicted the epiretinal position of the electrode array.

References

1. Iannaccone A. The genetics of hereditary retinopathies and optic neuropathies. *Comp Ophthalmol Update.* 2005;5:39–62.
2. Ferreira S, Pereira AC, Quendera B, Reis A, Silva ED, Castelo-Branco M. Primary visual cortical remapping in patients with inherited peripheral retinal degeneration. *Neuroimage Clin.* 2017;13:428–438.
3. Myers MH, Iannaccone A, Bidelman GM. A pilot investigation of audiovisual processing and multisensory integration in patients with inherited retinal dystrophies. *BMC Ophthalmol.* 2017 Dec 7;17(1):240.
4. Battaglia Parodi M, La Spina C, Triolo G, et al. Correlation of SD-OCT findings and visual function in patients with retinitis pigmentosa. *Graefes Arch Clin Exp Ophthalmol.* 2016;254(7):1275–1279.
5. Tee JJL, Carroll J, Webster AR, Michaelides M. Quantitative analysis of retinal structure using spectral-domain optical coherence tomography in RPGR-associated retinopathy. *Am J Ophthalmol.* 2017;178:18–26.
6. Walia S, Fishman GA, Edward DP, Lindeman M. Retinal nerve fiber layer defects in RP patients. *Invest Ophthalmol Vis Sci.* 2007;48(10):4748–4752.
7. Liu G, Liu X, Li H, Du Q, Wang F. Optical coherence tomographic analysis of retina in retinitis pigmentosa patients. *Ophthalmic Res.* 2016;56(3):111–122.
8. Boon CJF, den Hollander AI, Hoyng CB, Cremers FPM, Klevering BJ, Keunen JEE. The spectrum of retinal dystrophies caused by mutations in the peripherin/RDS gene. *Prog Retin Eye Res.* 2008;27 (2):213–235.
9. Berdia J, Iannaccone A. *Retinitis Pigmentosa.* Review No. 21. Danbury, CT: National Organization for Rare Disorders, Inc.; 2017.*www.rarediseases.org*

CHAPTER 24

Other Forms of Retinitis Pigmentosa— Usher Syndrome, Leber Congenital Amaurosis, and Bardet-Biedl Syndrome

Mohsin H. Ali ■ Alessandro Iannaccone ■ Lejla Vajzovic

Introduction

There are several other manifestations of retinitis pigmentosa (RP), including Usher syndrome, Leber congenital amaurosis (LCA), and Bardet-Biedl syndrome, among others.[1]

Usher syndrome is a genetically heterogeneous autosomal recessive form of RP that is characterized by its association with hearing loss. The age of onset and the degree of both hearing loss and retinopathy vary, depending on the subtype of Usher syndrome.

LCA, also sometimes referred to as *severe early childhood onset retinal dystrophy* (SECORD), is a heterogeneous group of disorders that is characterized by severe visual impairment that occurs at birth or in very early childhood. It is typically inherited in an autosomal recessive pattern, and mutations on several different genes have been identified. There may be systemic associations, such as intellectual disability, deafness, and renal disease, among others. For example, LCA may occur in combination with a variety of systemic abnormalities in Senior-Loken syndrome (nephronophthisis, polyuria, polydipsia, and anemia) and Joubert syndrome (breathing dysregulation, renal disease, cerebellar vermis hypoplasia, and other neurologic abnormalities).

Bardet-Biedl syndrome is characterized by a constellation of findings, including retinopathy, polydactyly, obesity, behavioral and cognitive abnormalities, renal disease, and hypogenitalism.

The Brain Connection

Usher syndrome is typically associated with variable degrees of neurosensory hearing loss and possibly absent vestibular function and delayed motor development. Rarer forms of the condition may also be accompanied by additional neurologic sequelae, such as ataxia. Senior-Loken syndrome is not associated with a primary neurologic abnormality.[2] LCA, in the absence of syndromic features, is thought to be infrequently associated with intellectual disability or autism.[3] Bardet-Biedl syndrome may be associated with cognitive and behavioral abnormalities as severe as severe intellectual disability and autism, learning disability, developmental delay, speech disorder, or ataxia.[4] Patients with Bardet-Biedl syndrome have also been noted to have impaired olfaction.[5]

Clinical Features

Patients with Usher syndrome have retinal changes that may be indistinguishable from typical RP (see Chapter 23).

Patients with LCA/SECORD typically have severe visual impairment, nystagmus, poor pupillary light reflexes, and eye rubbing (oculodigital sign of Franceschetti). The fundus features are variable and may include such findings as mottling or granularity of the retinal pigment epithelium (RPE), salt-and-pepper retinopathy, retinitis punctate albescens-like whitish deposits, and vascular attenuation.[3]

The ocular manifestations of Bardet-Biedl syndrome may be quite varied. Generally, affected patients often exhibit reduced visual acuity, impaired color vision, impaired ocular motility (i.e. strabismus or nystagmus), variable degrees of optic disc atrophy and macular atrophy, retinal vasculature attenuation, and variable degrees of peripheral pigmentary changes (typically developing later in life).[6–7] Swelling of the optic nerve has also been reported.[7]

OCT Features

Similar to typical RP (see Chapter 23), OCT imaging (Figs. 24.1 through 24.4) may show progressive attenuation of the outer segment of photoreceptors and outer nuclear layer, loss of the

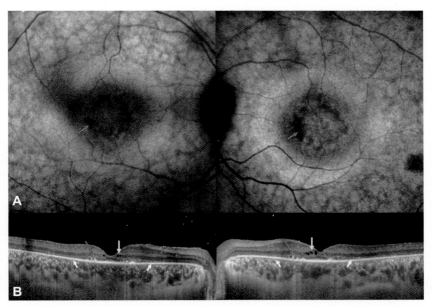

Fig. 24.1   (A) Fundus autofluorescence and (B) optical coherence tomography (OCT) image from a 16-year-old female with Usher syndrome type 1 (*MYO7A* gene mutation), showing bull's eye maculopathy (central mottled hypoautofluorescence surrounded by a ring of hyper-autofluorescence); mild cystoid intraretinal spaces *(yellow arrows)*; hyperreflective material above the retinal pigment epithelium (RPE), which corresponded to dark patches on autofluorescence *(red arrows)*; and severe loss of the parafoveal photoreceptor layers with the outer plexiform layer nearly touching the RPE (e.g., between *white arrows*). Note the thin photoreceptor layer at the foveal center with a poorly delineated ellipsoid zone. The visual acuity was 20/50 OU. The patient had cochlear implants for her sensorineural hearing loss. (Image courtesy of Alessandro Iannaccone, MD.)

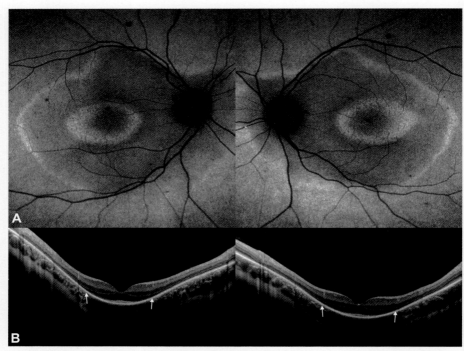

Fig. 24.2 (A) Fundus autofluorescence and (B) optical coherence tomography (OCT) image from a 9-year-old male with Leber congenital amaurosis (LCA) in conjunction with polyuria, polydipsia, nephronophthisis, and *NPHP1* gene mutations, consistent with a diagnosis of Senior-Loken syndrome type 1, reveals a bull's eye maculopathy and significant thinning of the parafoveal outer nuclear layer and loss of the ellipsoid zone *(white arrows)*, sparing only the subfoveal region. Photoreceptor loss is most severe between the two hyperautofluorescent rings on the fundus autofluorescence image. Visual acuity was 20/50 OU. (Image courtesy of Alessandro Iannaccone, MD.)

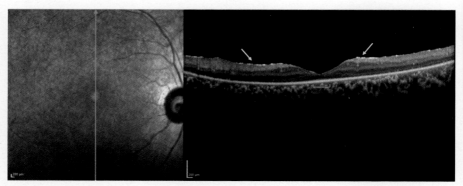

Fig. 24.3 Optical coherence tomography (OCT) image from an 11-year-old boy with Bardet-Biedl syndrome (*BBS6/MKKS* gene mutations), showing significant thinning of the outer nuclear layer and loss of the ellipsoid zone throughout the macula. There is a tiny area of preserved yet faint ellipsoid zone immediately subfoveally *(red bracket)*. A mild patchy epiretinal membrane is present *(yellow arrow)*. The en face infrared image also demonstrates vascular attenuation. The patient had polydactyly and obesity consistent with the diagnosis of Bardet-Biedl syndrome. Visual acuity was 20/64 in this eye and 20/126 in the fellow eye. (Image courtesy of Alessandro Iannaccone, MD.)

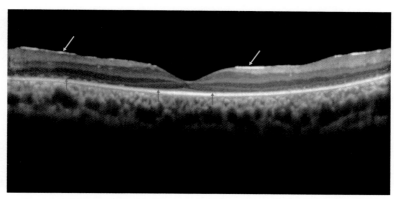

Fig. 24.4   Optical coherence tomography (OCT) image from a 15-year-old female with mild intellectual disability, obesity, polydactyly, retinopathy, and *BBS2* gene mutations, consistent with a diagnosis of Bardet-Biedl syndrome showing mild epiretinal membrane *(yellow arrows)*, extensive loss of the parafoveal ellipsoid zone (peripheral to the *red arrows*), and outer retinal hyperreflective deposits *(blue arrows)* at the level of the outer nuclear layer. Visual acuity was 20/70 OU. (Image courtesy of Alessandro Iannaccone, MD.)

external limiting membrane, and loss of the ellipsoid zone.[8-10] Intraretinal hyperreflective deposits (see Figs. 24.1 and 24.4) in the outer retina overlying the RPE/Bruch membrane complex have also been shown in various retinal degenerations, including Usher syndrome, Bardet-Biedl syndrome, and RP. The exact nature of these hyperreflective deposits remains unclear but may represent sequelae of photoreceptor cell death, with subsequent migration of the underlying RPE. Other OCT findings include cystoid intraretinal spaces (see Fig. 24.1) and epiretinal membrane (see Figs. 24.3 and 24.4).

As therapeutic options continue to advance, OCT will continue to play an important role in clinical trials because certain OCT structural markers (e.g., ellipsoid zone width, outer nuclear layer thickness, and others) will be used as clinical outcome measures to determine the efficacy of treatment.

Ancillary Testing

An abnormal electroretinography result is usually necessary to aide in the diagnosis of the previously mentioned conditions. As discussed with typical RP (see Chapter 23), fundus autofluorescence and visual field testing are important for disease monitoring (Fig. 24.5). Additionally, genetic testing and a thorough systemic evaluation by a pediatrician or geneticist are recommended, given the potential for serious systemic associations. Hearing testing is also necessary in Usher syndrome. Renal ultrasounds are usually recommended in patients with Bardet-Biedl and Senior Loken syndrome.

Treatment

There are currently no established treatments for the ocular manifestations of Usher syndrome, LCA/SECORD, or Bardet-Biedl syndrome, though gene replacement therapy, editing antisense oligonucleotide therapy, stem cell therapy, and drug-based therapy trials are ongoing. Dietary supplementation of vitamin A, docosahexaenoic acid (DHA), lutein, and zeaxanthin are proposed by some clinicians. Topical or oral carbonic anhydrase inhibitors may be beneficial for concurrent cystoid macular edema.

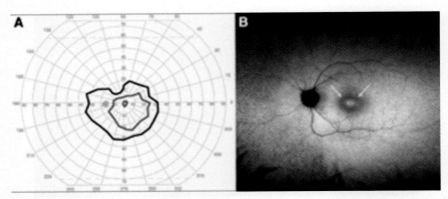

Fig. 24.5 A) Visual field testing of the same 15-year-old female with Bardet-Biedl syndrome depicted in Fig. 24.4, showing significant constriction of the visual field in both eyes with a small I4e central residue (green isopter) corresponding with the central ellipsoid zone residue seen on OCT and to the area of preserved foveal autofluorescence seen in (B). Note the bull's eye pattern of surrounding hypo-autofluorescence (yellow arrows) and the diffuse speckled hypo-autofluorescence seen in the periphery. (Image courtesy of Alessandro Iannaccone, MD.)

References

1. Iannaccone A. The genetics of hereditary retinopathies and optic neuropathies. *Comp Ophthalmol Update.* 2005;5:39–62.
2. Ronquillo CC, Bernstein PS, Baehr W. Senior-Løken syndrome: a syndromic form of retinal dystrophy associated with nephronophthisis. *Vision Res.* 2012;75:88–97.
3. Weleber RG, Francis PJ, Trzupek KM, Beattie C. Leber congenital amaurosis. In: Adam MP, Ardinger HH, Pagon RA, et al., eds. *GeneReviews®* [Internet]. Seattle, WA: University of Washington, Seattle; 1993. Available at http://www.ncbi.nlm.nih.gov/books/NBK1298/.
4. Forsythe E, Beales PL. Bardet-Biedl Syndrome. In: Adam MP, Ardinger HH, Pagon RA, et al., eds., *GeneReviews®* [Internet]. Seattle, WA: University of Washington, Seattle; 1993. Available at http://www.ncbi.nlm.nih.gov/books/NBK1363/.
5. Iannaccone A, Mykytyn K, Persico AM, Searby CC, Baldi A, Jablonski MM, et al. Clinical evidence of decreased olfaction in Bardet-Biedl syndrome caused by a deletion in the BBS4 gene. *Am J Med Genet A.* 2005;132A(4):343–346.
6. Iannaccone A, De Propris G, Roncati S, Rispoli E, Del Porto G, Pannarale MR. The ocular phenotype of the Bardet-Biedl syndrome. Comparison to non-syndromic retinitis pigmentosa. *Ophthalmic Genet.* 1997;18(1):13–26.
7. Cox KF, Kerr NC, Kedrov M, Nishimura D, Jennings BJ, Stone EM, et al. Phenotypic expression of Bardet-Biedl syndrome in patients homozygous for the common M390R mutation in the BBS1 gene. *Vision Res.* 2012;75:77–87.
8. Héon E, Westall C, Carmi R, et al. Ocular phenotypes of three genetic variants of Bardet-Biedl syndrome. *Am J Med Genet A.* 2005;132A(3):283–287.
9. Azari AA, Aleman TS, Cideciyan AV, et al. Retinal disease expression in Bardet-Biedl syndrome-1 (BBS1) is a spectrum from maculopathy to retina-wide degeneration. *Invest Ophthalmol Vis Sci.* 2006;47(11):5004–5010.
10. Gerth C, Zawadzki RJ, Werner JS, Héon E. Retinal morphology in patients with BBS1 and BBS10 related Bardet-Biedl Syndrome evaluated by Fourier-domain optical coherence tomography. *Vision Res.* 2008;48(3):392–399.

Albinism

Mohsin H. Ali ■ Lejla Vajzovic

Introduction

Oculocutaneous albinism (OCA) and *ocular albinism* (OA) are terms used to describe a group of congenital disorders characterized by variable degrees of depigmentation of the eyes, skin, and hair.[1]

OCA is typically inherited in an autosomal recessive manner and consists of several subtypes. Type 1 (or OCA1) is caused by a mutation in the *TYR* gene and is further subdivided into OCA1A, in which there is absent tyrosinase activity, and OCA1B, in which there is reduced tyrosinase activity. Types 2 through 7 (termed *OCA2, OCA3, OCA4, OCA5, OCA6,* and *OCA7*) are caused by genetic mutations in *OCA2, TYRP1, MATP/SLC45A2,* chromosome 4q24, *SLC24A5,* and *C10ORF11,* respectively.

OA is typically caused by an X-linked mutation in the *GPR143* gene (and sometimes referred to as *Nettleship-Falls type ocular albinism*). Ocular albinism has clinical manifestations isolated to the eyes, whereas oculocutaneous albinism also results in light-colored hair and skin.

Hemansky-Pudlak and Chédiak-Higashi syndromes are two important OCA subtypes with potentially life-threatening complications. Patients with Hemansky-Pudlak syndrome may have a bleeding diathesis, pulmonary fibrosis, granulomatous colitis, and renal failure. Patients with Chédiak-Higashi syndrome may have a bleeding diathesis, frequent and recurrent bacterial infections, lymphoproliferative disorder, and neurologic abnormalities.[2]

The Brain Connection

There is increased decussation of optic nerve fibers across the optic chiasm, though OCA and OA are not typically associated with other neurologic abnormalities.[1,3] The notable exception is Chédiak-Higashi syndrome, which is associated with a variety of central and peripheral nervous system defects such as intellectual disability, cranial nerve palsies, peripheral neuropathy, decreased deep tendon reflexes and nerve conduction velocities, tremor, seizures, and brain and spinal cord atrophy.[2]

The increased decussation across the optic chiasm in patients with albinism may be related to the lack of melanin in the retinal pigment epithelium, though the exact mechanism is unknown.[3] Additionally, patients with albinism have an increased occipital pole cortical thickness.[3] The thickness of the visual cortex may be inversely related to the thickness of the retinal pigment epithelium (the thickness of which is affected by the degree of melanin present within the RPE) – suggesting that the abnormal melanin pigmentation affects cortical structure in patients with albinism.[3] Magnetic resonance imaging has also found that the optic nerve, optic tracts, and optic chiasm are smaller in patients with albinism.[3]

Clinical Features

Ocular features of OCA and OA include misrouted optic nerve fibers (as described previously), nystagmus, strabismus, reduced stereopsis, refractive error, iris transillumination defects, photophobia, foveal hypoplasia, and hypopigmented fundi (Figs. 25.1 and 25.2). These features can be quite variable in severity. Female carriers of ocular albinism may have a mosaic pigmentation pattern of the fundus with patches of hypopigmented and pigmented areas (sometimes referred to as a "mud flung" or "mud splattered" pattern), likely caused by the lyonization (X-inactivation) phenomenon.

OCT Features

Optical coherence tomography (OCT) of children with OCA and OA is frequently challenging because of coexisting nystagmus. Newer, spectral domain–OCT (SD-OCT) devices allow for more rapid image acquisition and may therefore be able to acquire interpretable images even in the setting of nystagmus. Additionally, in these patients, handheld SD-OCT is particularly useful in that it allows OCT image acquisition during an examination with the patient under anesthesia.

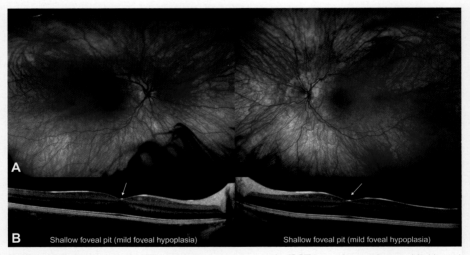

Fig. 25.1 (A) Fundus images and (B) optical coherence tomography (OCT) image from an 8-year-old white male with congenital nystagmus, iris transillumination defects, and lighter skin and hair color in comparison with his family members. His visual acuity was 20/32 in both eyes. Genetic testing revealed a heterozygous mutation in the *OCA2* gene, suggestive of a phenotypically mild form of oculocutaneous albinism (OCA). The fundi were very lightly pigmented, as evidenced by the striking prominence of the underlying choroidal vasculature. OCT of the macula showed mild foveal hypoplasia as evidenced by shallowing of the foveal pit and the persistence (or incursion) of the plexiform layers at the foveal center (the incomplete displacement of the inner retinal layers from the foveal center leads to an incomplete, shallow foveal pit formation).

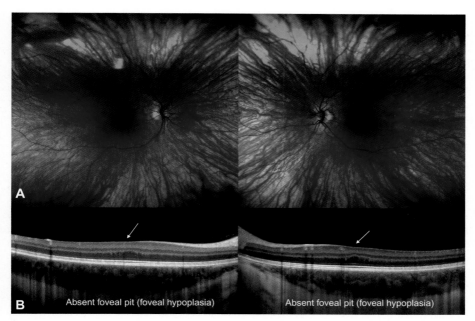

Fig. 25.2 (A) Fundus images and (B) optical coherence tomography (OCT) image of a 17-year-old white male with a history of strabismus, iris transillumination defects, and photophobia without hypopigmentation of the skin or hair—findings suggestive of ocular albinism (OA). The fundi were diffusely hypopigmented with prominent choroidal vasculature similar to the patient in Fig. 25.1. OCT of the macula demonstrates more severe foveal hypoplasia compared with the patient in Fig. 25.1 without a discernible foveal pit. Visual acuity was 20/50 OD and 20/32 OS.

Employing handheld OCT technology to image young children with suspected albinism may therefore allow for earlier detection of abnormal foveal morphology.

The main structural abnormality visible on OCT in patients with OCA or OA is the absence of the normal central foveal depression and the persistence of the inner retinal layers across the foveal depression, which may include persistence of the retinal nerve fiber layer (RNFL), ganglion cell layer, inner and outer plexiform layers, and inner nuclear layer (see Figs. 25.1 and 25.2).[3-5] It is important to recognize that patients without albinism may also have a blunted foveal depression and that there is a range of abnormal foveal morphology that may occur in albinism—including an entirely absent foveal depression (e.g., fovea plana) or a blunted but still partially depressed foveal contour. An individual's visual potential cannot be determined by the presence or absence of a pit— patients with absent foveal pits may have good visual acuity (even 20/20). Nonetheless, in patients with albinism, the degree of abnormal foveal morphology may correlate to some extent with visual acuity.

Additionally, the ellipsoid zone may not exhibit its normal subfoveal thickening or upward bulge in these patients. Because of the paucity of melanin pigment in the retinal pigment epithelium (RPE) of patients with albinism, there is enhanced light transmission through the RPE, leading to enhanced visualization of the choroidal details and enhanced definition of the sclera on OCT (see Fig. 25.1 and 25.2). Optic nerve thickening has also been described in some patients with albinism.

When assessing for an abnormal foveal depression in patients with albinism, it is important for clinicians to obtain macular volume scans and examine multiple cross-sectional images throughout the macula to capture the central foveal scan. This will help ensure that an image acquired from outside the foveal center is not mistaken as being representative of foveal hypoplasia.

The optic nerve head may also be abnormal in patients with albinism and the following observations have been noted:[4,7] (1) the optic nerve head may appear elevated; (2) the neuroretinal rim is thicker (the nasal rim is thicker than the temporal rim) than patients without albinism, and this may be related to an abnormal distribution of the nerve fibers entering the optic nerve; (3) the peripapillary RNFL is thinner (particularly in the temporal quadrant) than patients without albinism; and (4) horizontal elongation of the discs is more common in patients with albinism (in contrast to the typical vertical elongation seen in patients without albinism).

Ancillary Testing

Special attention should be paid to screen for features of Hemansky-Pudlak and Chédiak-Higashi syndromes in conjunction with a pediatrician or geneticist. Genetic testing for the previously mentioned gene defects may also be considered. Fundus photographs (see Figs. 25.1 and 25.2) may reveal a light-colored fundus, prominent choroidal markings, blunted foveal light reflex, and an absent or reduced capillary-free zone in the macula. The latter finding also may sometimes be seen on fluorescein angiography.

Treatment

There is currently no established cure for oculocutaneous or ocular albinism. Management typically consists of correcting refractive error, possible strabismus surgery to dampen the nystagmus, and minimizing photodysphoria with hats, dark glasses, tinted contact lenses (or artificial iris implants), and minimizing sun exposure to the skin given the higher rate of cutaneous malignancies in these patients.

References

1. Grønskov K, Ek J, Brondum-Nielsen K. Oculocutaneous albinism. *Orphanet J Rare Dis.* 2007;2:43.
2. Introne WJ, Westbroek W, Golas GA, Adams D. Chediak-Higashi syndrome. In: Adam MP, Ardinger HH, Pagon RA, et al., eds. *GeneReviews*® [Internet]. Seattle, WA: University of Washington, Seattle; 1993. Available at http://www.ncbi.nlm.nih.gov/books/NBK5188/.
3. Ather S, Proudlock FA, Welton T, Morgan PS, Sheth V, Gottlob I, et al. Aberrant visual pathway development in albinism: from retina to cortex. *Hum Brain Mapp.* 2019;40(3):777–788.
4. Chong GT, Farsiu S, Freedman SF, et al. Abnormal foveal morphology in ocular albinism imaged with spectral-domain optical coherence tomography. *Arch Ophthalmol.* 2009;127(1):37–44.
5. McCafferty BK, Wilk MA, McAllister JT, et al. Clinical insights into foveal morphology in albinism. *J Pediatr Ophthalmol Strabismus.* 2015;52(3):167–172.
6. Thomas MG, Kumar A, Mohammad S, et al. Structural grading of foveal hypoplasia using spectral-domain optical coherence tomography: a predictor of visual acuity? *Ophthalmology.* 2011;118(8):1653–1660.
7. Mohammad S, Gottlob I, Sheth V, Pilat A, Lee H, Pollheimer E, et al. Characterization of abnormal optic nerve head morphology in albinism using optical coherence tomography. *Invest Ophthalmol Vis Sci.* 2015;56(8):4611–4618.

CHAPTER 26

X-Linked Juvenile Retinoschisis

Mohsin H. Ali ■ Lejla Vajzovic

CHAPTER OUTLINE

Introduction

X-linked retinoschisis (XLRS) is an inherited retinal degeneration affecting males caused by a mutation in the *RS1* gene, which encodes the protein complex retinoschisin.

The Brain Connection

XLRS is not typically associated with neurologic abnormalities.

Clinical Features

Given the X-linked inheritance pattern, all affected patients are males. Patients with XLRS typically develop central vision deterioration within the first or second decade of life. The clinical manifestations and severity may be highly variable.[1,2] In general, most patients have bilateral (although possibly asymmetric) disease, with splitting of the inner retinal layers. In the majority of patients, this involves the fovea leading to the appearance of foveal cystoid spaces in a "wheel spokes" arrangement. Approximately half the patients have peripheral retinoschisis as well, often involving the inferotemporal quadrant. Foveal retinoschisis yields decreased central visual acuity, whereas peripheral retinoschisis causes absolute scotomas in the peripheral visual field. Severe complications of retinoschisis include vitreous hemorrhage, retinal detachment (which requires a retinal break in both the inner and outer layers of split retina), or hemorrhage within a schisis cavity.

OCT Features

Optical coherence tomography (OCT) findings in XLRS include splitting of the inner retinal layers in the macula or peripheral retina (Figs. 26.1 through 26.4).[3,4] The resulting schisis cavities most commonly involve the inner nuclear layer, but they may also involve the retinal nerve fiber, ganglion cell, inner plexiform, outer plexiform, and outer nuclear layers. Of these, the most commonly affected sites are likely to be the inner nuclear layer, followed by the outer plexiform and outer

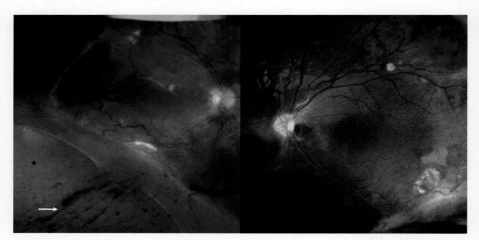

Fig. 26.1 Fundus image of the posterior pole in a 10-year-old male with an *RS1* gene mutation. The fundus image of the right eye depicts the peripheral retinoschisis that can be seen in these patients. Large inner retinal holes *(black asterisks)* can be seen just peripheral to the inferotemporal vascular arcade, leading to the presence of a large peripheral schisis cavity. A bridging retinal vessel *(white arrow)* is seen extending inferotemporally over the schisis cavity—serving as a reminder to clinicians for how susceptible these patients may be to vitreous hemorrhage. The left eye demonstrates the characteristic whitish stippling in the macula corresponding to the macular retinoschisis.

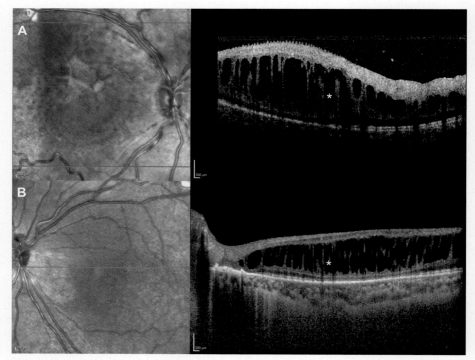

Fig. 26.2 Optical coherence tomography (OCT) image from the same patient shown in Fig. 26.1 demonstrates the characteristic splitting *(asterisks)* of the inner and outer retinal layers in the macula, with the right eye (A) appearing to be more severely affected than the left eye (B). The patient's visual acuity was 20/250 in both eyes. He was started on topical dorzolamide three times daily to both eyes, although without significant anatomic improvement.

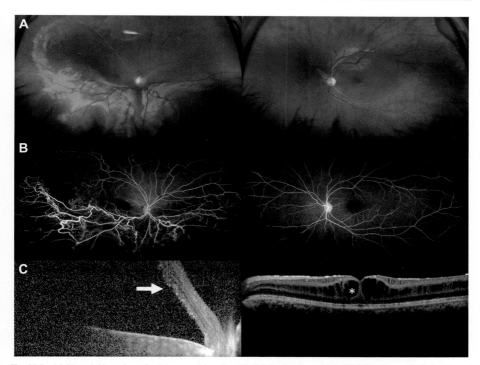

Fig. 26.3 Multimodal imaging of a 14-year-old male with X-linked retinoschisis (XLRS). The patient developed retinal detachment after being hit in the eye with an elbow while playing basketball. Visual acuity in the right eye was 20/320 OD and 20/40 OS. (A) Wide-field fundus imaging showed a macula-off retinal detachment of the right eye and an attached retina in the left eye without any apparent peripheral retinoschisis. (B) Wide-field fluorescein angiography demonstrated a large area of temporal nonperfusion in the right eye. There was no dye leakage in the macula of either eye. (C) Optical coherence tomography (OCT) confirmed the retinal detachment *(arrow)* in the left eye (as evidenced by the presence of subretinal fluid separating the neurosensory retina from the underlying retinal pigment epithelium [RPE]) and the macular retinoschisis *(asterisk)* in the left eye (as evidenced by splitting of retinal layers while outer retinal adhesion to the underlying RPE is maintained). These images are representative of the risks of minor trauma in patients with XLRS, including retinal detachment, the potential for asymmetric disease, and the potential for peripheral retinal ischemia.

nuclear layers. It is possible for schisis cavities to affect multiple layers within the same eye and for two eyes of the same patient to have dissimilar schisis cavities, both in location and severity. Other findings that may be seen on OCT include disruption of the ellipsoid zone and vitreoretinal attachment and/or traction.

Patients with retinoschisis may develop retinal detachment if there are both inner and outer retinal breaks (thereby allowing vitreous fluid to access the subretinal space). Schisis cavities, especially those that are larger and more bullous, can mimic retinal detachments ophthalmoscopically. In these situations, OCT can be particularly helpful in differentiating retinoschisis from retinal detachment—in areas of retinoschisis, there will be adhesion of the outer retina to the underlying retinal pigment epithelium (RPE), whereas in areas of retinal detachment, subretinal fluid will be

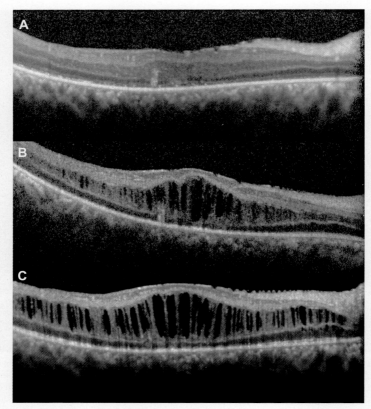

Fig. 26.4 Postoperative optical coherence tomography (OCT) image from the same patient shown in Fig. 26.3. The retinal detachment in the right eye was treated with scleral buckle with pars plana vitrectomy and silicone oil tamponade. No membrane or internal limiting membrane peeling was performed. The retina has remained attached, and visual acuity improved to 20/60. (A) At postoperative months 1 (B) and 2 (C). At postoperative months 1 and 2. This sequence of images illustrates the recurrence and persistence of macular retinoschisis despite initial improvement after vitrectomy.

seen separating the neurosensory retina from the underlying RPE (see Fig. 26.3). OCT may also be able to identify the locations of inner and outer retinal holes.

Ancillary Testing

Visual field testing may be useful to delineate the absolute scotomas that may be present in patients with peripheral retinoschisis. Electroretinography may show fairly normal a-wave amplitude with a reduced b-wave amplitude. Fluorescein angiography will fail to demonstrate leakage in the area of foveal schisis in XLRS, thereby eliminating potentially similar appearing etiologies of cystoid macular edema. Finally, genetic testing for the *RS1* mutation may be employed to confirm the diagnosis.

Treatment

There is currently no cure for retinoschisis. Carbonic anhydrase inhibitors, such as topical dorzolamide, have been found to be beneficial in improving visual acuity and OCT-derived structural parameters.[5] Gene replacement, stem cell, and drug-based therapies are in development.

References

1. Sieving PA, MacDonald IM, Chan S. X-Linked Juvenile Retinoschisis. In: Adam MP, Ardinger HH, Pagon RA, Wallace SE, Bean LJ, Stephens K, et al., eds. *GeneReviews® [Internet]*. Seattle (WA): University of Washington, Seattle; 1993. Available at: http://www.ncbi.nlm.nih.gov/books/NBK1222/.
2. Tantri A, Vrabec TR, Cu-Unjieng A, Frost A, Annesley WH, Donoso LA. X-linked retinoschisis: a clinical and molecular genetic review. *Surv Ophthalmol.* 2004;49(2):214–230.
3. Yu J, Ni Y, Keane PA, Jiang C, Wang W, Xu G. Foveomacular schisis in juvenile X-linked retinoschisis: an optical coherence tomography study. *Am J Ophthalmol.* 2010;149(6):973–978. e2.
4. Gregori NZ, Lam BL, Gregori G, et al. Wide-field spectral-domain optical coherence tomography in patients and carriers of X-linked retinoschisis. *Ophthalmology.* 2013;120(1):169–174.
5. Khandhadia S, Trump D, Menon G, Lotery AJ. X-linked retinoschisis maculopathy treated with topical dorzolamide, and relationship to genotype. *Eye (Lond).* 2011;25(7):922–928.

CHAPTER 27

Other Inherited Retinal Diseases

Mohsin H. Ali ■ Alessandro Iannaccone ■ Lejla Vajzovic

Introduction

Alagille syndrome, choroideremia, and neuronal ceroid lipofuscinosis (Batten disease) are inherited entities with retinal manifestations. This chapter describes the clinical features and optical coherence tomography (OCT) characteristics of other inherited retinal degenerations, such as Alagille syndrome, choroideremia, and neuronal ceroid lipofuscinosis (Batten disease).

The Brain Connection

Alagille syndrome—abnormalities of the nervous system in Alagille syndrome may include absent deep tendon reflexes and intellectual or learning disabilities.

Choroideremia—choroideremia is not associated with neurologic or systemic abnormalities.

Neuronal ceroid lipofuscinosis (Batten disease)—this is a neurodegenerative disorder, although neurologic manifestations may be highly variable.[1,2] Potential neurologic consequences include intellectual disability, seizures, motor function loss, myoclonic ataxia, depression, anxiety, pyramidal signs, spasticity, and Parkinsonism.

Clinical Features (Nonocular)

Alagille syndrome—Alagille syndrome is an autosomal dominant disorder that is caused by a mutation in the *JAG1* gene (type 1) or *NOTCH2* gene (type 2).[3] In addition to the ocular findings described in the next section, characteristic systemic findings include intrahepatic biliary duct hypoplasia with resulting cholestatic liver disease, pulmonic valve stenosis, peripheral arterial stenosis, butterfly vertebrae, and a distinct facies described as a prominent forehead and chin, deep-set and hyperteloric eyes, and a straight nose with flattened tip.[3,4]

Choroideremia—choroideremia is an X-linked disorder caused by a mutation in the *CHM* gene characterized by isolated chorioretinal degeneration primarily affecting the retinal pigment epithelium in the absence of systemic abnormalities.[5]

Neuronal ceroid lipofuscinosis (Batten disease)—this is a heterogeneous group of neurodegenerative lysosomal storage disorders caused by mutations in various genes and most commonly inherited in an autosomal recessive manner.[1,2] Clinical symptoms may begin in the infant, juvenile, or adult age groups and typically include severe central and peripheral visual loss accompanied by progressive neurologic dysfunction.

Clinical Features (Ocular)

Alagille syndrome—the ocular manifestations of Alagille syndrome may include posterior embryotoxon, iris abnormalities, pigmentary chorioretinal atrophy, chorioretinal folds, angulated or tortuous retinal vessels, and pseudopapilledema (so named because the elevated optic disc does not exhibit fluorescein leakage or optic nerve head drusen and is not associated with elevated intracranial pressure).[3,4]

Choroideremia—in affected male patients, night blindness and peripheral visual field constriction typically develop in the second and third decades of life, as well as decline in their central vision later in life. The fundus findings include atrophy of the retinal pigment epithelium (RPE) and choroid beginning in the midperiphery of the fundus.[5] Unlike retinitis pigmentosa, retinal vasculature narrowing, and optic nerve pallor are often noted only in late stages of the disease. Cystic intraretinal spaces may also be present. Importantly, female carriers may have pigmentary changes (e.g., mottling, granularity, or hypopigmentation of the RPE) in the midperiphery, most often without impact on the visual function.

Neuronal ceroid lipofuscinosis (Batten disease)—severe vision loss typically begins centrally and progresses rapidly, potentially leading to blindness within a few years.[1,2] The initial retinal phenotype can simulate Stargardt disease.

OCT Features

Alagille syndrome—the severity of chorioretinal manifestations in Alagille syndrome may be variable. Loss of the outer retinal bands, including the ellipsoid zone, in the parafoveal and perifoveal regions and peripheral retina, initially sparing the fovea, may be seen—reminiscent of a bull's eye maculopathy and peripheral retinal degenerations (Fig. 27.1).[3,4]

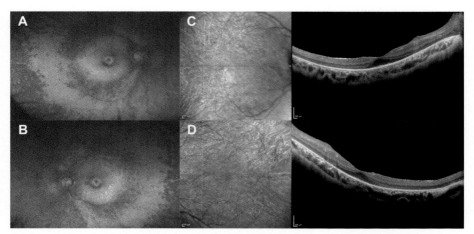

Fig. 27.1 Fundus autofluorescence and optical coherence tomography (OCT) in a 12-year-old female patient with Alagille syndrome caused by a mutation in *JAG1*. Visual acuity was 20/50 OD and 20/25 OS. (A, B) Fundus autofluorescence reveals rings of alternating hypo- and hyperautofluorescence with a bull's eye–like pattern involving the posterior pole and periphery. There is corresponding attenuation of the vessels. (C, D) Optical coherence tomography reveals significant parafoveal loss of the outer retinal bands including the ellipsoid zone with relative foveal-sparing in the right eye *(top)* and left eye *(bottom)*. (Image courtesy of Nathan Cheung, OD and Alessandro Iannaccone, MD.)

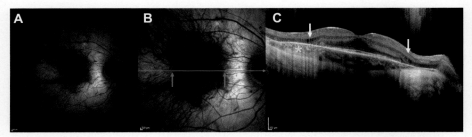

Fig. 27.2   (A, B) Infrared fundus imaging of a 20 year-old-male with choroideremia caused by a *CHM* gene muta-tion showing widespread atrophy of the retinal pigment epithelium (RPE) and choriocapillaris with relative sparing of the central macula in both eyes. (C) Optical coherence tomography (OCT) reveals parafoveal loss of the outer retinal bands, including the ellipsoid zone, along with loss of the RPE, as evidenced by the enhanced transmis-sion of light in affected areas (yellow asterisks). The transition between zones of intact and disrupted outer retina and RPE colocalizes with the transition between dark and light areas on the en face infrared image *(red arrows)*. Parafoveal cystic intraretinal spaces are also seen *(white arrows),* which are commonly found in choroideremia patients. Visual acuity was 20/20 OU. (Image courtesy of Alessandro Iannaccone, MD.)

OCT may also demonstrate an elevated optic nerve head, with or without peripapillary chorioretinal folds, in those patients with pseudopapilledema.

Choroideremia—when the disease progresses from the midperiphery to the macula, loss of the outer retinal bands and RPE, initially sparing the fovea, may be seen, similar to other inher-ited retinal degenerations (Fig. 27.2). Cystoid macular edema may also be seen (see Fig. 27.2). The most typical finding is the sharp transition from the central preserved areas to the sur-rounding areas overlying atrophic retinal pigment epithelium and markedly thinned chorio-capillaris, where marked hypertransmission defects are noted.

Neuronal ceroid lipofuscinosis (Batten disease)—in contrast to many other retinal degenera-tions, which progress centripetally from the retinal periphery, Batten disease may begin cen-trally and thus the macula may be affected severely early in the disease, simulating Stargardt disease.[1,2] Also, in contrast to other retinal degenerations (e.g., retinitis pigmentosa [RP]), which may show preferential loss of the outer retinal bands, in Batten disease, both the inner and outer retinal layers may become severely attenuated, with corresponding significant

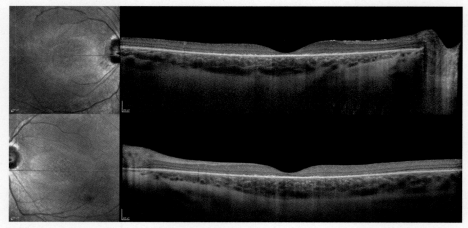

Fig. 27.3   Optical coherence tomography (OCT) image from a 9-year-old male patient with neuronal ceroid lipofuscinosis (Batten disease) secondary to a mutation in the *CLN3* gene. There is significant disruption of the ellipsoid zone, including subfoveally, and both the inner and outer retinal layers are attenuated and poorly defined. Visual acuity was 20/80 OD and 20/100 OS. (Image courtesy of Alessandro Iannaccone, MD.)

reduction in the central retinal thickness (Fig. 27.3).[1] In other presentations of Batten disease, a bull's eye pattern of maculopathy may be seen.

Ancillary Testing

Alagille syndrome—gonioscopy can help confirm the presence of posterior embryotoxon. Fundus autofluorescence, electroretinography, and visual field testing are often important in monitoring disease progression in cases of chorioretinal atrophy.[3,4] Referral to medical subspecialists (e.g., gastroenterologist and cardiologist) is warranted given the likelihood of coexisting systemic abnormalities.

Choroideremia—fundus autofluorescence and fluorescein angiography help highlight the extent of RPE and choroidal atrophy. Visual field testing is essential for monitoring disease progression. Abnormal dark adaptometry and electroretinography may also aide in the diagnosis.

Neuronal ceroid lipofuscinosis (Batten disease)—electroretinography and visual field testing are usually severely affected even when the clinical picture suggests macular disease only. All affected patients will require systemic ancillary testing and monitoring by other medical subspecialists (e.g., neurologist).

Treatment

Alagille syndrome—there is no known treatment for the ocular findings in Alagille syndrome. In the absence of chorioretinal degeneration, several of the remaining ocular manifestations, such as posterior embryotoxon and pseudopapilledema, are unlikely to significantly impact vision. Systemic treatment depends on the involvement and severity of other organ systems.

Choroideremia—there are currently no established treatments for choroideremia, though gene replacement therapy, stem cell therapy, and drug-based therapy are ongoing. Carbonic anhydrase inhibitors may be helpful in treating cystoid macular edema.[6]

Neuronal ceroid lipofuscinosis (Batten disease)—There are no established treatments for the chorioretinal degeneration in Batten disease. In April 2017, the FDA approved Brineura (cerliponase alfa) as the first treatment for Batten disease linked to mutations in the *CLN2* gene to slow ambulation loss in symptomatic pediatric patients 3 years of age and older. Brineura is an enzyme replacement therapy (a recombinant form of human TPP1, the enzyme deficient in patients with CLN2 disease) and is administered intrathecally. Systemic treatment focuses on addressing the variety of other organ systems affected in the other genetic subtypes of Batten disease.

References

1. Preising MN, Abura M, Jäger M, Wassill K-H, Lorenz B. Ocular morphology and function in juvenile neuronal ceroid lipofuscinosis (CLN3) in the first decade of life. *Ophthalmic Genet.* 2017;38(3):252–259.
2. Hansen MS, Hove MN, Jensen H, Larsen M. Optical coherence tomography in juvenile neuronal ceroid lipofuscinosis. *Retin Cases Brief Rep.* 2016;10(2):137–139.
3. Kim BJ, Fulton AB. The genetics and ocular findings of Alagille syndrome. *Semin Ophthalmol.* 2007;22(4):205–210.
4. Hingorani M, Nischal KK, Davies A, et al. Ocular abnormalities in Alagille syndrome. *Ophthalmology.* 1999;106(2):330–337.
5. Roberts MF, Fishman GA, Roberts DK, et al. Retrospective, longitudinal, and cross sectional study of visual acuity impairment in choroideraemia. *Br J Ophthalmol.* 2002;86(6):658–662.
6. Salvatore S, Fishman GA, Genead MA. Treatment of cystic macular lesions in hereditary retinal dystrophies. *Surv Ophthalmol.* 2013;58(6):560–584.

Vitreoretinal and Vascular Diseases

CHAPTER 28

Retinopathy of Prematurity

Cynthia A. Toth ■ Alexandria Dandridge ■ Xi Chen

Introduction

Retinopathy of prematurity (ROP) is the most common retinal cause of blindness in children in the developed world and has increased in prevalence around the world as more infants survive preterm birth. Despite this, over 80% of infants with ROP do not progress to a level of disease that warrants treatment, and the vast majority of these infants also develop excellent visual acuity. In the developed world, ROP is more common in infants of lower birthweight and younger gestational age who are born preterm. The birthweight is higher, gestational age greater, and oxygen exposure often less controlled in infants at risk for ROP in the developing world. Access to screening and treatment are important. Infrared optical coherence tomography (OCT) imaging is well tolerated by infants and is likely to play a role in future screening and management of care.

The Brain Connection

The immature retina and brain are both in rapid development and refinement in the final months of pregnancy. Abnormalities of this development may arise from shared risk factors. This is reflected in more severe stages of ROP being associated with brain abnormalities and poorer neurodevelopment. Macular edema in premature infants with ROP has been associated with poorer neurodevelopment,[1] and a thinner retinal nerve fiber layer (RNFL) in these infants has been associated with brain abnormalities on magnetic resonance imaging (MRI).[2,3]

Clinical Features

ROP is identified clinically by a pattern of incomplete and abnormal retinal vessel development in preterm infants. Assessment is centered on determining whether retinal findings indicate a course of disease that requires treatment. The international classification uses five stages to classify the

129

vascular–avascular junction in ROP, with the most posterior location of the junction designated as in zone I, II, or III of the retina. Severity of dilation and tortuosity of the retinal vasculature in a posterior region near the optic nerve is described as none, pre-plus, and plus disease, based on severity of the features relative to reference photographs. Plus disease is the most common indicator of a need for treatment, although in certain cases, extent of neovascularization may also be an indicator for treatment. In late disease, retinal vessels may be dragged and elevated, and there may be vitreous hemorrhage and retinal detachment.

OCT Features

As in adult vitreoretinal and neurovascular disease, OCT imaging reveals features in ROP that are difficult to identify by using any other examination and imaging modalities.[4]

Classic OCT findings of immature retinal (foveal) development are found in preterm infants (see Chapter 10), and relate to age at birth, current age, and ROP. Although imaging is typically limited to the posterior zones, the en face retinal view, the three-dimensional (3D) view, and cross-sectional B-scans provide unique perspectives of the developing retinal structures and vasculature, extraretinal neovascularization, fluid, traction, and retinal detachment.[4-7] OCT angiography (OCTA) is especially useful to distinguish abnormalities of retinal vascular development and flow in extraretinal neovascularization[8] and to distinguish vascular flow across areas of laser.[9] OCT may be limited by preretinal hemorrhage or a very prominent tunica vasculosa lentis.

The stages of ROP are currently based on clinical examination and fundus photographs. Within these stages, we describe the distinct retinal appearances from OCT imaging.

Stage 1—there is no distinct boundary between vascularized and avascular retina in cross-section, with a gradual slope of inner retinal thinning in the avascular retina, comparable with stage 0.[10] The inner retinal surface is bland in volumetric (3D) view.

Stage 2—the inner retina thickens in a bulge at the vascular–avascular junction, and the avascular inner retina peripheral to the junction may remain thin (Fig. 28.1). Small neovascular buds may be visible on OCT over the vascularized retina, even though they are not visible on clinical examination.[10] The retinal surface is otherwise bland in 3D.

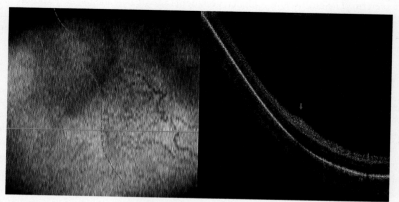

Fig. 28.1 Optical coherence tomography (OCT) retinal view *(left)* and B-scan *(right)* in a 36-week postmenstrual age (PMA) infant with stage 2 retinopathy of prematurity (ROP) in zone I. At the retinal vascular–avascular junction *(red dashed line)* there is localized hyperreflective thickened ridge of the inner retina. The inner retina is thinner in the avascular retina, whereas the outer retinal layers do not vary across the junction. (Right, Image courtesy of Isaac Bleicher.)

Stage 3—preretinal neovascularization is present at and behind the vascular–avascular junction and may appear as sessile or pedunculated buds (Figs. 28.2 and 28.3), which may develop into bridging networks and thicker placoid lesions. Buds are often present posterior to bridging networks or placoid lesions. The inner retinal surface is often no longer bland, with peripheral retinal vessel dilation, tortuosity, and bulging along the inner retinal surface. The inner retina may be elevated with split inner retinal layers with a cleft of fluid from either vitreous traction or fluid leakage[10] (see Fig. 28.3).

Regressed Stage 3—a distinct decrease in the neovascular structure is evident, and this may lift away from the retina. Effects of vitreous traction on inner retina may stabilize, increase, or decrease[10] (Fig. 28.4), and subclinical schisis may be only detected on OCT.[11]

Stage 4—retinal schisis, microcystic changes across the posterior pole in eyes with peripheral RD, and retinal detachment are distinguished by OCT.[4,5,12] The photoreceptor layer is present over the retinal pigment epithelium (RPE) in retinal schisis (Fig. 28.5) and separated from the retinal pigment epithelium by fluid in a retinal detachment (Fig. 28.6). The posterior extent of schisis or detachment can be localized with OCT, which enables a clear distinction between presence (stage 4B) or absence of retinal detachment at the fovea (stage 4A).[4,5]

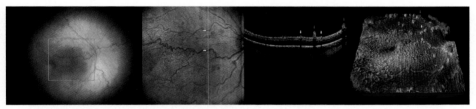

Fig. 28.2   A color photograph *(left)*, Optical coherence tomography (OCT) retinal view *(mid-left)*, OCT B-scan *(mid-right)*, and 3D-thickness map *(right)* of an infant with aggressive posterior retinopathy of prematurity (ROP). The en face OCT retinal view shows a high-resolution image of the macula similar to the Retcam fundus photograph. Multiple posterior extraretinal neovascular buds are visible on the B-scan, on the three-dimensional (3D) thickness map and as focal dark patches (shadowing from the blood) on the retinal view. Note the tortuosity and dilation of distinct large and small vessels on OCT.

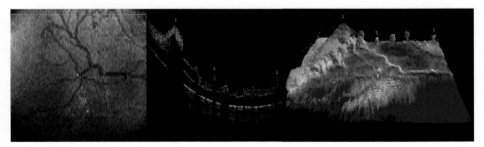

Fig. 28.3   Optical coherence tomography (OCT) retinal view (left), B-scan *(middle)*, and three-dimensional (3D)-thickness map *(right)* in a 33-week postmenstrual age (PMA) female (born at 24 weeks) with stage 3 retinopathy of prematurity (ROP) in zone I. Note the elevation of and shadowing from buds and placoid neovascular tissue *(arrows)*. Retinal vessels also bulge up from the inner retinal surface *(yellow* on 3D map) and produce a wavy pattern within the retina on the B-scan; these findings in small peripheral retinal vessels are similar to OCT findings of posterior plus disease (see Fig. 28.7). The retinal vascular–avascular junction is marked with red dashed line on en face view, and inner layers of the avascular retina are thickened peripheral to this junction *(left margin* of the B-Scan) while inner retinal cystoid spaces are present posterior to the neovascular structures. Reflective foci are seen within the vitreous over the neovascularization. (Right, Image courtesy of Isaac Bleicher.)

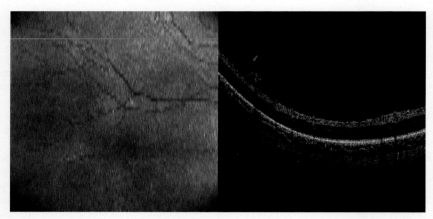

Fig. 28.4 Optical coherence tomography (OCT) retinal view *(left)* and B-scan *(right)* of regression of the placoid extraretinal neovascularization and buds from Fig. 28.3, several weeks after intravitreal bevacizumab. The neovascular tissue appears more attenuated on cross-sectional view (of the same location as in the b-scan in Fig. 28.5). Progressive vascularization of the previous avascular retina is visible on the OCT retinal view *(left)*.

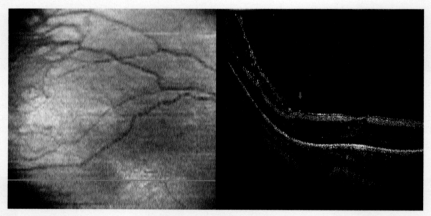

Fig. 28.5 Optical coherence tomography (OCT) retinal view *(left)* and B-scan *(right)* demonstrate dilated vessels and retinoschisis in nerve fiber layer and ganglion cell layer in temporal retina outside of the foveal center *(stopping at arrow)*. This infant was diagnosed with 4A retinopathy of prematurity (ROP) based on ophthalmoscopic examination, but retinoschisis and not retinal detachment is present in the areas imaged with OCT. Posterior to the schisis, vertically aligned cystoid spaces extend evenly across the inner nuclear layer. The evenly distributed macular cystoid spaces contiguous with peripheral inner schisis appear to be from traction, although they could be from leakage or both. A few hyperreflective foci are visible in the inner retina and in the vitreous over the schisis.

Hyperreflective spots or bands may occur within vitreous, retina or even beneath the retina and may reflect vitreous organization with traction, exudates, or inflammation.[13]

Stage 5—thickness and attachments of preretinal fibrovascular tissue and spaces of separation from the detached retina may be seen. It may be difficult to image when there is a high or steep detachment because of the shallow depth of focus of OCT.

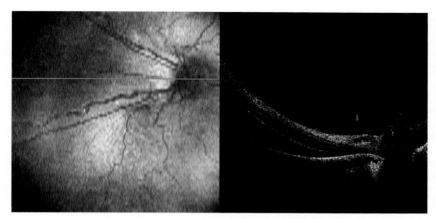

Fig. 28.6 Optical coherence tomography (OCT) retinal view and B-scan demonstrating region of subretinal fluid extending almost to the optic nerve head in an infant clinically diagnosed with stage 4B retinopathy of prematurity (ROP) in zone II at 45 weeks' postmenstrual age (PMA) (born at <25 weeks' gestational age). Cystoid structures within the retinal nerve fiber layer (RNFL) surround the optic nerve head, and the nerve head appeared slightly elevated and without a cup suggesting traction. The infant had previous laser photocoagulation of the avascular periphery.

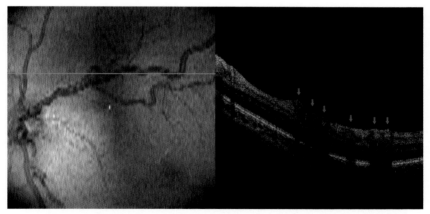

Fig. 28.7 A 37-week postmenstrual age (PMA), ex-25 weeks female infant with zone II stage 3 retinopathy of prematurity (ROP) with plus disease. Retinal vessels appear dilated and tortuous in the en face view *(left)* and on the corresponding cross-sectional view *(right),* where anteroposterior retinal vessel tortuosity deformed the retinal surface *(right, arrows)* and plexiform layers.

PRE-PLUS AND PLUS DISEASE

Tortuosity of retinal vessels and enlargement of retinal vessel diameter are visible in 3D on OCT. The tortuous vessels both bulge out of the inner retinal surface and also deform the adjacent and underlying retina (Fig. 28.7). The retina is split or has pockets of fluid in eyes with more severe tortuosity. Together, vascular dilation, elevation of the retinal surface, and distortion of the retinal layers and adjacent spaces comprise the Vascular Abnormality Score on OCT (VASO).[14] A higher VASO score has been associated with plus disease.[12]

LASER SCARS

The retina is hyperreflective and thickened immediately after laser treatment and thinned at sites of older laser scar. Areas of hyperreflectivity of the choroid and sclera are caused by loss of the RPE, and pigment clumping will shadow.

MACULAR EDEMA

Intraretinal cystoid spaces are common on OCT in preterm infants and have been found in from one-third to over one-half of infants with ROP (whether of very low gestational age and birthweight, or whether of higher birthweight and gestational age but at ROP risk because of oxygen exposure).[1,4,6,7,15-17] The cystoid spaces are found in the inner nuclear layer and often produce an upward bulge at the foveal center and may also deform the immature foveal photoreceptors[15] (Fig. 28.8). This may range from small cystoid spaces in perifovea with a preserved foveal depression (Vinekar "pattern B") to massive vertical spaces elevating the foveal center (Vinekar "pattern A").[16] Central foveal thickness or fovea-to-parafoveal ratio provides a reproducible measure of severity of edema.[18] Macular edema has been associated with fluorescein leakage in some cases[19] and with developmental delay.[1]

RETINAL NERVE FIBER LAYER THINNING

RNFL thinning has been found on OCT in infants with ROP, although this may reflect hypoxic injury in utero or at birth, or be associated with causes of periventricular leukomalacia (which may occur in the infants at risk for ROP). Brain abnormalities on MRI have been associated with the RNFL thinning in infants with ROP[2] (Fig. 28.9).

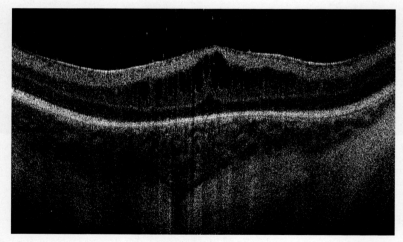

Fig. 28.8 Optical coherence tomography (OCT) of macular edema of prematurity in a 37-week postmenstrual age (PMA) infant who was born at 25 weeks. Cystoid spaces in the inner nuclear layer increase in size with an upward deformation of the foveal center and an upward pinched elevation of the outer plexiform layer and photoreceptors. A tractional component to the macular findings cannot be ruled out. The inner aspect of the nerve fiber layer in highly reflective and there is profound thinning of the nerve fiber and ganglion cell layers. There are reflective foci in the vitreous. The photoreceptor layer has not yet developed an ellipsoid zone at the foveal center (Chapter 10), and the ellipsoid zone and the external limiting membrane are visible outside the central macula on the left side of the scan.

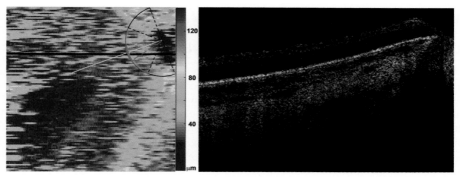

Fig. 28.9 Retinal nerve fiber layer (RNFL) thickness map *(left)* are derived from inner retina segmented from spectral domain–optical coherence tomography (SD-OCT) scans (B-scan with thin retinal layers on *right*) in a preterm infant. This infant has severe thinning of all retinal layers and of the choroid. The thick pink arc marks the papillomacular bundle and extends 15 degrees on either side of the organizing axis from the optic nerve center to the fovea. The thin pink arc corresponds to the temporal quadrant RNFL which extends 45 degrees above and below the organizing axis. The thick black line corresponds to the representative B-scan location.

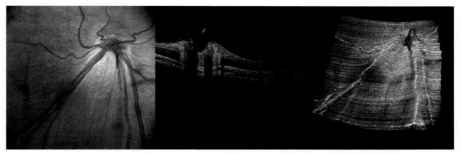

Fig. 28.10 The en face retinal view *(left)*, cross-sectional view *(middle)* and three-dimensional (3D) volume view in grayscale *(right)* of the optic nerve head in a 37-week postmenstrual age (PMA) (born at <25 weeks' gestational age) male infant with stage 4A retinal detachment. The macula is not in this volume because the retina is dragged toward neovascular tissue in the temporal periphery (producing straightened and elevated vessels on the retinal and volume views). Vitreous bands are elevated over the optic nerve head, and old blood in the vitreous produces dark shadows with blurred margins on the retinal view.

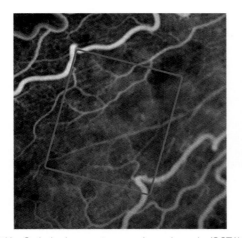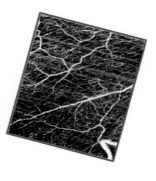

Fig. 28.11 Optical coherence tomography angiography (OCTA) image from a portable handheld investigational research system used to image a young child with retinopathy of prematurity (ROP). In the fluorescein angiogram *(left)*, dragged vessels nasal to the fovea are visible. The handheld OCTA image of the same region *(right)* reveals these small vascular structures and loops, and these can be depth resolved, without the need for fluorescein dye injection.

DRAGGED RETINA, RETINAL VESSELS, AND OPTIC NERVE HEAD

RNFL thickening and elevation and straightening of large retinal vessels has been found associated with tractional dragging of retina or of the optic nerve head, from advanced stages of ROP with extraretinal neovascularization (Fig. 28.10). Abnormalities in smaller vessels, secondary to ROP and premature birth, have been evident on fluorescein angiograms (Fig. 28.11, left). Novel OCTA imaging has enabled visualization of fine retinal vasculature in young children, without the need for fluorescein dye (see Fig. 28.11, right). With this imaging, the failure of development of the foveal avascular zone has been shown to parallel the persistence of inner retinal layers at the fovea after preterm birth[20] and in ROP.[21]

VITREOUS ORGANIZATION, CELLS, AND HEMORRHAGE

Hyperreflectivities within the vitreous gel may reflect hemorrhage or vitreous organization with traction and may precede a more active or advanced disease stage.[13] Vitreous hemorrhage may limit the view of the underlying retina.

Ancillary Testing

Retinal photography has been used for screening and documentation, and fluorescein angiography has been used to evaluate nonperfusion and leakage from neovascularization. B-scan ultrasonography has been useful to examine for detachment when there is vitreous hemorrhage.

Treatment

Prevention and management center on controlling oxygen exposure, optimizing early infant health and development, examining the eyes of infants at risk, and intervention if indicated by severity of disease. Treatment of ROP includes laser photocoagulation of nonvascular areas of the retina and/or injection of anti–vascular endothelial growth factor (anti-VEGF) agents into the vitreous cavity (a treatment not cleared by the U.S. Food and Drug Administration [FDA] as of 2018). Vitreoretinal surgery is used to remove nonclearing hemorrhage or release tractional retinal detachment, especially when the central retina is at risk. We do not have a clear indication as to when vitreoretinal surgery is indicated for OCT findings of retinal schisis rather than detachment, although progression of schisis on OCT may contribute to this determination.[12]

References

1. Rothman AL, Tran-Viet D, Gustafson KE, et al. Poorer neurodevelopmental outcomes associated with cystoid macular edema identified in preterm infants in the intensive care nursery. *Ophthalmology.* 2015;122(3):610–619.
2. Rothman AL, Mangalesh S, Chen X, Toth CA. Optical coherence tomography of the preterm eye: from retinopathy of prematurity to brain development. *Eye Brain.* 2016;8:123–133.
3. Rothman AL, Sevilla MB, Mangalesh S, et al. Thinner retinal nerve fiber layer in very preterm versus term infants and relationship to brain anatomy and neurodevelopment. *Am J Ophthalmol.* 2015;160 (6):1296–1308.
4. Lee AC, Maldonado RS, Sarin N, et al. Macular features from spectral-domain optical coherence tomography as an adjunct to indirect ophthalmoscopy in retinopathy of prematurity. *Retina.* 2011;31 (8):1470–1482.
5. Chavala SH, Farsiu S, Maldonado R, Wallace DK, Freedman SF, Toth CA. Insights into advanced retinopathy of prematurity using handheld spectral domain optical coherence tomography imaging. *Ophthalmology.* 2009;116(12):2448–2456.

6. Maldonado RS, Toth CA. Optical coherence tomography in retinopathy of prematurity: looking beyond the vessels. *Clin Perinatol.* 2013;40(2):271–296.
7. Vinekar A, Mangalesh S, Jayadev C, Maldonado RS, Bauer N, Toth CA. Retinal imaging of infants on spectral domain optical coherence tomography. *Biomed Res Int.* 2015;2015:782420.
8. Campbell JP, Nudleman E, Yang J, et al. Handheld optical coherence tomography angiography and ultra-wide-field optical coherence tomography in retinopathy of prematurity. *JAMA Ophthalmol.* 2017;135 (9):977–981.
9. Chen X, Viehland C, Carrasco-Zevallos OM, et al. Microscope-integrated optical coherence tomography angiography in the operating room in young children with retinal vascular disease. *JAMA Ophthalmol.* 2017;135(5):483–486.
10. Chen X, Mangalesh S, Dandridge A, Tran-Viet D, Wallace DK, Freedman SF, Toth CA. Spectral-domain optical coherence tomography imaging of retinal vascular-avascular junction in infants with retinopathy of prematurity. *Ophthalmol Retina.* 2018;2(9):963–971.
11. Muni RH, Kohly RP, Charonis AC, Lee TC. Retinoschisis detected with handheld spectral-domain optical coherence tomography in neonates with advanced retinopathy of prematurity. *Arch Ophthalmol.* 2010;128(1):57–62. https://doi.org/10.1001/archophthalmol.2009.361.
12. Patel CK. Optical coherence tomography in the management of acute retinopathy of prematurity. *Am J Ophthalmol.* 2006;141(3):582–584.
13. Zepeda EM, Shariff A, Gillette TB, et al. Vitreous bands identified by handheld spectral-domain optical coherence tomography among premature infants. *JAMA Ophthalmol.* 2018;136(7):753–758.
14. Maldonado RS, Yuan E, Tran-Viet D, et al. Three-dimensional assessment of vascular and perivascular characteristics in subjects with retinopathy of prematurity. *Ophthalmology.* 2014;121(6):1289–1296.
15. Maldonado RS, O'Connell R, Ascher SB, et al. Spectral-domain optical coherence tomographic assessment of severity of cystoid macular edema in retinopathy of prematurity. *Arch Ophthalmol.* 2012;130(5):569–578.
16. Vinekar A, Avadhani K, Sivakumar M, et al. Understanding clinically undetected macular changes in early retinopathy of prematurity on spectral domain optical coherence tomography. *Invest Ophthalmol Vis Sci.* 2011;52:5183–5188.
17. Erol MK, Ozdemir O, Turgut Coban D, et al. Macular findings obtained by spectral domain optical coherence tomography in retinopathy of prematurity. *J Ophthalmol.* 2014;2014:468653.
18. Lee H, Proudlock FA, Gottlob I. Pediatric optical coherence tomography in clinical practice-recent progress. *Invest Opthalmol Vis Sci.* 2016;57(9):OCT69–79.
19. Chen X, Mangalesh S, Tran-Viet D, Freedman SF, Vajzovic L, Toth CA. Fluorescein angiographic characteristics of macular edema during infancy. *JAMA Ophthalmol.* 2018;136(5):538–542.
20. Falavarjani KG, Iafe NA, Velez FG, Schwartz SD, Sadda SR, Sarraf D, Tsui I. Optical coherence tomography angiography of the fovea in children born preterm. *Retina.* 2017;37(12):2289–2294
21. Chen YC, Chen YT, Chen SN. Foveal microvascular anomalies on optical coherence tomography angiography and the correlation with foveal thickness and visual acuity in retinopathy of prematurity. *Graefes Arch Clin Exp Ophthalmol.* 2019;257(1):23–30. https://doi.org/10.1007/s00417-018-4162-y.

CHAPTER 29

Familial Exudative Vitreoretinopathy and Norrie Disease

Cynthia A. Toth

Introduction

Familial exudative vitreoretinopathy (FEVR), Norrie disease, and other retinal diseases with a FEVR-like appearance are diseases of abnormal vascular development with peripheral retinal vascular nonperfusion as a predominant feature. FEVR is identified clinically by a pattern of incomplete and abnormal retinal vessel development in full-term infants. These mimic, in part, the vascular abnormalities of retinopathy of prematurity (ROP) but occur in full-term infants and can progress further. Assessment is centered on determining status of peripheral retinal vascularization, presence of neovascularization, and leakage and tractional effects. In Norrie disease (and osteoporosis pseudoglioma), retinal dysgenesis and fibrovascular tissue growth are severe.

The Brain Connection

Developmental delay, intellectual impairment, and psychosis may be prominent in Norrie disease. Developmental delay is also found in osteoporosis pseudoglioma and *KIF11*-related disease.

Common Clinical Features

Common clinical features include avascular retina, preretinal neovascularization, fibrovascular tissue (Fig. 29.1), macular pucker, exudates, retinal folds, retinal malformation/dysgenesis, partial or complete retinal detachment and vitreous hemorrhage, and other nonocular features discussed later.[1]

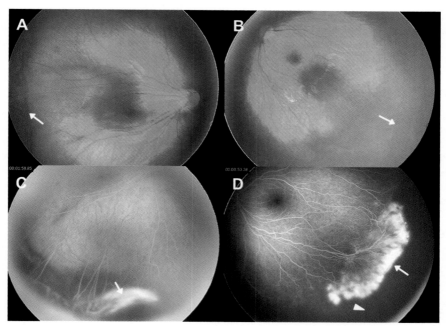

Fig. 29.1   A 5-year-old girl with familial exudative vitreoretinopathy (FEVR). (A, B) Color photos show temporal dragging of the macula and vessels in the right eye greater than the left, with peripheral neovascularization (white arrows) and a low fold in the right eye periphery. (C, D) Fluorescein angiography illustrates late leakage consistent with neovascularization in each eye (arrow) and peripheral non-perfusion (arrowhead).

Familial Exudative Vitreoretinopathy

FEVR mimics the vascular abnormalities of ROP but occurs in full-term infants or even in preterm ones, in whom the progression of disease does not follow a typical ROP time course. FEVR can progress in childhood and later. The disease may have highly variable severity, be asymmetric between eyes, and identified at birth or many years later. Most severe disease is often evident in early childhood. Differential diagnoses for these conditions include ROP (Chapter 28) and incontinentia pigmenti (Chapter 30).

FEVR may be of autosomal dominant, autosomal recessive, or X-linked inheritance, and genetic mutations have been found in NDP, LRP5, FZD4, and TSPAN12 (which affect the proteins in the Norrin/Frizzled4 signaling pathway), as well as in ZNF408 and KIF11.[2]

NDP gene–related retinopathies may range in severity from FEVR to Norrie disease, which involves very severe retinal malformation or dysgenesis and fibrovascular tractional detachment at birth or early in life. Patients with Norrie disease also often have progressive hearing loss and may have developmental delay in motor skills, intellectual disability, behavioral abnormalities, or psychosis.

LRP5 gene–related retinopathies may range in expression and severity from FEVR to FEVR with juvenile primary osteoporosis to osteoporosis pseudoglioma (severe retinal malformation with FEVR). These patients may have reduced bone density, fractures, and, less commonly, microphthalmia or developmental delay.

Patients with *KIF11* gene–related chorioretinopathies may also have microcephaly, lymphedema, and intellectual disability. Other rare systemic conditions with vascular complications may also present with retinal findings comparable with those in FEVR: dyskeratosis congenita, a telomere biology disorder, and FEVR-type or Coats-type retinopathy. An infant with hemophagocytic lymphohistiocytosis and hypercoagulable state demonstrated FEVR and OCT revealed tractional retinal schisis and detachment.[3]

OCT Features

Optical coherence tomography (OCT) reveals many aspects of disease that may not be fully appreciated on conventional clinical examination. OCT findings vary from mild disease, which may include early stages prior to neovascularization, to more severe disease, where neovascularization, retinal malformation, and tractional elevation with schisis and detachment are all more severe.[4] These are detailed in the following sections. Posttreatment monitoring includes assessment of persistence, progression or resolution of the OCT features, especially retinal folds, epiretinal membrane, subretinal fluid, exudates, and schisis (Fig. 29.2).[1,4]

OCT ANGIOGRAPHY

OCT angiography (OCTA) provides a unique view into perfusion defects, abnormal vascular density, vascular layer abnormalities, and deviations in the foveal avascular zone, some of which cannot be determined from fluorescein angiography.[5]

OPTIC NERVE HEAD

Deformation of the optic nerve caused by vitreous or retinal traction or both may be mild or severe with herniation of the nerve head, and may progress over months to years. (Fig. 29.3).[6]

EPIRETINAL PROLIFERATION AND ORGANIZED POSTERIOR HYALOID

Cellular infiltration and elevation/traction of the posterior hyaloid may be evident across the retina and at the optic nerve head and may be associated with lamellar or full thickness macular hole.

RETINAL LAYER THINNING AND RETINAL THINNING

As with other retinal vascular diseases, widespread thinning of the retina may be evident with loss of the foveal pit. This may also be seen in incontinentia pigmenti (see Chapter 30).

NEOVASCULARIZATION

Fronds of preretinal neovascularization at and behind the vascular–avascular junction are characteristic. The effects of vitreous traction are often seen elevating the retina and split inner retinal layers. In regressed neovascularization, neovascular structures may lift away from the retina and appear as sheets or bands, whereas retinal deformation from vitreous traction may increase or decrease (Fig. 29.4).

MACULAR CYSTOID SPACES

These occur most commonly in the inner nuclear layer, outer plexiform layer, and Henle fiber layer and may be caused by traction or fluid leakage or both. These are often associated with flattened foveal pit or diffuse or focal elevation of the central macula. Central foveal thickness provides a measure of severity of edema (see Fig. 29.2).

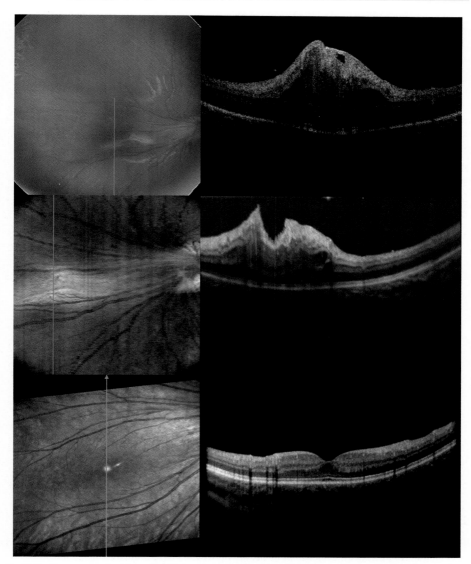

Fig. 29.2 The same patient from Fig. 29.1 underwent bilateral peripheral laser photocoagulation, and subsequently a retinal fold in the right eye developed, distorting the fovea and affecting visual acuity, which dropped to 20/80. (A) Color photo shows membrane and dragging. Optical coherence tomography (OCT) demonstrates the grossly thickened retina with posterior hyaloid/epiretinal membrane bridging from superior to inferior arcades with a retinal fold and intraretinal cystoid spaces. (B) At the completion of pars plana vitrectomy with membrane/hyaloid release, handheld OCT reveals release of the bridging traction, although intraretinal cystoid spaces and thickening persist. (C) Five years after surgery, the macular architecture and foveal contour appear preserved, and visual acuity is 20/30.

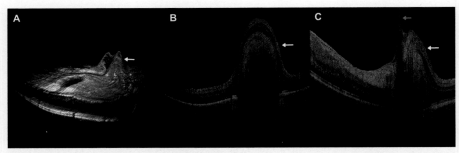

Fig. 29.3   Elevation of optic nerve head (white arrows) from axial vitreous traction in familial exudative vitreoretinopathy (FEVR). In an 11-month-old boy with FEVR, the axial elevation is readily apparent on three-dimensional (A) and cross-sectional (B) optical coherence tomography (OCT) scans. OCT of the optic nerve from a 5-year-old girl with FEVR demonstrates vitreopapillary attachment (red arrow) with tractional deformation and elevation of the optic nerve head.

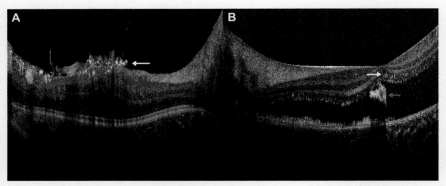

Fig. 29.4   Optical coherence tomography (OCT) image of the location of exudates and fluid in familial exudative vitreoretinopathy (FEVR). (A) In a 6-month-old boy, on OCT imaging, exudates are visible within preretinal fibrovascular tissue over and within the inner macula and appear as hyperreflective foci (white arrow) with posterior shadowing. Larger hyperreflective exudates are visible in the inner retina temporal to the macula. (B) Hyperreflective exudates are visible in the outer nuclear layer (white arrow) and in the subretinal space (red arrow) along the undersurface of the retina and heaped over the retinal pigment epithelium in a 2-year-old boy with FEVR.

EXUDATES

Preretinal, intraretinal, and subretinal exudates may be visible as hyperreflective foci on OCT and may be found in eyes with evidence of or history of neovascularization (see Fig. 29.4).[7]

TRACTIONAL RETINAL SCHISIS AND RETINAL DETACHMENT

Vitreoretinal traction may produce retinal schisis and retinal detachment are distinguished by photoreceptor layer presence over the retinal pigment epithelium (RPE) in schisis and subretinal fluid in detachment. The posterior extent of schisis or detachment can be identified with OCT. OCT enables a clear distinction between presence or absence of retinal detachment at the fovea (Fig. 29.5). There may be difficulties in imaging when there is a high or steep detachment because of the shallow depth of focus of OCT. There is often greater difficulty in imaging the neovascular lesions and areas with traction in FEVR because of the peripheral location of the disease process, overlying vitreous hemorrhage, and severe retinal elevation and malformation.

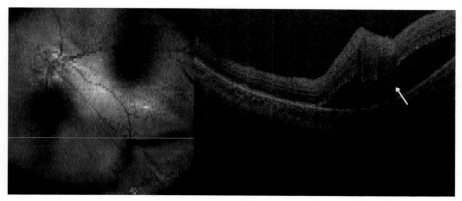

Fig. 29.5 Tractional retinal detachment in a 3-year-old boy with Norrie disease. Cross-sectional optical coherence tomography (OCT) image demonstrates presence of subretinal fluid (white arrow).

RETINAL FOLDS

The "taco fold" may occur with epiretinal membranes, and high fold with peripheral traction, or combinations of malformation and severe folds (Fig. 29.6).

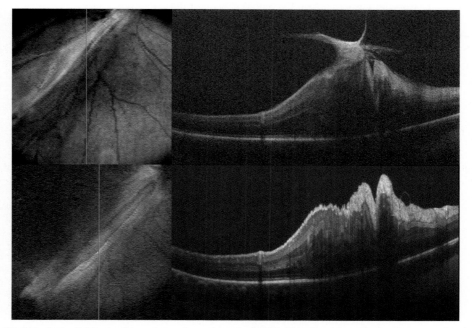

Fig. 29.6 Retinal fold in familial exudative vitreoretinopathy (FEVR). (A) En face infrared (left) and cross-sectional optical coherence tomography (OCT) image (right) shows a thick fibrotic membrane (red arrow) with traction and a retinal fold (white arrow) in the right eye of a 4-year-old boy with FEVR. The green line on the left infrared image corresponds to the horizontal OCT section on the right. (B) After the traction is surgically released, handheld OCT reveals thickened retinal structures with intact inner retinal layers.

LASER SCARS

The retina is hyperreflective and thickened immediately after laser treatment and thinned at sites of the older laser scar.

Ancillary Testing

Fluorescein angiography is an integral test used to evaluate the extent of peripheral nonperfusion (in contrast to the limited peripheral capture of current OCTA systems), active neovascularization with leakage, vascular abnormalities, and macular edema. Wide-field angiography may be especially useful for the examination of patients and other family members. Fundus autofluorescence does not provide unique information; however, hypoautofluorescence would be found in areas of retinal detachment, edema, or retinal folds or absent after laser treatment. Ultrasonography provides lower-resolution imaging of vitreoretinal traction and schisis or detachment with a useful overview across the eye.

Treatment

Management centers on examination of the eyes of infants at risk, intervening to prevent neovascular complications and evaluation for the systemic associations described previously. Treatment includes laser treatment of the avascular areas of the retina and/or injection of antivascular endothelial growth factor (anti-VEGF) agents into the vitreous cavity (a treatment not cleared by the U.S. Food and Drug Administration). Vitreoretinal surgery may be applied in cases of tractional retinal detachment, especially when the central retina is at risk.

References

1. Kashani AH, Brown KT, Chang E, Drenser KA, Capone A, Trese MT. Diversity of retinal vascular anomalies in patients with familial exudative vitreoretinopathy. *Ophthalmology*. 2014;121(11):2220–2227.
2. Seo SH, Yu YS, Park SW, et al. Molecular characterization of FZD4, LRP5, and TSPAN12 in familial exudative vitreoretinopathy. *Invest Ophthalmol Vis Sci*. 2015;56(9):5143–5151.
3. Finn AP, Roehrs P, Grace SF, Vajzovic L. Ischemic retinal vascular disease in an infant with hemophagocytic lymphohistiocytosis. *JAMA Ophthalmol*. November 1, 2017;135(11):1277–1279.
4. Yonekawa Y, Thomas BJ, Drenser KA, Trese MT, Capone Jr A. Familial exudative vitreoretinopathy: spectral-domain optical coherence tomography of the vitreoretinal interface, retina, and choroid. *Ophthalmology*. 2015;122(11):2270–2277.
5. Chen X, Viehland C, Carrasco-Zevallos OM, et al. Microscope-integrated optical coherence tomography angiography in the operating room in young children with retinal vascular disease. *JAMA Ophthalmol*. May 1, 2017;135(5):483–486.
6. Lee J, El-Dairi MA, Tran-Viet D, et al. Longitudinal changes in the optic nerve head and retina over time in very young children with familial exudative vitreoretinopathy. *Retina November*. 2017;22 [Epub ahead of print].
7. Day S, Maldonado RS, Toth CA. Preretinal and intraretinal exudates in familial exudative vitreoretinopathy. *Retina*. 2011;31(1):190–191.

Incontinentia Pigmenti

Cynthia A. Toth

Introduction

Incontinentia pigmenti (*IKBKG/NEMO* gene–related retinopathy, Bloch-Sulzberger syndrome) is an X-linked dominant disorder characterized by abnormalities of the skin, teeth, nails, hair, retina, and central nervous system (CNS) and usually lethal before birth in males. Ocular disease severity depends on the extent of abnormal retinal vascularization, presence of neovascularization, and secondary complications.

The Brain Connection

Neurologic changes are found in up to 30% and range from early childhood encephalopathy, stroke or seizures in infancy, microcephaly, to intellectual disability. Some have suggested that the brain abnormalities occurred in children with retinal findings.

Clinical Features

Ocular disease is found in 20% and is typically of the retina and includes avascular retina, preretinal neovascularization, fibrovascular tissue, macular pucker, exudates, retinal folds, retinal malformation/dysgenesis, partial or complete retinal detachment, and vitreous hemorrhage (Fig. 30.1). Optic nerve atrophy or occipital infarct may rarely occur. Ocular features are generally unilateral or asymmetric, and this may relate to cells where the mutant X chromosome is inactivated, thus being more viable. Early erythematous, blistering skin lesions are followed by verrucous patches, then by pigmentation, and finally by depigmented skin lesions following the Blaschko lines. Abnormalities of teeth, nails, and hair may also occur. Neurologic effects are described previously.

OCT Features

Optical coherence tomography (OCT) imaging reveals many aspects of disease that may not be fully appreciated on conventional clinical examination. OCT findings vary from mild disease, which may

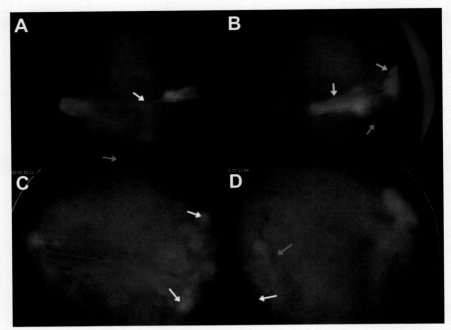

Fig. 30.1 An 11-year-old girl with incontinentia pigmenti presented with retinal fold and temporal dragging in the left eye. (A) Color photo shows retinal fold *(white arrow)*, temporal dragging of the vessels and macula, and inferior vitreous hemorrhage *(red arrow)*. (B) Color photo of the temporal periphery demonstrates subretinal exudates *(yellow arrow)*, tractional membranes with retinal detachment *(green arrow)*, and neovascular tufts with hemorrhage *(red arrow)*. (C) Fluorescein angiography shows late leakage from neovascular tufts *(white arrows)* in the temporal periphery. (D) Fluorescein angiography also illustrates areas of nonperfusion *(white arrow)* and blockage from hemorrhage *(red arrow)* in the nasal periphery.

include retinal thinning and avascularity that may extend into the macula, to more severe disease, where neovascularization and tractional elevation with schisis and detachment are all more severe.[1-3] Loss of inner retinal layers and patchy loss of the outer plexiform layer have been observed in children. OCT features may be similar to those in familial exudative vitreoretinopathy (FEVR), as described in Chapter 29. OCT angiography (OCTA) of the macula reveals areas of macular flow loss and decrease in vascular density in superficial and deep plexuses along with anastomoses. Macular vascular abnormalities do not necessarily match the severity of those in the periphery.[3] Posttreatment OCT monitoring includes assessment of persistence, progression, or resolution of OCT features, such as retinal folds, epiretinal membrane, subretinal fluid, exudates, and schisis (Fig. 30.2).

Macular Cystoid Spaces

These are less common in incontinentia pigmenti but can occur in the inner nuclear layer, outer plexiform layer, and Henle fiber layer and may be caused by traction, fluid leakage, or both. These may be associated with flattened foveal pit or diffuse or focal elevation of the central macula. Central foveal thickness provides a measure of severity of edema (see Fig. 30.2).

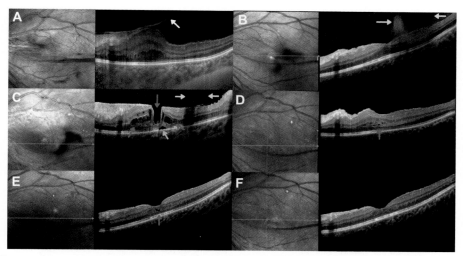

Fig. 30.2 Horizontal spectral-domain optical coherence tomography (SD-OCT) line scans across the fovea for the same patient in Fig. 30.1. (A) On presentation, there was a thick epiretinal membrane *(white arrow)* with traction, elevation, and thickening of the underlying retina. Visual acuity was 20/200. (B) Ten months after treatment of peripheral neovascularization and nonperfusion with laser photocoagulation, the posterior hyaloid and the epiretinal membrane had become detached, causing flattening of the retina and restoration of the foveal contour. Note the posterior shadowing caused by the detached membrane floating in the vitreous *(yellow arrows)*. Visual acuity improved to 20/60. (C) Five months later, the child returned to clinic with decline in vision (20/200), and there was a new lamellar hole *(red arrow)* with surrounding intraretinal cystoid spaces *(blue arrow)* and subretinal fluid *(light blue arrow)*. There was again posterior shadowing from the detached membrane in the vitreous *(yellow arrows)*. (D) One month after vitreoretinal surgery with pars plana vitrectomy, membrane peel, and fluid air exchange, the lamellar hole and subretinal fluid resolved, although some intraretinal cystoid spaces remained *(blue arrow)*. (E) Eight months after vitreoretinal surgery, the intraretinal cystoid spaces continued to improve *(blue arrow)*, and there was restoration of normal foveal contour. Visual acuity was 20/100. (F) At the most recent follow-up (3 years postoperatively), there were no remaining intraretinal cystoid spaces, and visual acuity was 20/60.

Retinal Layers and Retinal Thinning

There may be profound loss of the inner retinal layers and some loss of the outer retinal layer in the posterior pole, which may reflect transient retinal vascular impairment in infancy and the mosaicism of this disease expression in cells. Widespread thinning of the retina may also be evident (Fig. 30.3).

Other Imaging

Fluorescein angiography is an integral test used to evaluate the extent of retinal nonperfusion, active neovascularization with leakage, vascular abnormalities, and macular edema. Ultrasonography provides lower-resolution imaging of vitreoretinal traction and schisis or detachment, with a useful overview across the eye.

Treatment

Ocular management centers on early assessment of infants at risk through eye examination soon after birth, typically prior to leaving the hospital. Intervention is then focused on preventing ocular neovascular complications. Treatment includes laser treatment of the avascular areas of the retina

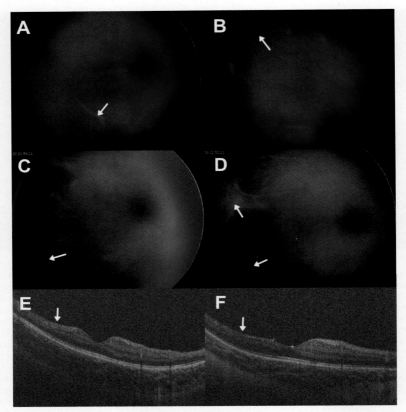

Fig. 30.3 A 7-month-old girl with incontinentia pigmenti presented with temporal vessel dragging in the right eye. (A, B) Color photos demonstrate areas of focal tractional retinal detachment temporally *(white arrows)*. (C, D) Fluorescein angiograms reveal temporal nonperfusion *(white arrows)* and late leakage from neovascularization *(red arrow)*. (E) Vertical spectral-domain optical coherence tomography (SD-OCT) across the fovea demonstrates inner retinal thinning in the inferior macula *(white arrow)*. (F) Horizontal SD-OCT across the fovea shows inner retinal thinning in the temporal macula *(white arrow)*.

and/or injection of anti–vascular endothelial growth factor (anti-VEGF) agents into the vitreous cavity (a treatment not cleared by the U.S. Food and Drug Administration [FDA]). Vitreoretinal surgery may be applied in cases of tractional retinal detachment, especially when the central retina is at risk.

References

1. Basilius J, Young MP, Michaelis TC, Hobbs R, Jenkins G, Hartnett ME. Structural abnormalities of the inner macula in incontinentia pigmenti. *JAMA Ophthalmol.* 2015;133(9):1067–1072.
2. Mangalesh S, Chen X, Tran-Viet D, Viehland C, Freedman SF, Toth CA. Assessment of the retinal structure in children with incontinentia pigmenti. *Retina.* 2017;37(8):1568–1574.
3. Liu TYA, Han IC, Goldberg MF, Linz MO, Chen CJ, Scott AW. Multimodal retinal imaging in incontinentia pigmenti including optical coherence tomography angiography: findings from an older cohort with mild phenotype. *JAMA Ophthalmol.* 2018;136:467–472.

CHAPTER 31

Coats Disease and Coats Plus Syndrome

Sally S. Ong ■ Cynthia A. Toth

Summary

Coats disease, or Leber multiple miliary aneurysm disease, is characterized by idiopathic retinal vascular telangiectasias that can occur with retinal exudates and exudative retinal detachments.[1-3] It is a rare, sporadic, and nonhereditary condition. It is usually unilateral and predominantly affects males in their first two decades of life. An adult form occurs in older patients.[4] Depending on the severity of disease, vision can range from being unaffected to being extremely limited. The overwhelming majority of patients with Coats disease are otherwise in good health. In rare cases, Coats disease has been associated with systemic disorders, such as facioscapulohumeral muscular dystrophy, a genetic disorder that is characterized by muscle weakness and wasting.

The Brain Connection

Patients with Coats plus syndrome (mutations in *CTC1*) also have cerebral microangiopathy with brain cysts, intracranial calcifications, leukodystrophy, gastrointestinal vascular ectasias with risk of bleeding, and osteopenia.

Clinical Features

Coats disease has been classified into stages by several groups. The Shields classification includes five stages of disease.[4] Stage 1 is defined by retinal telangiectasias only; stage 2 by the presence of telangiectasias and exudates (2A: extrafoveal exudates and 2B: foveal exudates); stage 3 by retinal detachment without glaucoma (3A: subtotal and 3B: total), with subtotal detachment distinguished

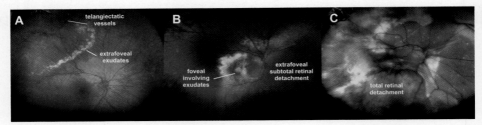

Fig. 31.1   (A) Extrafoveal exudates with telangiectatic vessels in a 6-year-old boy with stage 2A disease. (B) Foveal exudates and extrafoveal subtotal retinal detachment in a 13-year-old boy with stage 3A1 disease. (C) Exudates and total retinal detachment in a 16-year-old girl with stage 3B disease.

by the presence (3A2) or the absence (3A1) of foveal involvement; stage 4 by total retinal detachment with glaucoma; and stage 5 by advanced end-stage disease[4] (Fig. 31.1). In late-stage disease, it is important to differentiate Coats disease from retinoblastoma, von Hippel-Lindau syndrome, late-stage retinopathy of prematurity (ROP), familial exudative vitreoretinopathy, and incontinentia pigmenti (IP). The presence of Coats disease has been reported in less than 5% of eyes with retinitis pigmentosa.

OCT Features

OCT imaging is especially useful in distinguishing the presence or absence of foveal involvement with subretinal fluid, exudates, or fibrosis.

Vascular Lesions

Aneurysmal dilatations can be visualized on OCT as enlarged circular structures that span from the ganglion cell layer to the outer retina, cast a shadow posteriorly, and may deform the retina, which can then bulge upward into the vitreous cavity (Fig. 31.2A). These lesions are surrounded by exudates and occasionally by fluid.

Intraretinal Cystoid Spaces

Cystoid hyporeflective spaces representing intraretinal fluid are also seen in some cases and are often associated with severe intraretinal exudation. The cystoid spaces are seen in the outer and inner nuclear layers and may cover broad regions (see Fig. 31.2B). Macular intraretinal fluid can occur in the absence of macular telangiectasia, aneurysms, and leakage and likely originate from peripheral vascular anomalies.

Exudates and Crystals

Both intraretinal and subretinal exudates are common, appearing as bright hyperreflective opacities that can cast a shadow and obscure details of underlying retina. Intraretinal exudates accumulate predominantly in the Henle fiber layer and outer plexiform layer but are also observed in the outer nuclear layer, inner nuclear layer, inner plexiform layer, ganglion cell layer, and nerve fiber layer. Well-defined linear hyperreflective structures may also be found in subretinal fluid and appear to correspond to cholesterol crystals.

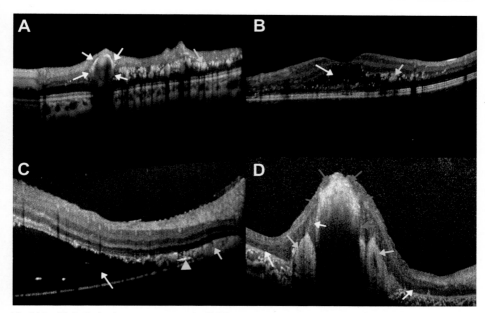

Fig. 31.2   (A) Optical coherence tomography (OCT) image of a vascular lesion in an 18-year-old male patient demonstrates a large circular structure *(white arrows)* representing a dilated vessel surrounded by exudates *(yellow arrow)*. The aneurysm creates a bulging elevation of the retina, and the central blood-filled lesion shadows the underlying retina, retinal pigment epithelium (RPE), and choroid. (B) OCT in a 4-year-old boy shows intraretinal cystoid spaces in both the inner and outer nuclear layers *(white arrows)* and exudates in the outer plexiform and outer nuclear layers *(yellow arrow)*. (C) OCT in a 17-year-old male patient demonstrates subretinal fluid *(white arrow)* with hyperreflective crystals *(yellow arrowhead)* as well as exudates *(yellow arrow)* in the sub-retinal space. (D) OCT image of a fibrotic nodule *(red arrows)* in a 6-year-old boy. The nodule is protruding through all layers of the neurosensory retina, and there is atrophy of the outer retinal layers overlying and adjacent to the nodule *(white arrows)*. There are also subretinal exudates *(yellow arrow)* around the nodule.

Retinal Detachment

Subretinal fluid is seen in eyes with more advanced disease (see Fig. 31.2C).

Retinal Layers and Retinal Thinning

Outer retinal atrophy involving the outer nuclear layer, ellipsoid zone, and retinal pigment epithelium (RPE) has been observed in eyes after prolonged subretinal exudation and fluid. Diffuse retinal thinning is seen overlying fibrotic nodules, and there may even be a full-thickness macular hole.

Fibrotic Nodule

A subretinal nodule (also referred to as *macular fibrosis*) may be seen at the first examination or may develop later. A nodule appears as heterogeneously hyperreflective material in the subretinal/sub-RPE space with overlying atrophic retina (see Fig. 31.2D). The pathophysiology of nodule formation is thought to be associated with chronic exudation, inflammation, retinal vascular anastomoses, or neovascularization. Nodules typically persist despite treatment, and when present within the fovea they portend a poor visual prognosis.

After Treatment

Intra- and subretinal exudates and fluid often resolve after treatment of vascular abnormalities, and the retinal appearance on OCT after treatment can be unremarkable, with intact layers and minimal or no retinal thinning (Fig. 31.3A–B). When exudation and fluid accumulation have been severe, outer retinal atrophy and thinning may be observed after treatment with resolution of exudates (see Fig. 31.3C–D).

Ancillary Testing

Conventional retinal photography, wide-field imaging, and fluorescein angiography can be helpful in diagnosing the disease and monitoring response to treatment. Photography may document the extent of detachment, peripheral versus macular exudates, and vascular abnormalities, with wide-field photography especially being useful for documenting these in the peripheral retina. Fluorescein angiography reveals characteristic dilated bulblike aneurysms and telangiectatic vessels, as well as retinal nonperfusion.[5] In late frames, aneurysmal vascular lesions and neovascular complexes also show leakage (Fig. 31.4A). Ultrasonography provides lower-resolution imaging of retinal detachment and highly reflective cholesterol foci moving within the subretinal fluid (see Fig. 31.4B).

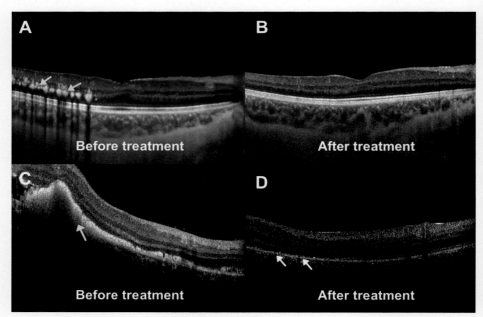

Fig. 31.3 (A) In an 18-year-old male patient with Coats disease, before treatment, optical coherence tomography (OCT) demonstrates intraretinal exudates *(yellow arrows)*. (B) After treatment, OCT demonstrates resolution of exudates and subretinal fluid, as well as preserved retinal architecture. (C) In a 4-year-old boy with Coats disease, before treatment, thick subretinal exudates *(yellow arrow)* and subretinal fluid *(blue arrow)* were observed. (D) After treatment, OCT demonstrates resolution of exudates and subretinal fluid but new atrophy of ellipsoid zone and thinning of retinal pigment epithelium and outer nuclear layer *(white arrows)*.

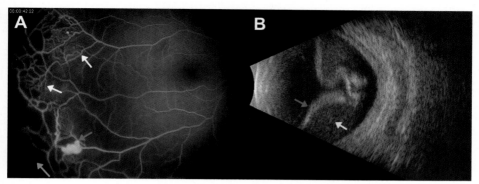

Fig. 31.4 (A) In a 2-year-old boy with Coats disease, telangiectatic vessels *(white arrows)*, aneurysmal dilatation *(red arrow)*, and areas of peripheral nonperfusion *(green arrow)* are observed on fluorescein angiography. (B) Ultrasonography in a 1-year-old boy with Coats disease shows total retinal detachment *(blue arrow)* with highly reflective cholesterol deposits *(white arrow)* in the subretinal fluid.

Treatment

Conventionally, the goal of treatment is to eliminate exudation by destruction of anomalous retinal vessels. Laser photocoagulation is applied to telangiectatic vessels in the early stages of the disease. When severe exudation or subretinal fluid prevents laser uptake, cryotherapy is used to ablate abnormal blood vessels. In advanced disease, when there is extensive retinal detachment, cryotherapy may not be able to ablate the retinal vascular lesions in the presence of bullous subretinal fluid. These cases are treated with intravitreal triamcinolone or anti–vascular endothelial growth factor (VEGF) injections or with vitreoretinal surgical approaches, such as vitrectomy, scleral buckling, or external subretinal fluid drainage. Although visual prognosis is poor in advanced disease, failure to treat these patients may result in progression to secondary angle closure or neovascular glaucoma, resulting in a blind and painful eye requiring enucleation.

References

1. Coats G. Forms of retinal disease with massive exudation. *R Lond Ophthalmic Hosp Rep.* 1908;17:440–525.
2. Leber T. Ueber eine durch Vorkommen multipler Miliar aneurysmen charakterisierte Form von Retinal degeneration. *Von Graefe's Arch Ophthalmol.* 1912;81:1–14.
3. Reese AB. Telangiectasis of the retina and Coats' disease. *Am J Ophthalmol.* 1956;42(1):1–8.
4. Shields JA, Shields CL, Honavar SG, Demirci H, Cater J. Classification and management of Coats disease: the 2000 Proctor Lecture. *Am J Ophthalmol.* 2001;131(5):572–583.
5. Otani T, Yamaguchi Y, Kishi S. Serous macular detachment secondary to distant retinal vascular disorders. *Retina.* 2004;24(5):758–762.

CHAPTER 32

Sickle Cell Retinopathy

Marguerite O. Linz ■ Adrienne W. Scott

Summary

Although children with sickle cell disease (SCD) are generally visually asymptomatic, associated changes in retinal vasculature are prevalent in this population. Proliferative sickle cell retinopathy (PSR) is the most commonly observed cause of vision loss in SCD. The incidence and prevalence of PSR increases with age of patient and disease duration, and thus is not typically observed in the pediatric population. PSR may be observed in all genotypes of patients with SCD, but PSR risk is typically higher in hemoglobin SC (HbSC) and hemoglobin S–β-thalassemia than in homozygous hemoglobin SS (HbSS) disease (also called sickle cell anemia).

The Brain Connection

Children with SCD are prone to a variety of neurologic complications, including stroke, silent cerebral infarcts, transient ischemic attack, intracranial blood flow abnormalities, headaches, reduced cognitive function, acute coma, and seizures,[1] as well as "soft neurologic signs," such as slight motor impairments of the upper and lower limbs,[2] among other manifestations.

Clinical Features

Common sequelae of nonproliferative sickle cell retinopathy include salmon patch retinal hemorrhages, refractile or iridescent spots, and black sunburst lesions (Figs. 32.1 and 32.2), as well as retinal vascular changes, such as tortuosity of retinal vessels, areas of peripheral vascular dropout (see Fig. 32.2), retinal vascular occlusions, or arteriovenous anastomoses. Clinicians should carefully monitor patients with SCD for signs of PSR, such as sea fan neovascularization, vitreous hemorrhage, and tractional or tractional–rhegmatogenous retinal detachment.

OCT Features

The most notable OCT feature in sickle cell retinopathy regardless of SCD genotype is macular thinning (Fig. 32.3). Focal macular thinning is most characteristically noted in the

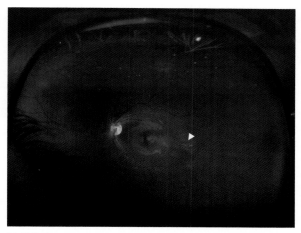

Fig. 32.1   Ultrawide-field (UWF) color fundus photograph of the left eye of a 10-year-old female with Hemoglobin SS sickle cell disease shows black sunburst *(arrow)*.

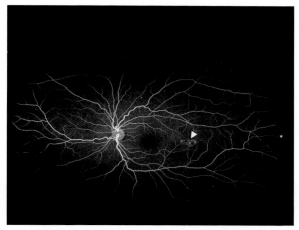

Fig. 32.2   Ultrawide-field (UWF) fluorescein angiography (FA; corresponding to Fig. 31.1) image shows vessel tortuosity, a sunburst lesion *(arrow)*, and peripheral ischemia in the nasal and temporal regions.

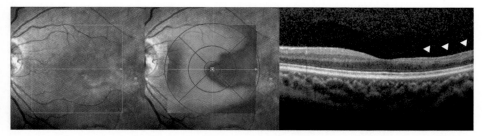

Fig. 32.3   Macular spectral-domain optical coherence tomography (SD-OCT) (corresponding to the patient's macula in Figs. 32.1 and 32.2) B scan shows temporal macular thinning involving the central subfield *(arrows, far right)*. The thickness map *(middle)* and infrared image *(right)* are also shown.

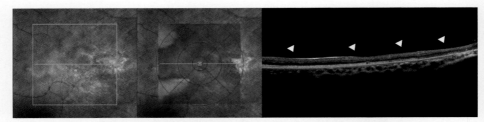

Fig. 32.4 ETDRS Field 3 (SD-OCT) (corresponding to Fig. 32.3) image shows extent of temporal thinning (*arrows*). The thickness map (*left*) and infrared image (*middle*) are also shown.

temporal outer subfields, a known watershed zone for the macular vasculature (Early Treatment Diabetic Retinopathy Study (ETDRS) Field 3) (Fig. 32.4). Patients with SCD also have decreased overall macular thickness measurements compared with controls.[3] This retinal thinning may be more common in the HbSS genotype,[3,4] and retinal thickness in SCD decreases with increasing age.[3] One hypothesis for this finding is that repetitive vascular occlusions within the macular microvasculature may lead to chronic ischemia and tissue loss over time.[3,5] The degree of macular thinning can be variable and does not necessarily correlate with the stage of sickle cell retinopathy.[3] Although there does not appear to be an association with decreased distance visual acuity, macular thinning on OCT has been associated with decreased retinal sensitivity in adult patients with SCD.[6] OCT angiography (OCTA) in individuals with SCD may show pathologic decreased vascular flow loss (the absence of flow or decreased vessel density relative to reported normative data) in the superficial plexus, deep plexus, or both (Figs. 32.5 and 32.6). These areas of vascular flow loss may be more frequently observed in the deep retinal plexus in adult patients with SCD.[7,8] The correlation between OCT thinning and loss of retinal vascular flow on OCTA and peripheral retinal nonperfusion on FA has been described.[8,9] There may be an association between subclinical decline in distance visual acuity and decreased vascular flow measured on OCTA in patients with SCD.[8] Further prospective studies of a larger cohort of patients are necessary to determine the visual consequences of the prognostic implications of these imaging findings.

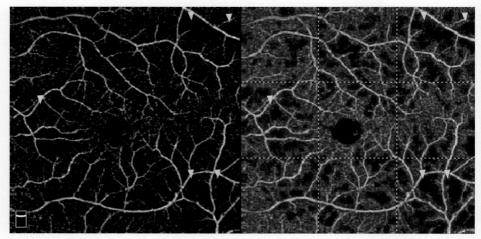

Fig. 32.5 A 6 × 6 mm optical coherence tomography angiography (OCTA) (corresponding to Fig. 32.3) image shows areas of loss of macular flow (*arrows*) in the superficial plexus (*arrows*). Areas of decreased macular vascular density are most easily noted on the density map (*right*) in blue.

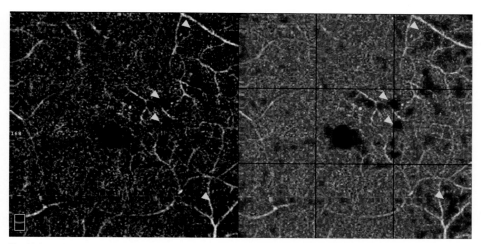

Fig. 32.6 A 6 × 6 mm optical coherence tomography angiography (OCTA) (corresponding to Fig. 32.3) image shows regions of loss of macular flow (*arrows*) in the deep plexus. Areas of decreased macular vascular density are most easily noted on the density map (*right*) in blue.

Ancillary Testing

FA is the most commonly utilized ancillary test for evaluating patients with SCD to identify neo-vascularization and to assess retinal perfusion. FA is typically reserved for older pediatric patients because of the invasive nature of the test and the low prevalence of proliferative disease in younger patients. Fundus photography may be useful in documenting the presence of sickle cell retinopathy and monitoring the retinopathy and peripheral retinal ischemia for progression over time. Ultrawide-field (UWF) fundus imaging is particularly useful in the evaluation of sickle cell retinopathy because peripheral retinal pathology is commonly observed. Pathology within the far peripheral retina would be difficult to capture on most OCT imaging systems, although this may improve with wide-field OCT imaging in the future.

Treatment

Current guidelines based on expert consensus recommend retinopathy surveillance examinations every 1 to 2 years in children with SCD starting at age 10 years.[10] Typically, no treatment is required for nonproliferative sickle cell retinopathy. If small areas of retinal neovascularization occur, observation and monitoring may be considered, given the known tendency for spontaneous regression, or autoinfarction, in up to 32% to 60% of sea fan neovascular lesions, resulting in a fibrotic appearance that often remains stable over time.[11,12] Treatment regimens for PSR have not been standardized. However, when neovascular lesions enlarge, increase in number, or result in progressive retinal traction or vitreous hemorrhage, retinal scatter laser photocoagulation treatment is typically considered. Based on studies which have identified retinal location of proangiogenic factors such as hypoxia-inducible growth factor-1 alpha (HIF-1α) and vascular endothelial growth factor (VEGF) in eyes with PSR, application of sectoral or circumferential scatter laser photocoagulation to areas of ischemic retina is recommended. Laser should be centrally applied at the border of ischemic and non-ischemic retina, and broadly applied peripheral to this border.[13] Scatter laser may also be applied as a barricade surrounding sea fan neovascular complexes.[13]

Intravitreal anti-VEGF injection may also be considered as adjunctive therapy to retinal laser photocoagulation to achieve regression of active sea fan neovascular lesions.[14] Pars plana vitrectomy may be indicated for nonclearing vitreous hemorrhage and in cases of tractional and/or tractional–rhegmatogenous retinal detachment. It is as yet unclear which, if any, systemic associations, such as hemoglobin levels and frequency of occlusive pain crises, and systemic therapies, such as hydroxyurea and regular exchange transfusions, are correlated with the degree or stage of sickle cell retinopathy. In addition to treatment compliance and regular hematology and ophthalmology evaluations, individuals with SCD should avoid dehydration, overexertion, high altitudes, smoking, temperature extremes, stress, and infection.[15]

References

1. Kirkham FJ. Therapy insight: stroke risk and its management in patients with sickle cell disease. *Nat Clin Pract Neurol.* 2007;3:264–278.
2. Mercuri E, Faundez JC, Roberts I, et al. Neurological 'soft' signs may identify children with sickle cell disease who are at risk for stroke. *Eur J Pediatr.* 1995;154(2):150–156.
3. Lim JI, Cao D. Analysis of retinal thinning using spectral-domain optical coherence tomography imaging of sickle cell retinopathy eyes compared to age- and race-matched control eyes. *Am J Ophthalmol.* 2018;192:229–238. https://doi.org/10.1016/j.ajo.2018.03.013 S0002-9394.
4. Lim WS, Magan T, Mahroo OA, Hysi PG, Helou J, Mohamed MD. Retinal thickness measurements in sickle cell patients with HbSS and HbSC genotype. *Can J Ophthalmol.* 2018;53(4):420–424. https://doi.org/10.1016/j.jcjo.2017.10.006.
5. Stevens TS, Busse B, Lee CB, Woolf MB, Galinos SO, Goldberg MF. Sickling hemoglobinopathies: macular and perimacular vascular abnormalities. *Arch Ophthalmol.* 1974;92(6):455–463.
6. Chow CC, Genead MA, Anastasakis A, Chau FY, Fishman GA, Lim JI. Structural and functional correlation in sickle cell retinopathy using spectral-domain optical coherence tomography and scanning laser ophthalmoscope microperimetry. *Am J Ophthalmol.* 2011;152(4):704–711.
7. Han IC, Tadarati M, Scott AW. Macular vascular abnormalities identified by optical coherence tomographic angiography in patients with sickle cell disease. *JAMA Ophthalmol.* 2015;133(11):1337–1340.
8. Han IC, Tadarati M, Pacheco KD, Scott AW. Evaluation of macular vascular abnormalities identified by optical coherence tomography angiography in sickle cell disease. *Am J Ophthalmol.* 2017;177:90–99.
9. Han IC, Linz MO, Liu TYA, Zhang AY, Tian J, Scott AW. Correlation of ultra-widefield fluorescein angiography and OCT angiography in sickle cell retinopathy. *Ophthalmol Retina.* 2018;2(6):599–605.
10. Yawn BP, Buchanan GR, Afenyi-Annan AN, et al. Management of sickle cell disease: summary of the 2014 evidence-based report by expert panel members. *JAMA.* 2014;312(10):1033–1048.
11. Downes SM, Hambleton IR, Chuang EL, Lois N, Serjeant GR, Bird AC. Incidence and natural history of proliferative sickle cell retinopathy: observations from a cohort study. *Ophthalmology.* 2005;112 (11):1869–1875.
12. Condon PI, Serjeant GR. Behaviour of untreated proliferative sickle retinopathy. *Br J Ophthalmol.* 1980;64:404–411.
13. Rodrigues M, Kashiwabuchi F, Deshpande M, et al. Expression pattern of HIF-1α and VEGF supports circumferential application of scatter laser for proliferative sickle retinopathy. *Invest Ophthalmol Vis Sci.* 2016;57(15):6739–6746.
14. Cai CX, Linz MO, Scott AW. Intravitreal bevacizumab for proliferative sickle retinopathy: a case series. *J Vitreoretin Dis.* 2018;2(1):32–38.
15. National Health Service. *Sickle cell disease.* The National Health Service UK website. Updated May 15, 2016. Available at: https://www.nhs.uk/conditions/sickle-cell-disease/living-with/. Accessed March 1, 2018.

Epiretinal Membrane

Adam L. Rothman

Introduction

Although the etiology of the adult epiretinal membrane (ERM) is most often idiopathic, pediatric ERM typically develops secondary to vitreoretinal pathology, such as retinopathy of prematurity (ROP), retinal detachment, retinoschisis, trauma, familial exudative vitreoretinopathy, combined hamartoma of retina and retinal pigment epithelium, toxocariasis, and uveitis.[1-5] Although less common in the pediatric population than in adults, ERM can also cause significant decrease and distortion of vision, which would require thorough assessment.

The Brain Connection

There is no brain connection for pediatric ERM.

Clinical Features

Pediatric ERM more commonly appears as opaque preretinal fibrotic ingrowth into the condensed posterior hyaloid and adherent to the inner retinal surface, with associated vessel dragging, in contrast to the more typical translucent cellophane macular reflex morphology in adults.[1-3] Pediatric ERM also may spare the fovea, unlike ERM in adults. The posterior hyaloid attachment varies according to the underlying etiology. Pediatric ERM may occur secondary to other pediatric retinal conditions such as: combined hamartoma of the retina and retinal pigment epithelium, familial exudative vitreoretinopathy, retinopathy of prematurity, uveitis or trauma.

OCT Features

Compared with adult ERM, pediatric ERM more frequently grows confluently to the inner retinal surface (Fig. 33.1), and they lack the fibrillary retinal-ERM attachment which is common in adult cases with partial vitreous separation. OCT can also help visualize retinal folding caused by ERM,

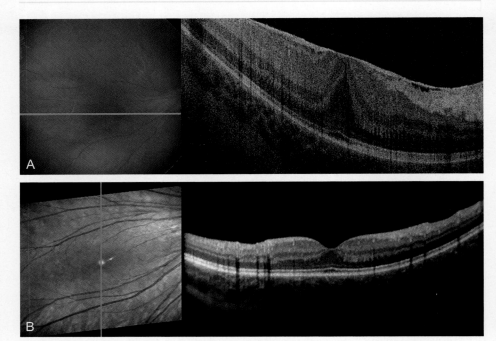

Fig. 33.1 (A) Handheld optical coherence tomography (OCT) image and corresponding fundus photograph of a 4-year-old male with epiretinal membrane (ERM) secondary to familial exudative vitreoretinopathy, obtained during examination under anesthesia. Note the broad, confluent attachment of the ERM to the retina, with resultant foveal thickening and a distorted yet intact ellipsoid zone. The patient underwent subsequent pars plana vitrectomy with membrane peel. (B) OCT image and corresponding scanning laser fundus image obtained during most recent clinic visit of patient at age 9 years and with 20/30 visual acuity demonstrates appropriate foveal contour without recurrent ERM.

which, in children, tends to cause deeper retinal folds or "taco" folds, with apposition of the inner retinal layers and invagination into the outer retinal layers (Fig. 33.2). OCT helps characterize the vitreo–retinal interface and sites of separation and attachment may be helpful in surgical planning.[4]

Ancillary Testing

A detailed examination should assess for concurrent pathology, because idiopathic pediatric ERMs are uncommon. A thorough peripheral examination and wide-field fluorescein angiography are thus commonly utilized in pediatric evaluation.

Treatment

Pediatric ERM causing significant decline in vision or metamorphopsia can be removed surgically with vitrectomy and membrane/hyaloid removal, along with management of other disease processes, when present (e.g., familial exudative vitreoretinopathy).[3,5] Preoperative integrity of the photoreceptors on OCT may correlate with potential for postoperative visual improvement. OCT images obtained before, during, and at the end of surgery can confirm the extent of removal of ERM and configuration of the retina.[4]

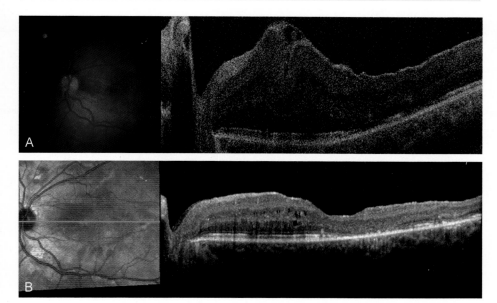

Fig. 33.2 (A) Optical coherence tomography (OCT) image and corresponding fundus photograph of a 16-year-old male referred for persisting epiretinal membrane (ERM) after vitrectomy. The patient had preoperative visual acuity of 20/250. Note the deep "taco" retinal fold, with apposition of the inner retinal layers and invagination into the outer retinal layers and underlying disruption of the photoreceptor layers. (B) OCT image and corresponding scanning laser fundus image obtained 5 months after recurrent ERM peel with resultant visual acuity 20/160. Note the persistent parafoveal thickening nasally with an abnormal foveal contour and temporal degradation of the ellipsoid zone.

References

1. Smiddy WE, Michels RG, Gilbert HD, Green WR. Clinicopathologic study of idiopathic macular pucker in children and young adults. *Retina.* 1992;12:232–236.
2. Khaja HA, McCannel CA, Diehl NN, Mohney BG. Incidence and clinical characteristics of epiretinal membranes in children. *Arch Ophthalmol.* 2008;126:632–636.
3. Fang X, Chen Z, Weng Y, et al. Surgical outcome after removal of idiopathic macular epiretinal membrane in young patients. *Eye.* 2008;22:1430–1435.
4. Rothman AL, Folgar FA, Tong AY, Toth CA. Spectral domain optical coherence tomography characterization of pediatric epiretinal membranes. *Retina.* 2014;34:1323–1334.
5. Ferrone PJ, Chaudhary KM. Macular epiretinal membrane peeling treatment outcomes in young children. *Retina.* 2012;32:530–536.

Uveitis and Infectious Diseases

CHAPTER 34

Infectious Retinitis: TORCH Syndrome

Dilraj S. Grewal

Introduction

TORCH syndrome (Toxoplasmosis, Other infections [syphilis, varicella-zoster virus, parvovirus B19), Rubella, Cytomegalovirus [CMV] infection, and Herpesvirus infection) usually causes mild maternal morbidity, but fetal consequences are serious. Infectious retinitis in children, although rare, can have devastating long-term ocular sequelae. Despite advances in therapy, infectious retinitis continues to be prevalent. Congenital syphilis is still a burden on the public health care system, and ocular syphilis, known as the great masquerader, may occur during any stage of congenital syphilis. Approximately 85% of women of childbearing age in the United States are susceptible to acute infection with the protozoan parasite *Toxoplasma gondii*. Zika virus, a mosquito-borne flavivirus, has now been designated by the World Health Organization as a public health emergency. Recent clusters of CMV retinitis in pediatric allogeneic hematopoietic stem cell transplant recipients have been reported.[1] There has been success with vaccination, however, in reducing the incidence of rubella retinitis and congenital rubella syndrome.

The Brain–Eye Connection

In all cases of infectious retinitis, there may be neurologic involvement, so appropriate screening is important. Congenital Zika syndrome comprises ocular abnormalities, microcephaly, hearing loss, and limb anomalies.[2] The mechanism of chorioretinal atrophy is thought to be similar to that by which Zika causes microcephaly.[3] Congenital cerebral toxoplasmosis may cause cerebral abscesses, calcifications in the basal ganglia, and hydrocephalus. Depending on the severity, these conditions may cause symptoms ranging from behavioral changes to seizures.

Clinical Features

Ocular findings depend on the severity of involvement. Although syphilis may affect any part of the eye, posterior segment involvement includes vitritis, optic neuritis, and "ground glass" retinitis often associated with retinal vasculitis. Syphilitic retinitis may be a patchy multifocal chorioretinitis early on, becoming more confluent over time and may result in a bilateral "salt and pepper" fundus.

CMV retinitis causes progressive necrotizing retinitis and may also cause occlusive retinal vasculopathy. Zika virus infection may cause optic nerve hypoplasia with the "double ring" sign, pallor, increased cup-to-disc ratio, macular pigment mottling and lacunar maculopathy, chorioretinal scarring, and congenital glaucoma. Typically, no intraocular inflammation is seen in Zika virus infection.

Ocular toxoplasmosis can cause focal necrotizing retinochoroiditis, punctate outer retinitis, vitritis, and optic nerve edema. Complications include choroidal neovascularization, vitreous hemorrhage, and tractional retinal detachment. Ocular toxocariasis is mostly unilateral, usually presenting as a posterior pole granuloma seen as an elevated, well-demarcated white mass. There may be dense vitreous inflammation mimicking endophthalmitis. Exudative or tractional retinal detachment, epiretinal membrane (ERM), and choroidal neovascularization may be present.

OCT Features

Ventura et al. first described the OCT characteristics of congenital Zika syndrome.[3] They reported neurosensory retinal and choroidal thinning, discontinuation of the ellipsoid zone, hyperreflectivity underlying the atrophic retinal pigment epithelium (RPE), and coloboma-like excavation involving the neurosensory retina, RPE, and choroid (Fig. 34.1). Thinning of the ganglion cell layer and the inner nuclear layer has been reported in Zika syndrome, even in the areas of unaffected retina, suggesting a causal relationship between the central nervous system malformations and chorioretinal degeneration.[4] Depending on the severity of the ocular involvement in congenital Zika syndrome, the neurosensory retina may be solely affected, whereas in more severe cases both the retina and the choroid are affected.

OCT findings in *Toxoplasma* (Fig. 34.2) and *Toxocara* (Fig. 34.3) chorioretinitis are characterized acutely by thickening and disorganization of the retina and the choroid, often with a subretinal granuloma seen as subretinal hyperreflective material. After scar formation, there may be thinning, irregular elevation, RPE elevation, and persistent loss of the outer retinal layers, depending on the severity of retinitis. Deeper scars in toxoplasmosis may show an excavated structure, with atrophy of the neurosensory retina, RPE, and outer retinal bands. Persistent retinal disorganization limits visual recovery, and the extent and location of disorganization are important factors in determining oral versus intravitreal therapy. Hyperreflective dots are often seen in the vitreous overlying the lesion and resolve with treatment; thus they may be used to monitor improvement of inflammatory response.[5] Choroidal thickening occurs during the active phase of ocular toxoplasmosis but reduces with treatment.[6]

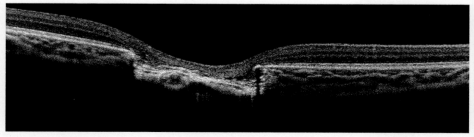

Fig. 34.1 Optical coherence tomography (OCT) image in 3-month-old infant with congenital Zika syndrome demonstrates a chorioretinal scar with neurosensory retinal thinning, discontinuation of the ellipsoid zone, and hyperreflectivity underlying the retinal pigment epithelium (RPE). A slight excavation with a colobomatous aspect is seen in the affected neurosensory retina, RPE, and choroid. (Image courtesy of Camila Ventura, MD, PhD.)

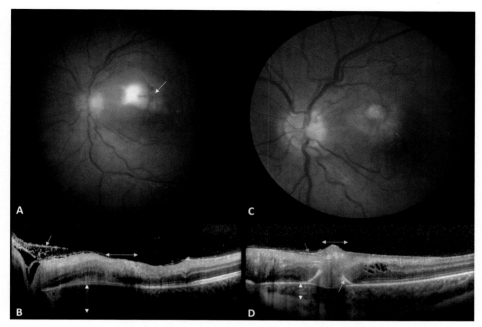

Fig. 34.2 Fundus photograph (A) in a 14-year-old girl showing a macular *Toxoplasma* lesion with the presence of neovascularization intrinsic to it *(white arrow)*. Optical coherence tomography (OCT) image through the lesion (B) shows hyperreflective foci in the vitreous *(yellow arrow)* consistent with inflammatory cells and severely disorganized retina with full-thickness necrosis *(yellow double-ended arrow)*. Following treatment (C), there is consolidation of the area of *Toxoplasma* chorioretinitis and development of epiretinal membrane (ERM) with striae in the macula. OCT image obtained after treatment (D) shows development of ERM *(orange arrow)*, resolution of hyperreflective vitreous opacities, partial restoration of retinal laminar architecture, and outer retinal bands, but there is an area of persistent full-thickness disorganization *(yellow dotted double-ended arrow)* along with a few intraretinal cysts *(red arrow)*, and hyperreflectivity of the underlying RPE *(yellow dotted arrow)*. There is also reduction of choroidal thickness underlying the area of retinitis after treatment *(double ended arrows; B and D)*.

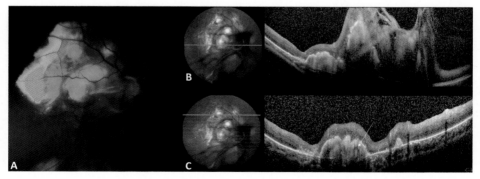

Fig. 34.3 Optos retinal image showing a large *Toxocara* subretinal granuloma in an 8-year-old female, involving nearly the entire macula with overlying preretinal fibrosis and dragged vessels. Wide-field optical coherence tomography (OCT) image through the fovea (B) shows subretinal hyperreflective material *(white arrow)* consistent with the granuloma with a large amount of retinal elevation, severely disorganized retinal architecture, and overlying tractional bands. OCT through the superior macula (C) shows the subretinal granuloma extending superiorly, with disorganization of the inner retinal layers and loss of the outer retinal bands.

In ocular syphilis, depending on the area of involvement, there may be cystoid macular edema, loss of outer retinal layers, and ERM formation. After resolution of retinitis, usually retinal thinning occurs, with disorganization of the inner retina and loss of outer retinal bands. A secondary choriocapillaritis may be seen. CMV retinitis causes disorganization of the inner retina (Fig. 34.4), and serial OCT can be used to monitor response to treatment, with thinning and atrophy occurring after the retinitis is consolidated and inactive.

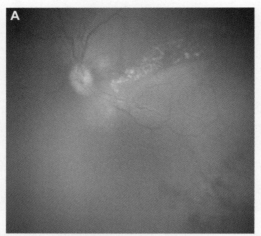

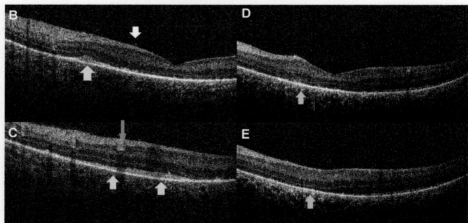

Fig. 34.4 A 4-month-old female patient with cytomegalovirus (CMV) retinitis in the left eye. (A) Color photograph shows active disease with vitreous haze, retinal whitening and focal exudates in the inferior macula, and peripheral retinal hemorrhages inferiorly. (B) OCT image of fovea shows focal vitreous hyperreflectivity (white arrow), diffuse and focal hyperreflective areas in retina, RPE deposits, and subretinal hyperreflective material (yellow arrows in B & C), and the inferior macula (C) shows hyperreflective retinal vasculature (orange arrow) and disorganization of retinal inner layers. OCT image obtained 4 weeks after initiation of treatment at the fovea (D) and inferior macula (E) show interval resolution of inner retinal layer disorganization but persistent photoreceptor layer and retinal pigment epithelium (RPE) thinning (pale blue arrows) and focal hyperreflective scars.

Ancillary Testing

Neuroimaging should be performed in cases of Zika syndrome and *Toxoplasma* infection because of the high incidence of cerebral involvement. Cerebrospinal fluid sampling is recommended when ocular syphilis is suspected. Testing for concomitant human immunodeficiency virus (HIV) infection is also warranted.

Treatment

Early treatment of conditions that are treatable reduces long-term sequelae. Neonatal screening is important to identify asymptomatic children, and teleophthalmic screening can play a vital role. Treatment for *Toxoplasma* chorioretinitis consists of pyrimethamine with sulfadiazine and folinic acid. In older children, azithromycin or clindamycin may be used as an alternative. In severe cases with macular involvement, intravitreal clindamycin may be administered. Patients with small areas of retinitis that are extramacular may be observed without treatment. *Toxocara* chorioretinitis is treated with one of the benzimidazole derivatives (albendazole, thiabendazole, and mebendazole) in conjunction with local and/or systemic corticosteroids, depending on the severity of inflammation. Ocular syphilis should be treated as neurosyphilis with 10 to 14 days of aqueous penicillin G or procaine penicillin G. CMV retinitis is treated with a course of intravenous valganciclovir, and depending on the severity of involvement, intravitreal ganciclovir may be administered.

References

1. Larochelle MB, Phan R, Craddock J, et al. Cytomegalovirus retinitis in pediatric stem cell transplants: report of a recent cluster and the development of a screening protocol. *Am J Ophthalmol.* 2017;175:8–15.
2. Ventura CV, Maia M, Bravo-Filho V, Góis AL, Belfort Jr R. Zika virus in Brazil and macular atrophy in a child with microcephaly. *Lancet.* 2016;387:228.
3. Ventura CV, Ventura LO, Bravo-Filho V, et al. Optical coherence tomography of retinal lesions in infants with congenital Zika syndrome. *JAMA Ophthalmol.* 2016;134:1420–1427.
4. Aleman TS, Ventura CV, Cavalcanti MM, et al. Quantitative assessment of microstructural changes of the retina in infants with congenital zika syndrome. *JAMA Ophthalmol.* 2017;135:1069–1076.
5. Goldenberg D, Goldstein M, Loewenstein A, Habot-Wilner Z. Vitreal, retinal, and choroidal findings in active and scarred toxoplasmosis lesions: a prospective study by spectral-domain optical coherence tomography. *Graefes Arch Clin Exp Ophthalmol.* 2013;251:2037–2045.
6. Freitas-Neto CA, Cao JH, Oréfice JL, et al. Increased submacular choroidal thickness in active, isolated, extramacular toxoplasmosis. *Ophthalmology.* 2016;123:222–224. e221.

White Dot Syndromes

Dilraj S. Grewal

Introduction

White dot syndromes are a group of posterior uveitis disorders of unknown cause and share a characteristic appearance of multiple whitish-yellow inflammatory lesions located at the level of the outer retina, retinal pigment epithelium (RPE), and choroid.[1] They include multiple evanescent white dot syndrome (MEWDS), placoid diseases (including acute posterior multifocal placoid pigment epitheliopathy [APMPPE], serpiginous choroiditis, and relentless placoid chorioretinitis), multifocal choroiditis (MFC) with panuveitis, punctate inner choroidopathy (PIC), acute zonal occult outer retinopathy (AZOOR), acute macular neuroretinopathy (AMN), and birdshot chorioretinopathy (BCR). These are rare in children, and the relative frequency of white dot syndromes in pediatric patients with uveitis is estimated to be between 1% and 5%.[2,3] It is, however, possible that increased access to pediatric retinal imaging evaluations will lead to greater detection at younger ages and that the current incidence may be underestimated. Some of the youngest cases of white dot syndrome were of MEWDS reported in a 4-year-old.[4] Given their overlapping clinical and imaging features, white dot syndromes and their masqueraders may represent a diagnostic challenge for clinicians, and more precise anatomic localization of the lesions with multimodal imaging with optical coherence tomography (OCT), enhanced-depth OCT, fluorescein angiography (FA), indocyanine green angiography (ICGA), and autofluorescence can be helpful to better characterize them.[1,2,5,6]

The Brain Connection

APMPPE may rarely be associated with cerebral vasculitis, which involves small and large arteries and may cause lacunar and territorial strokes, and also with meningoencephalitis.[7] These complications usually occur within a few weeks of onset of ocular symptoms. Cases presenting with such symptoms as headaches should undergo neuroimaging. The presence of cerebral vasculopathy also warrants aggressive steroid and immunosuppressive treatments, as for primary central nervous system vasculitis.

Clinical Features

White dot syndromes have distinct features and yet share some common symptoms, including blurred vision, photopsias, scotomas and visual field changes, floaters, and changes in contrast sensitivity.

APMPPE consists of multifocal, cream-colored, placoid lesions at the level of the choriocapillaris, RPE, and outer retina. MEWDS is typically unilateral and shows multifocal, small, deep, white dots involving the posterior pole, often with mild vitritis, macular edema, and vasculitis and usually associated with preceding flulike symptoms.[8] PIC consists of small, yellow-white lesions (usually <300 microns diameter) at the level of the choroid and the RPE in the posterior pole. MFC usually involves some anterior segment inflammation and vitritis, an important feature that distinguishes it from PIC. AMN presents as wedge-shaped, reddish brown, deep retinal lesions that are often best seen on near-infrared imaging. APMPPE, MEWDS, and AMN are usually seen in older children, typically girls in their teenage years. In AZOOR, the fundus is initially normal, and there are no visible white dots. Areas of peripheral and peripapillary retina may develop mottled pigmentation, vascular narrowing, and sheathing, and these pigmentary changes may resemble retinitis pigmentosa. Serpiginous choroiditis shows geographic peripapillary patches of creamy yellow placoid lesions that progress in a centrifugal manner. The etiology of white dot syndromes is not completely understood, but several of these are seen in myopes, and it has been suggested that the fragility of the myopic choriocapillaris may have a role to play.

OCT Features

MEWDS shows focal irregularities in the external limiting membrane (ELM) and the ellipsoid zone (EZ) and thinning of the outer nuclear layer. APMPPE shows a hyperreflective area above the RPE corresponding to the placoid lesions, with disruption of the outer retina and rarely the presence of subretinal or intraretinal fluid. Serpiginous choroiditis shows outer retinal atrophy in the affected areas, with disruption of the ELM and the EZ and increased reflectance of the choroid and deeper retinal layers. MFC shows irregularities at the level of the RPE or deeper in the choroid, sometimes with the presence of subretinal hyperreflective material and older lesions that are atrophic (Fig. 35.1). PIC shows sub-RPE hyperreflective material, patches of loss of the ELM and the EZ, and subretinal or intraretinal fluid if there is an associated choroidal neovascular membrane (CNVM) (Fig. 35.2). In AZOOR, there is ELM and EZ loss in the areas of involvement, with thinning of the inner and outer nuclear layers (Fig. 35.3). AMN shows irregularities in the ELM and the EZ and focal areas of outer nuclear layer thinning.[9]

Ancillary Testing

FA and OCT characteristics of APMPPE, MEWDS, PIC, MFC, serpiginous choroiditis, AMN, and AZOOR are summarized in Table 35.1. CNV is an uncommon complication. Fundus autofluorescence imaging shows areas of hyper- and hypoautofluorescence corresponding to RPE abnormalities, which vary with disease activity. Visual field testing is helpful to monitor the scotoma size.

Treatment

MEWDS and AMPPE are usually self-limiting, but APMPPE with cerebral involvement needs aggressive treatment with steroids and immunomodulatory argents. Serpiginous choroiditis and relentless placoid also warrant immunomodulatory therapy. PIC and MFC can cause CNVMs, which need to be treated with a combination of anti–vascular endothelial growth factor and anti-inflammatory therapies, followed by immunomodulatory therapy.

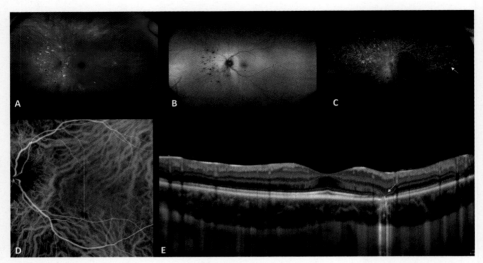

Fig. 35.1 Fundus photograph (A) of a 17-year-old with multifocal choroiditis showing multiple, small, yellow-pigmented spots, which are mostly nasal to the optic nerve and are hypoautofluorescent on autofluorescence imaging (B). They demonstrate late staining on fluorescein angiography, with mild perivascular leakage in the periphery (*white arrow*, C), hypocyanescence on indocyanine green angiography (D). On a vertical optical coherence tomography (OCT) scan (corresponding to the white dotted line in image D), there is a focal area of disruption of the external limiting membrane (ELM) and the ellipsoid zone (EZ), with thinning of the outer plexiform layer (OPL) and underlying choroidal hypertransmission (*yellow arrow*, E).

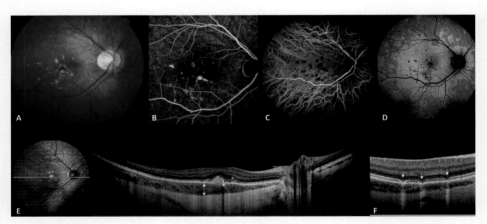

Fig. 35.2 Fundus photograph in 16-year-old with punctate inner choroidopathy (A). Right eye shows multiple small round lesions throughout the macula. Fluorescein angiography (FA) (B) shows late staining of the lesions. Indocyanine green angiography (C) shows hypocyanescence of the lesions, and there are more lesions visible than seen on FA. Fundus autofluorescence (D) shows hypoautofluorescence corresponding to the lesions with diffuse hyperfluorescence throughout the macula and extending beyond the arcades. Enhanced-depth imaging optical coherence tomography (OCT) shows sub–retinal pigment epithelium (sub-RPE) hyperreflective material (*yellow arrow*) with overlying loss of the ELM and the EZ, surrounding decreased reflectivity of the ELM and the EZ (*orange arrow*), and underlying choroidal thickening (*dotted double arrow*). Cross-sectional scan superior to the fovea shows smaller lesions, in earlier stages of evolution, with multiple areas of EZ and ELM loss and underlying signal hypertransmission (*white arrows*, F).

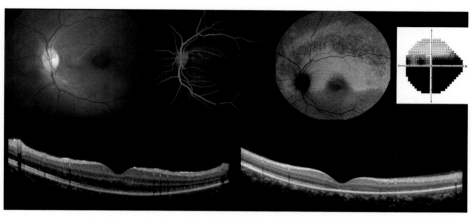

Fig. 35.3   Fundus photograph (A) in 17-year-old girl with acute zonal occult outer retinopathy with mild pigmentary changes in the superior macula. Fluorescein angiography (FA) (B) was unremarkable. Fundus autofluorescence (C) showed a well-demarcated area of hyperautofluorescence in the superior macula, sparing the fovea and extending beyond the arcades with a superior arc of stippled hypoautofluorescence, and there was a corresponding inferior scotoma on visual field (D). Vertical optical coherence tomography (OCT) scan through the macula (E, corresponding to vertical dotted white line on image A) shows ELM and EZ loss with outer nuclear layer (ONL) thinning in the superior macula *(white dotted double arrow)*. OCT on follow-up 2 years later (F) shows increased area of ELM and EZ loss, with increased ONL thinning as well as reduction in retinal thickness *(white dotted double arrow)* and progression into the fovea. The fellow eye was unremarkable.

TABLE 35.1 ■ Fluorescein Angiography and OCT Characteristics of the White Dot Syndromes

Imaging	APMPPE	MEWDS	PIC	MFC	Serpiginous Choroiditis	AMN	AZOOR
FA	Early hypofluorescence, late hyperfluorescence, and staining; window defects in the quiescent stage	Early and late hyperfluorescence of the white dots in a wreathlike pattern. May have optic nerve leakage	Early hypofluorescence, late hyperfluorescence, late leakage from CNVM, if present	Early hypofluorescence, late hyperfluorescence	Early hypofluorescence of the central portion of the lesion with hyperfluorescence at the margins	Usually normal	Normal in early stages, later may have window defects corresponding to RPE attenuation
OCT	Hyperreflective area above RPE with disruption of ELM and EZ corresponding to the placoid lesions Rare: presence of subretinal or intraretinal fluid	Focal irregularities in ELM and EZ, focal thinning of the ONL, usually resolves.	Patches of loss of ELM and EZ with sub-RPE hyperreflective material If CNV, then subretinal or intraretinal fluid may be seen	Irregularities at the level of the RPE or deeper in the choroid Sometimes with presence of subretinal hyperreflective material Older lesions are atrophic	Outer retinal atrophy in the affected areas with disruption of ELM and EZ and increased reflectance of the choroid and deeper retinal layers	Acutely with patchy ONL and OPL hyperreflectivity, ELM and EZ loss, and RPE attenuation Long term with partial restoration of ELM, EZ, and RPE changes but persistent focal ONL thinning	Demarcating line, loss of ELM and EZ, thinning of ONL, RPE and choroid Long term with inner retinal thinning, ELM, EZ, RPE, and choroidal thinning

AMN, Acute macular retinopathy; APMPPE, acute posterior multifocal placoid pigment epitheliopathy; AZOOR, acute zonal occult outer retinopathy; CNVM, choroidal neovascular membrane; ELM, external limiting membrane; EZ, ellipsoid zone; FA, fluorescein angiography; MEWDS, multiple evanescent white dot syndrome; MFC, multifocal choroiditis; OCT, optical coherence tomography; ONL, outer nuclear layer; OPL, outer plexiform layer; PIC, punctate inner choroidopathy; RPE, retinal pigment epithelium.

References

1. Mirza MR RG, Jampol LM. Posterior uveitis of unknown cause—white spot syndromes. In: Yanoff DJ M, ed. *Ophthalmology*. Philadelphia: Elsevier-Health Sciences Division; 2014:778–787.
2. Spital G, Heiligenhaus A, Scheider A, Pauleikhoff D, Herbort CP. "White dot syndromes" in childhood. *Klin Monbl Augenheilkd*. 2007;224:500–506.
3. Smith JA, Mackensen F, Sen HN, et al. Epidemiology and course of disease in childhood uveitis. *Ophthalmology*. 2009;116:1544–1551. 1551. e1541.
4. BenEzra D, Cohen E, Maftzir G. Uveitis in children and adolescents. *Br J Ophthalmol*. 2005;89:444–448.
5. Zarranz-Ventura J, Sim DA, Keane PA, et al. Characterization of punctate inner choroidopathy using enhanced depth imaging optical coherence tomography. *Ophthalmology*. 2014;121:1790–1797.
6. Pichi F, Sarraf D, Arepalli S, et al. The application of optical coherence tomography angiography in uveitis and inflammatory eye diseases. *Prog Retin Eye Res*. 2017;59:178–201.
7. Hsu CT, Harlan JB, Goldberg MF, Dunn JP. Acute posterior multifocal placoid pigment epitheliopathy associated with a systemic necrotizing vasculitis. *Retina*. 2003;23:64–68.
8. Olitsky SE. Multiple evanescent white-dot syndrome in a 10-year-old child. *J Pediatr Ophthalmol Strabismus*. 1998;35:288–289.
9. Makino S, Tampo H. Acute macular neuroretinopathy in a 15-year-old boy: optical coherence tomography and visual acuity findings. *Case Rep Ophthalmol*. 2014;5:11–15.

CHAPTER 36

Choroidal Granulomas: Tuberculosis and Sarcoidosis

Dilraj S. Grewal

Introduction

Choroidal granulomas are round nodular lesions in the vascular choroid, often seen during the active phase of sarcoidosis and tuberculosis (TB), among others. Ocular TB is rare ($\approx$1% of all cases of TB), may occur without evidence of systemic TB, and may involve any part of the eye. A choroidal tuberculoma often appears as a well-defined, yellow, subretinal mass on examination. Mycobacteria spread hematogenously, and this may explain its propensity for the highly vascular choroid. Sarcoid choroidal granulomas are also a rare manifestation, occurring in approximately 5% of patients with ocular sarcoidosis.[1] A detailed review of systems is important to elicit the history of systemic symptoms.

The Eye–Brain Connection

Although there is no established correlation of choroidal granulomas with cerebral involvement in sarcoidosis or TB, it is important to remember that both these diseases may involve any part of the body. A high index of clinical suspicion must be maintained, and brain magnetic resonance imaging (MRI) and angiography should be considered in patients with neurologic symptoms or in those with optic nerve edema (Chapter 66). Both central nervous system (CNS) TB and neurosarcoidosis may cause nonspecific and variable symptoms simulating many other conditions. Visual symptoms are associated with the location of granuloma formation and related inflammatory sequelae and may include decreased vision, floaters, visual field defects, nystagmus, and cranial neuropathy.

Clinical Features

Multiple choroidal tubercles are more common than a single, large tuberculoma (usually a solitary yellowish or grayish white, large lesion, generally located in the posterior pole). There may be overlying vitritis and sometimes an associated serous retinal detachment and vitreous hemorrhage as well. A tuberculoma may also be the presenting sign in a patient with no evidence of systemic disease.

OCT Features

Choroidal granulomas are seen as distinct areas of hyporeflectivity compared with the surrounding healthy choroid. There may be subretinal fluid overlying the granuloma. In cases with severe vitritis, good-quality imaging of the retinal pigment epithelium (RPE), Bruch membrane, choriocapillaris, and choroid may not be possible. Optical coherence tomography (OCT) allows for early recognition and quantitative assessment of the choroidal granulomas as well as assessment of response to treatment. Enhanced-depth imaging (EDI) (Fig. 36.1) allows for evaluation of various anatomic and tomographic features, such as extent of choroidal involvement, shape, reflectivity, internal pattern and margins.[2,3] It also allows for quantitative monitoring of such parameters as area, lateral and anteroposterior extent, and volume. Repeat scanning of the same location allows for accurate quantitative assessment of changes in size. In contrast, indocyanine green angiography (ICG) provides only two-dimensional information and may be less sensitive in detecting variations in lesion size. OCT is, however, limited in its ability to easily and reproducibly assess granulomas located beyond the equator. Swept-source OCT (SS-OCT) and wide-field imaging may be more helpful to better characterize these lesions.

Lesions involving the full thickness of the choroid (Fig. 36.2) initially decrease in size to become partial-thickness lesions, with a reduction in the anteroposterior dimension more than in the lateral

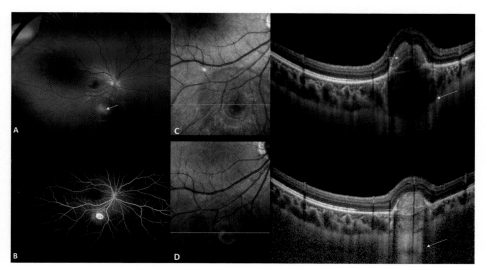

Fig. 36.1 Choroidal granuloma with overlying neovascularization. (A) Fundus photograph in a 7-year-old girl with tuberculosis demonstrates a large, solitary, yellow, deep, subretinal mass (*white arrow*) consistent with a choroidal granuloma. (B) Fluorescein angiography (FA) image shows leakage in the area of the choroidal granuloma resulting from an overlying choroidal neovascular membrane (CNVM). (C and D) Serial registered enhanced-depth imaging optical coherence tomography (OCT) scans show a choroidal granuloma (*white arrow*) and the overlying CNVM seen as subretinal hyperreflective material (*yellow arrow*). Following injection of anti–vascular endothelial growth factor (VEGF), tapering course of prednisone, and completion of antitubercular therapy, there is significant consolidation of the subretinal hyperreflective material (D) as well as resolution of the choroidal granuloma (*white arrow*). There is also an overall reduction in choroidal thickness. There is persistent loss of the retinal pigment epithelium (RPE), external limiting membrane (ELM), and ellipsoid zone (EZ) over the choroidal granuloma, resulting in signal hypertransmission (*white arrow*, D).

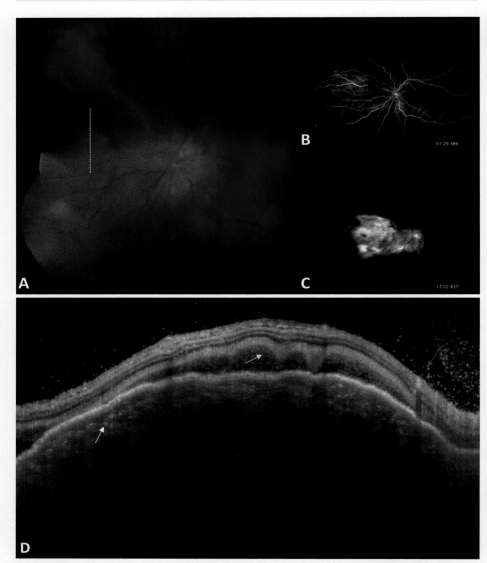

Fig. 36.2 Choroidal granuloma. (A) Fundus photograph in an 11-year-old girl with tuberculosis demonstrates a large, yellow, deep, subretinal mass (*white dotted line*) consistent with a choroidal granuloma. (B and C) Fluorescein angiography (FA) shows diffuse leakage both in mid (B) and late (C) phases of the FA, in the area of the granuloma. (D) Optical coherence tomography (OCT) scan obtained through the granuloma (corresponding to white dotted line in image A) shows a large choroidal granuloma with choroidal thickening and elevation with hyperreflective foci in the choroid *(white arrow)*, overlying thickened and undulating retinal pigment epithelium (RPE), subretinal fluid, and subretinal hyperreflective material *(yellow arrow)*, and overlying vitreous hyperreflective foci consistent with vitritis *(red arrow)*. Unlike in the case in Figure 36.1, there is no associated choroidal neovascular membrane (CNVM). (Image courtesy Aniruddha Agarwal, MD).

extent.[2] This could suggest that healing occurs in the outer choroid first and then in the inner choroid, whereas the inner choroid may be the first area to be affected by choroidal granulomas.[2] Large and long-standing granulomas can induce atrophic changes in the overlying RPE as well as in the external limiting membrane (ELM) and ellipsoid zone (EZ), and these changes result in increased signal penetration.

Ancillary Testing

Fluorescein angiography (FA) and ICG angiography are helpful in detecting other signs of inflammation, such as retinal vasculitis and the presence of choroidal neovascular membrane (CNVM), and in determining areas of choroidal involvement. In cases where inflammation or cataract limits the view of the fundus, B-scan ultrasonography is useful because the A-scan shows low to medium internal reflectivity of the granuloma, which may help differentiate it from other entities, such as a hemangioma. Testing for TB includes a QuantiFERON-TB test and a purified protein derivative skin test. Chest radiography should be performed, followed by high-resolution CT (with pediatric radiation dose calculation) if suspicious features are seen on the radiograph. Testing for sarcoid includes chest radiography, angiotensin-converting enzyme and lysozyme, and conformation with biopsy and histologic analysis demonstrating noncaseating granuloma.

Treatment

When a choroidal granuloma is noted, a systemic evaluation needs to be performed to identify the underlying cause. In cases with a positive TB test result, pulmonary and systemic evaluations are needed to determine whether the TB is active or latent. For TB, treatment is often initiated in conjunction with an infectious disease specialist for TB, treatment antitubercular therapy. For sarcoidosis, treatment is often initiated with the input from a rheumatologist when systemic immunosuppression is warranted. Sarcoid granulomas are usually very sensitive to steroids, often demonstrating a rapid response to a course of prednisone. In patients with TB, steroids should be initiated only in conjunction with antitubercular therapy. Parallel treatment for refractive error and amblyopia is important in affected children.

References

1. Desai UR, Tawansy KA, Joondeph BC, Schiffman RM. Choroidal granulomas in systemic sarcoidosis. *Retina.* 2001;21:40–47.
2. Invernizzi A, Agarwal A, Mapelli C, Nguyen QD, Staurenghi G, Viola F. Longitudinal follow-up of choroidal granulomas using enhanced depth imaging optical coherence tomography. *Retina.* 2017;37:144–153.
3. Ishihara M, Shibuya E, Tanaka S, Mizuki N. Diagnostic and therapeutic evaluation of multiple choroidal granulomas in a patient with confirmed sarcoidosis using enhanced depth imaging optical coherence tomography. *Int Ophthalmol.* 2018;38:2603–2608.

CHAPTER 37

Pediatric Intermediate Uveitis

Dilraj S. Grewal

Introduction

Cystoid macular edema (CME) and retinal vasculitis are common complications of pediatric uveitis but do not, of themselves, define the anatomic location of uveitis based on the Standardization of Uveitis Nomenclature (SUN) criteria. The annual incidence of pediatric uveitis is low (4.3–6.9 per 100,000 children ages <16 years), but there is often a delay in diagnosis and referral, resulting in a higher percentage of complications compared with adults.[1]

Juvenile idiopathic arthritis (JIA)–associated anterior uveitis is the most common cause of pediatric anterior uveitis in the United States and is often clinically silent.[2] Although rare, multiple sclerosis (MS) may cause intermediate uveitis (IU), whereas pars planitis is a type of IU that has no associated systemic disease or infectious etiology and comprises the large majority of pediatric IU cases.[3]

Multisystem autoimmune syndromes, such as tubulointerstitial nephritis and uveitis (TINU), Behçt syndrome, and systemic lupus erythematosus, are rare causes of pediatric uveitis with retinal vasculitis.

The Brain Connection

Pediatric IU may rarely be associated with MS, a demyelinating disease. Pediatric MS is believed to be underdiagnosed because symptoms are not easily recognized in children. In IU, it is important to obtain a brain magnetic resonance imaging (MRI) scan to rule out demyelinating disease, especially when considering immunomodulatory therapy, such as tumor necrosis factor–alpha (TNF-α) inhibitors. Neurologic associations in Behçet syndrome include headaches and aseptic meningitis, and white matter lesions may be seen on MRI.[4]

Clinical Features

Ocular findings depend on the severity and anatomic location of involvement. The most frequent complications are optic disc edema, CME, and glaucoma, which are caused by both steroids and inflammation. Anterior segment findings include cell, keratic precipitates (Fig. 37.1), corneal edema, pupillary membrane, posterior synechiae, and band keratopathy. Intermediate uveitis typically has vitritis, snowballs, and/or snowbanks and often retinal vasculitis with sheathing and of the vessels (mostly periphlebitis) that may result in ischemia and neovascularization (Figs. 37.2 and 37.3). Chronic snowbanks may evolve into a fibrotic, cyclitic membrane, leading to vitreous traction and retinal detachment. Inferior peripheral retinoschisis may also be seen.[5] Traction on areas of neovascularization can result in vitreous hemorrhage. Optic disc edema and hyperemia are also common.

TINU typically has bilateral, nongranulomatous, anterior uveitis accompanied by tubulointerstitial nephritis, and rarely posterior uveitis with hypopigmented chorioretinal scars. The renal

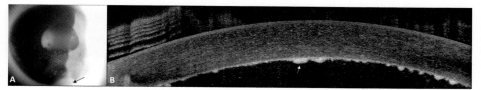

Fig. 37.1 Slit-lamp photograph (A) in an 8-year-old boy showing keratic precipitates, inferior iris nodules (black arrow), and posterior synechiae in sarcoid uveitis. Anterior-segment optical coherence tomography (OCT) image (B) shows the keratic precipitates as hyperreflective deposits on the corneal endothelium (white arrow).

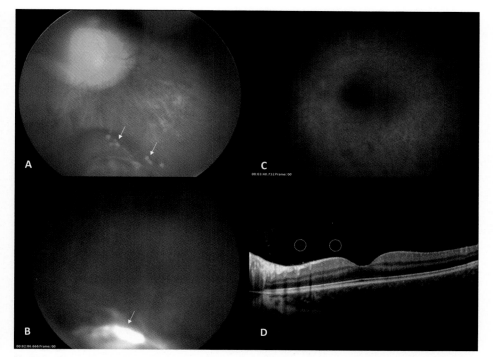

Fig. 37.2 Fundus photograph (A) in a 6-year-old boy. Scleral depression demonstrates inferior snowballs. Fluorescein angiography (FA) image shows leakage corresponding to the inferior snowballs (B) and area of snowbanks anterior to it. There is no leakage in macula (C), and OCT image through the fovea shows no macular edema, but there are few overlying hyperreflective vitreous opacities (circle, D).

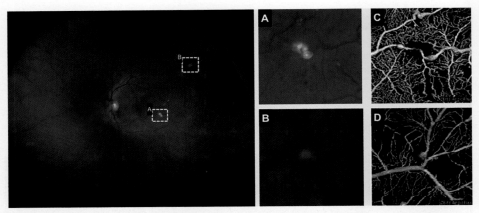

Fig. 37.3 Aneurysmal retinal vasculitis in a 7-year-old boy with sarcoid panuveitis (A and B) with optical coherence tomography angiography (OCTA) showing areas of retinal ischemia in the superficial capillary plexus in the region surrounding the area of retinal vasculitis with aneurysms (C and D).

course is independent from ocular disease.[6] Behçet syndrome can cause severe retinal vasculitis (Fig. 37.4), and diagnosis is based on international consensus clinical criteria.[7]

OCT Features

Although the association between central subfield thickness and visual acuity is well established in uveitic CME, several other OCT variables have also been evaluated and include integrity of the external limiting membrane, ellipsoid zone (EZ), hyperreflective foci, subretinal fluid, pattern of CME (cystoid versus diffuse; Figs. 37.5 and 37.6), and disorganization of retinal inner layers that may persist even after resolution of CME (see Fig. 37.6). Often, there are no cystic spaces visible on the cross-sectional B-scan, but noncystic thickening may be seen, especially on thickness maps, which can be used to monitor disease activity and response to treatment (Fig. 37.7). Perivascular

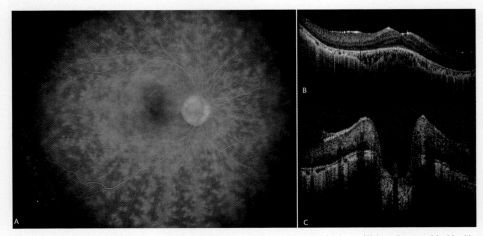

Fig. 37.4 Fluorescein angiography (FA) image shows diffuse perivascular leakage (A) in a 5-year-old girl with suspected Behçet syndrome. Optical coherence tomography (OCT) shows no cystoid macular edema, but there is an overlying epiretinal membrane (B). The patient developed steroid-induced glaucoma as a result of frequent periocular steroid injections, before being transitioned to immunomodulatory therapy; OCT image through the nerve shows an enlarged cup (C).

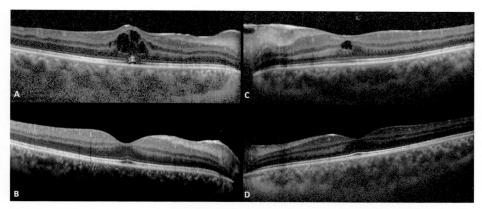

Fig. 37.5 Serial optical coherence tomography (OCT) scans in a 10-year-old boy show focal cystoid macular edema (CME) with cystoid spaces in both eyes (A and C) and subretinal fluid in the right eye (A), which resolved with treatment. After resolution, there is restoration of the normal retinal laminar architecture, with no disorganization of retinal inner layers.

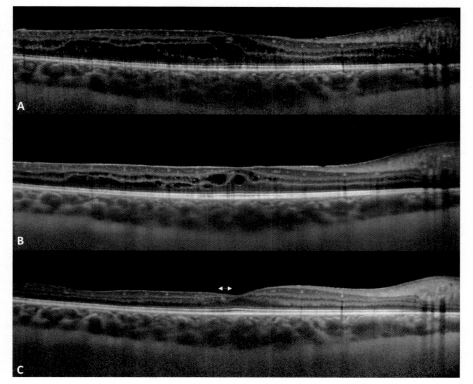

Fig. 37.6 Serial optical coherence tomography (OCT) scans in a 16-year-old girl with intermediate uveitis show diffuse cystoid macular edema (CME) with cystoid spaces (A), which improved (B) and then resolved with treatment. After resolution (C), there is persistent thinning of the inner and outer plexiform layers temporally, with a small area of persistent disorganization of retinal inner layers just temporal to the fovea *(arrow)*.

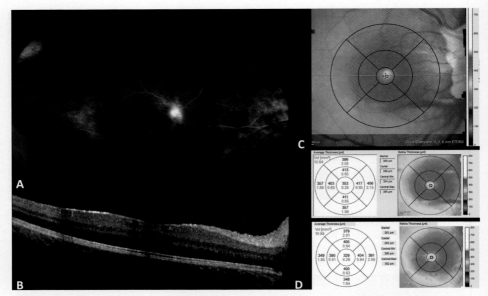

Fig. 37.7 Fluorescein angiography (FA) image shows disc and diffuse perivascular leakage in a 5-year-old boy with intermediate uveitis (A). Optical coherence tomography (OCT) shows no cystoid macular edema (CME), but there is noncystic thickening (B). This is more easily quantified on the thickness map (C), which is a color-coded volume map. Serial OCT scans with thickness maps (D) can be used to monitor response to treatment, even when there may not be much anatomic change visible on foveal B-scans.

thickness may also be monitored in vasculitis. Thickness of the retinal nerve fiber layer can be used to monitor optic nerve edema (Fig. 37.8) or atrophy. Overlying vitreous cells are also an inflammatory marker (see Fig. 37.2). There are ongoing efforts for developing automated imaging biomarkers for the quantification of anterior chamber cells, vitreous haze, retinovascular leakage, and chorioretinal infiltrates using OCT.[8] OCT angiography (OCTA) also has a role in assessment of microvascular capillary level flow abnormalities associated with both CME and retinal vasculitis, which are often seen in regions adjacent to large vessel inflammatory infiltrates as shown in Fig. 37.3.

Ancillary Testing

Laboratory testing and imaging should be performed to rule out associated systemic or infectious causes. Typical testing may include complete blood count with a differential, chest radiography (for sarcoidosis and tuberculosis), serum angiotensin-converting enzyme (sarcoidosis; although this enzyme is typically elevated in children), antinuclear antibody test (juvenile idiopathic arthritis), tuberculosis testing (skin or serum), syphilis testing via monoclonal antibody testing for *Treponema pallidum* (syphilis immunoglobulin) or fluorescent treponemal antibody absorption test with reflex rapid plasma reagin, urinary b2-microglobulin levels (TINU; renal biopsy is, however, considered gold standard for diagnostic interstitial nephritis) and human leukocyte antigen-B51 (when suspecting Behçet syndrome).

Treatment

Treatment depends on the severity of inflammation, and options range from topical corticosteroids, often used as the first-line treatment for anterior segment inflammation; regional steroids (periocular or intraocular steroids, sustained release dexamethasone or fluocinolone acetonide implants);

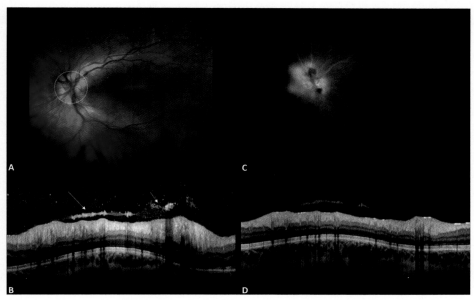

Fig. 37.8 Optic nerve edema in a 16-year-old with juvenile idiopathic arthritis (JIA) uveitis (A) with leakage at the optic disc on fluorescein angiography (FA) (C). Optical coherence tomography (OCT) obtained in a peripapillary circle around the optic disc (corresponding to white dotted circle in image A) shows thickening of the retinal nerve fiber layer (B) with overlying hyperreflective vitreous opacities *(white arrows)* consistent with inflammatory cells. After treatment, there is resolution of optic nerve edema (D) and overlying vitreous opacities.

and systemic steroids. In cases where long-term systemic steroids are needed, the children are transitioned to steroid-sparing immunomodulatory therapy, often in conjunction with pediatric rheumatologic treatment. Complications of uveitis, such as cataract and glaucoma refractory to medical therapy, may need surgical intervention. Areas of retinal ischemia may require panretinal photocoagulation, and vitrectomy may be indicated in some cases of nonclearing vitreous hemorrhage or tractional retinal detachment. Amblyopia management needs to be performed in parallel. Early diagnosis and strict control of inflammatory activity lead to a dramatic reduction in vision-threatening secondary complications.

References

1. Edelsten C, Reddy MA, Stanford MR, Graham EM. Visual loss associated with pediatric uveitis in English primary and referral centers. *Am J Ophthalmol.* 2003;135:676–680.
2. Ferrara M, Eggenschwiler L, Stephenson A, et al. The challenge of pediatric uveitis: tertiary referral center experience in the United States. *Ocul Immunol Inflamm.* 2018;1:1–8.
3. Majumder PD, Biswas J. Pediatric uveitis: an update. *Oman J Ophthalmol.* 2013;6:140–150.
4. Kone-Paut I. Behcet's disease in children, an overview. *Pediatr Rheumatol Online J.* 2016;14:10.
5. Guest S, Funkhouser E, Lightman S. Pars planitis: a comparison of childhood onset and adult onset disease. *Clin Exp Ophthalmol.* 2001;29:81–84.
6. Pakzad-Vaezi K, Pepple KL. Tubulointerstitial nephritis and uveitis. *Curr Opin Ophthalmol.* 2017;28:629–635.
7. Koné-Paut I, Shahram F, Darce-Bello M, et al. Consensus classification criteria for paediatric Behçet's disease from a prospective observational cohort: PEDBD. *Ann Rheum Dis.* 2016;75:958–964.
8. Denniston AK, Keane PA, Srivastava SK. Biomarkers and surrogate endpoints in uveitis: the impact of quantitative imaging. *Invest Ophthalmol Vis Sci.* 2017;58:BIO131–BIO140.

Vogt-Koyanagi Harada Syndrome

Dilraj S. Grewal

Introduction

Vogt-Koyanagi-Harada (VKH) syndrome refers to chronic, bilateral, granulomatous panuveitis and exudative retinal detachment associated with poliosis, vitiligo, alopecia, and central nervous system (CNS) and auditory signs. Approximately 3% of VKH syndrome cases are seen in patients under age 16 years.[1] Although the exact cause of VKH syndrome remains unknown, there is some evidence to suggest that it involves a T lymphocyte–mediated autoimmune process directed against melanocyte tyrosinase–related proteins, which are present in the uvea, retina, and leptomeninges.[2,3] Pediatric VKH syndrome can be more aggressive than that in adults, with high incidences of cataract (up to 61.5%), glaucoma (up to 46%), and choroidal neovascular membranes (up to 54%)[4] in the chronic, recurrent phase. If untreated or inadequately treated in the acute stage, VKH syndrome may progress to widespread bullous retinal detachment, accompanied by choroidal detachment and anterior segment inflammation with severe posterior iris synechia and iris bombe.

The Brain–Eye Connection

VKH syndrome is a multisystem disorder, and CNS symptoms, such as meningismus, headache, tinnitus, and aseptic meningitis, may manifest first followed by uveitis.[2] Brain magnetic resonance imaging (MRI) has demonstrated ischemic lesions in the territory of lenticulostriate and thalamic arteries.[5] If neither meningismus nor tinnitus is present, pleocytosis on cerebrospinal fluid (CSF) examination is required as confirmation of neurologic involvement. Although visual impairment is often an early sign in children, neurologic and auditory signs are usually the first signals of meningeal involvement in the prodromal stage. Diagnosis of complete VKH syndrome requires the absence of prior trauma, surgery, or other ocular diseases, along with bilateral ocular involvement, neurologic or auditory findings, and integumentary findings (alopecia, poliosis, or vitiligo).[6]

Clinical Features

Depigmentation of the fundus may result in the characteristic "sunset glow" fundus. In addition, multiple small, yellow, well-circumscribed areas of chorioretinal atrophy may develop in the midperiphery.

The clinical course classically consists of four stages: prodromal stage (lasts 3–5 days); acute uveitic stage (lasts several weeks); chronic stage, and chronic–recurrent stage (the last two may last for months or even years). In the last three stages, especially in the chronic and chronic– recurrent stages, small, isolated, hemispherical, yellowish Dalen-Fuchs nodules may develop in the peripheral retina.

OCT Features

In the acute phase, optical coherence tomography (OCT) shows thickening of the choroid, undulation of the retinal pigment epithelium (RPE), subretinal fluid accumulation, and loss of the normal reflectivity of the ellipsoid zone (EZ). In late-stage VKH syndrome, there is progression to RPE atrophy, loss of EZ, loss of the external limiting membrane (ELM), loss of the outer nuclear layer (ONL), and choroidal thinning. The goal of treatment is to prevent progression to this late stage. The clinical response with systemic corticosteroids is seen as resolution of exudative retinal detachment and subretinal fluid and absence of inflammatory vitreous cells. There is reduction in choroidal thickness and choroidal remodeling (Fig. 38.1), with reduction in RPE undulation and retinal thickness and restoration of the reflectivity of the EZ and ELM.[7,8]

Ancillary Testing

Fluorescein angiography (FA) may show leakage, especially at the nerve, and indocyanine green angiography (ICG) may show multifocal dark spots of choroidal hypocyanescence (Fig. 38.2); these features persist up to the late angiographic phase. Dalen-Fuchs nodules also show hypocyanescence on ICG angiography.

Treatment

The aim of therapy of VKH syndrome is suppression of the initial intraocular inflammation with early and aggressive use of systemic corticosteroids, followed by slow tapering and possible transition to steroid-sparing immunomodulatory therapy. Prompt and aggressive treatment may shorten the duration of the disease, prevent progression to the chronic stage, prevent severe ocular complications, and may reduce the incidence of extraocular manifestations.[1,4]

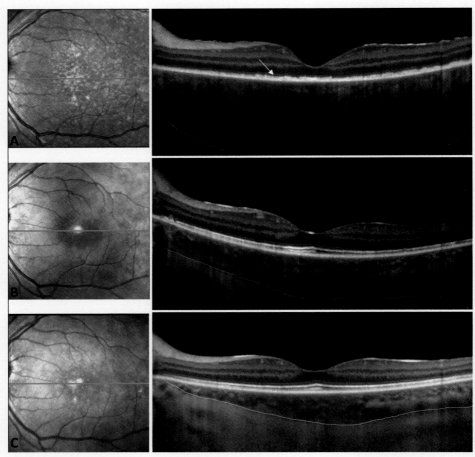

Fig. 38.1 Serial enhanced depth imaging optical coherence tomography (OCT) scans in a 14-year-old female with Vogt-Koyanagi-Harada (VKH) syndrome (A–C), showing progressive reduction in choroidal thickness *(posterior border indicated by white dotted line)* after initiation of steroids and transition to steroid-sparing immuno-modulatory therapy. There is patchy loss of the ellipsoid zone (EZ) at presentation (A, *white arrow*) and corresponding white discoloration on the near infrared image. After treatment, there is gradual restoration of the reflectivity of the EZ and normalization of the near infrared image (C).

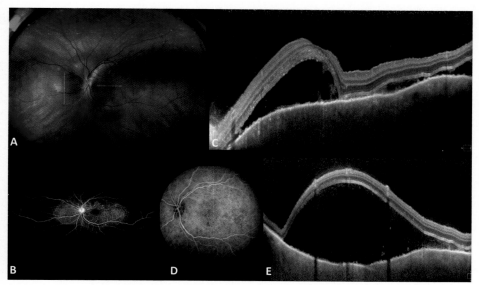

Fig. 38.2 Fundus photograph of a 17-year-old female with Vogt-Koyanagi-Harada (VKH) syndrome demonstrates acute phase of VKH syndrome with multifocal serous retinal detachments (A). Fluorescein angiography (B) shows multiple diffuse large areas of hyperfluorescence corresponding to the serous retinal detachment, along with multiple pinpoint areas of hyperfluorescence and leakage at the optic nerve. Indocyanine green (ICG) angiography (D) shows multiple small hypocyanescent spots throughout the posterior pole. Optical coherence tomography (OCT) through the macula (C, *corresponding to horizontal dotted white line on color photograph*) shows retinal pigment epithelium (RPE) undulation, choroidal thickening with hyperreflective dots in the choroid, subretinal fluid with hyperreflective dots in the outer retina, and loss of the normal reflectivity of the ellipsoid zone. Similar findings are seen through the area of serous retinal detachment nasal to the optic nerve (E, *corresponding to vertical dotted white arrow on color photograph*).

References

1. Soheilian M, Aletaha M, Yazdani S, Dehghan MH, Peyman GA. Management of pediatric Vogt-Koyanagi- Harada (VKH)-associated panuveitis. *Ocul Immunol Inflamm.* 2006;14:91–98.
2. Moorthy RS, Inomata H, Rao NA. Vogt-Koyanagi-Harada syndrome. *Surv Ophthalmol.* 1995;39:265–292.
3. Weisz JM, Holland GN, Roer LN, et al. Association between Vogt-Koyanagi-Harada syndrome and HLA-DR1 and -DR4 in Hispanic patients living in southern California. *Ophthalmology.* 1995;102:1012–1015.
4. Tabbara KF, Chavis PS, Freeman WR. Vogt-Koyanagi-Harada syndrome in children compared to adults. *Acta Ophthalmol Scand.* 1998;76:723–726.
5. Ryan SJ, Pettigrew LC. Cranial arteriopathy in familial Vogt-Koyanagi-Harada syndrome. *J Neuroimaging.* 1995;5:244–245.
6. Read RW, Holland GN, Rao NA, et al. Revised diagnostic criteria for Vogt-Koyanagi-Harada disease: report of an international committee on nomenclature. *Am J Ophthalmol.* 2001;131:647–652.
7. Jaisankar D, Raman R, Sharma HR, et al. Choroidal and retinal anatomical responses following systemic corticosteroid therapy in Vogt-Koyanagi-Harada disease using swept-source optical coherence tomography. *Ocul Immunol Inflamm.* 2017;1–9.
8. Nakayama M, Keino H, Okada AA, et al. Enhanced depth imaging optical coherence tomography of the choroid in Vogt-Koyanagi-Harada disease. *Retina.* 2012;32:2061–2069.

CHAPTER 39

Inflammatory and Idiopathic Choroidal Neovascularization

Dilraj S. Grewal ■ Cynthia A. Toth

Introduction

Choroidal neovascular membrane (CNVM), which is characterized by the growth of new blood vessels that originate from the choroid through a break in the Bruch membrane into the subretinal pigment epithelium (sub-RPE) or the subretinal space, is a rare but potentially sight-threatening event in children. CNVM may be idiopathic or may occur as a complication of trauma (Chapters 43 and 44), optic nerve head drusen (Chapter 69), or inflammatory and infectious pediatric posterior and panuveitis.[1] Neovascular proliferation develops as a response to both chronic inflammation and to inflammatory cytokines and vascular endothelial growth factor (VEGF) production. Histopathologic examinations of excised pediatric CNVM have previously shown that the most common components were RPE, fibrocytes, vascular endothelium, and collagen.[2] Diagnosis of the underlying cause is important because it is critical to rule out infectious causes before initiating antiinflammatory steroid therapy or initiating off-label use of anti-VEGF in idiopathic cases.

The Brain Connection

Although there is no known direct correlation between CNVM and brain abnormalities, in uveitis, CNVM may indicate more aggressive and active disease and warrant appropriate neurosurveillance, depending on the underlying etiology.

Clinical Features

CNVM may be located in the macula, in the subfoveal, juxtafoveal, or extrafoveal areas, or in the peripapillary area. Its subfoveal location carries the worst visual prognosis. On examination, there is a yellowish or gray-appearing subretinal lesion, often associated with subretinal hemorrhage and intraretinal and subretinal fluid. Over time, especially if undertreated, this may progress to fibrotic scar tissue and pigmentation resulting from RPE hyperplasia. Children do not have the same extent of calcification and Bruch membrane thickening as in adults, and with pediatric idiopathic or inflammatory CNVM, there is usually a solitary break in the Bruch membrane, unlike the multiple sites of breaks in adults.[2-6] This may be one of the reasons for the high rate of spontaneous regression of CNVM in children.

OCT Features

Optical coherence tomography (OCT) demonstrates increased retinal thickness with the presence of intraretinal fluid, subretinal fluid, or both (Figs. 39.1 through 39.4). There is often the presence of subretinal hyperreflective material, which may be associated with a classic type 2 CNVM and/or a fibrovascular pigment epithelial detachment, which is more typical of a type 1 lesion. In disorders with a choroidal inflammatory component, such as punctate inner choroidopathy, there is often associated choroidal thickening when the CNVM is active and reduction in choroidal thickness with treatment (see Fig. 39.2). Serial OCT enables monitoring of response to treatment, photoreceptor loss, or loss of the ellipsoid zone (EZ) or external limiting membrane (ELM), which may indicate localized loss of visual function. OCT angiography (OCTA) permits anatomic segmentation to quantify the CNVM dimensions, provide flow overlay information, and determine the location of the CNVM relative to the RPE (see Fig. 39.3).[7]

Ancillary Testing

Fluorescein angiography (FA; see Figs. 39.1 and 39.3) and indocyanine green angiography (ICGA) show leakage with the "classic" appearance of the CNVM. OCTA also allows for the identification and potential monitoring of the CNVM, but it may be challenging to obtain good-quality scans with adequate fixation in young children in the clinic.

Treatment

Anti-VEGF injections, less commonly photodynamic therapy (PDT), and rarely surgical removal are sometimes combined with steroid therapy for the treatment of idiopathic CNVM. For inflammatory CNVM, these are usually used in conjunction with steroids or steroid-sparing

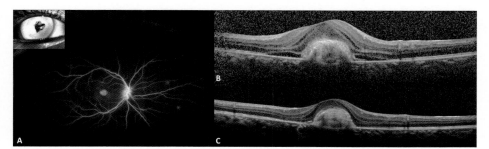

Fig. 39.1 (A) Fluorescein angiography (FA) shows a few areas of perivascular leakage, classic pattern of parafoveal leak, and optic disc hyperfluorescence in an 8-year-old girl with sarcoid panuveitis. Optical coherence tomography (OCT) scan through the fovea (B) shows an active choroidal neovascular membrane (CNVM) with subretinal hyperreflective material and subretinal fluid. After a single anti–vascular endothelial growth factor (VEGF) injection in conjunction with a course of prednisone and transition to steroid-sparing immunomodulatory therapy (adalimumab), there is resolution of the subretinal fluid and consolidation of the subretinal hyperreflective material (C). There is still persistence of the fibrotic lesion, which is likely to impact vision over the long term. Image A shows extensive posterior synechiae limiting the view for a clinical examination. In such cases, it is often possible to still obtain good-quality wide-field FA and OCT images, which are critical to clinical management.

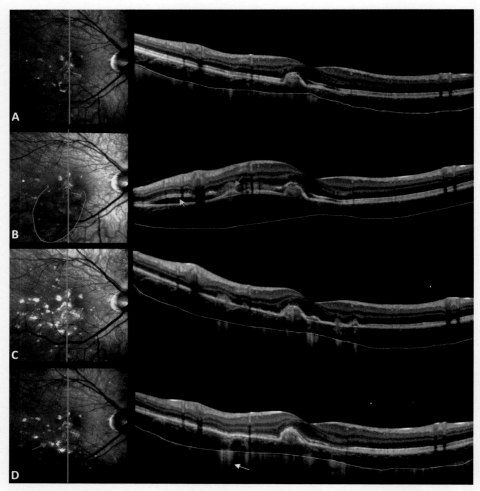

Fig. 39.2 Serial registered enhanced-depth optical coherence tomography (OCT) scans in a 15-year-old girl with punctate inner choroidopathy, initially seen with an inactive choroidal neovascular membrane (CNVM) (A) with normal choroidal thickness *(white dotted arrow)*. The patient then presented with recurrence of CNVM (B), with the hyporeflective area on the near infrared image *(yellow dotted line)* showing the extent of subretinal fluid. There was thickening of the choroid underlying the CNVM *(white dotted line)* with subretinal fluid *(yellow arrow)* and subretinal hyperreflective material *(orange arrow)*. After anti–vascular endothelial growth factor (VEGF) and steroid treatment and initiation of immunomodulatory therapy, there is resolution of the subretinal fluid (C) and a gradual reduction in the subretinal hyperreflective material and choroidal thickness. Once the CNVM was quiescent, there was improvement in the hyperreflective spots seen on the near infrared image (D, *red arrow)*. There was partial restoration of the external limiting membrane and ellipsoid zone, but despite resolution of fluid and normalization of choroidal thickness, there were increased hypertransmission defects consistent with small areas of persistent retinal pigment epithelium atrophy *(white arrow, D)*.

immunomodulatory therapy.[5] There is still, however, no consensus about the first-line immunomodulatory therapy in cases with inflammation. Adjunctive local steroids, such as subtenons triamcinolone injection, are a valuable option, with careful monitoring of side effects such as cataract and glaucoma. Anti-VEGFs cause rapid regression of the CNVM, and immunomodulatory therapy treats the underlying inflammatory disease. In general, pediatric inflammatory CNVM does not

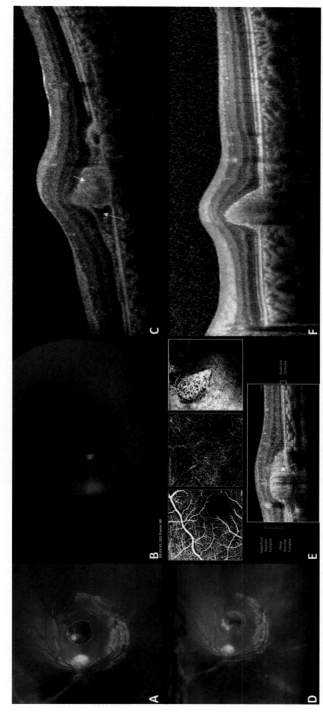

Fig. 39.3   Color photograph (A) from a 5-year-old girl with idiopathic panuveitis with choroidal neovascular membrane (CNVM) with subretinal hemorrhage (*yellow dotted area*). Fluorescein angiography (B) shows leakage from the CNVM, with blockage from the surrounding subretinal hemorrhage. Optical coherence tomography (OCT) (C) through the area corresponding to the white dotted line in image A shows subretinal hyperreflective material (*white arrow*) and subretinal fluid (*yellow arrow*). After treatment with anti-vascular endothelial growth factor (VEGF), steroids, and initiation of immunomodulatory therapy, there is resolution of the subretinal hemorrhage (D), subretinal fluid and consolidation of subretinal hyperreflective material (F). OCT angiography (OCTA) (E) at this visit shows a normal superficial and deep vascular complex (*red and blue bounding box*) and the avascular complex between the outer plexiform layer and the Bruch membrane (*yellow bounding box*) shows the CNVM lesion on the enface image (*yellow arrow*) with the OCTA flow overlay on the structural OCT (*white box*) showing high flow through the lesion (*white arrow highlights yellow speckled flow signal*).

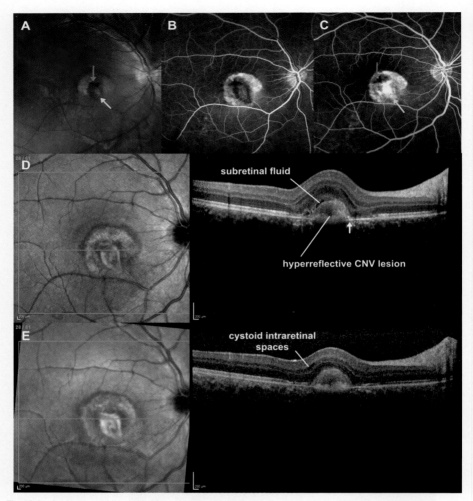

Fig. 39.4   A 10-year-old boy with idiopathic choroidal neovascular membrane (CNVM) *(yellow arrow)* and few dots of subretinal hemorrhage *(red arrow)* as shown on color photograph (A). No signs of vitritis or chorioretinal lesions suggestive of an underlying inflammatory process are observed. Visual acuity is 20/1250. Early (B) and late (C) frames of fluorescein angiography demonstrate circumferential staining with late leakage from the CNVM, and blocked fluorescence from the adjacent subretinal hemorrhage. OCT image (C) shows a sub–retinal pigment epithelium (RPE) hyperreflective lesion with ill-defined margins. The elevated RPE is denoted by the white arrow. There is also overlying subretinal fluid. After treatment with anti-VEGF injections, the CNV lesion appears inactive, as shown on OCT (D). Subretinal fluid has resolved, but minimal cystoid intraretinal spaces remain. The hyperreflective CNVM lesion also appears more consolidated with sharper margins. Visual acuity improves to 20/20.

need the same frequency of anti-VEGF treatment as in adults because the CNVM often involutes with much fewer anti-VEGF injections once the underlying inflammatory process is controlled. It is important to recognize that VEGF has an important role in normal angiogenesis, regulation of vessel permeability, and maintenance of the blood–brain barrier. Although there have been no adverse events reports with the use of anti-VEGF agents in children, long-term results of inhibiting the functions of VEGF, especially in younger children, need to be further evaluated.[8]

References

1. Sivaprasad S, Moore AT. Choroidal neovascularisation in children. *Br J Ophthalmol.* 2008;92:451–454.
2. Sears J, Capone Jr A, Aaberg Sr T. Surgical management of subfoveal neovascularization in children. *Ophthalmology.* 1999;106:920–924.
3. Spraul CW, Grossniklaus HE. Characteristics of Drusen and Bruch's membrane in postmortem eyes with age-related macular degeneration. *Arch Ophthalmol.* 1997;115:267–273.
4. Gass JD. Biomicroscopic and histopathologic considerations regarding the feasibility of surgical excision of subfoveal neovascular membranes. *Trans Am Ophthalmol Soc.* 1994;92:91–111; discussion 111-116.
5. Rishi P, Gupta A, Rishi E, Shah BJ. Choroidal neovascularization in 36 eyes of children and adolescents. *Eye (Lond).* 2013;27:1158–1168.
6. Daniels AB, Jakobiec FA, Westerfeld CB, Hagiwara A, Michaud N, Mukai S. Idiopathic subfoveal choroidal neovascular membrane in a 21-month-old child: ultrastructural features and implication for membranogenesis. *J AAPOS.* 2010;14(3):244–250.
7. Veronese C, Maiolo C, Huang D, et al. Optical coherence tomography angiography in pediatric choroidal neovascularization. *Am J Ophthalmol Case Rep.* 2016;2:37–40.
8. Kozak I, Mansour A, Diaz RI, et al. Outcomes of treatment of pediatric choroidal neovascularization with intravitreal antiangiogenic agents: the results of the KKESH International Collaborative Retina Study Group. *Retina.* 2014;34:2044–2052.

Trauma and Retial Detachment

CHAPTER 40

Nonaccidental Trauma

Wenlan Zhang ■ Lejla Vajzovic

Introduction

Nonaccidental trauma (NAT) or abusive head trauma, formerly referred to as *shaken baby syndrome*, occurs in the setting of head trauma in child abuse.[1-3] It occurs in an infant or child younger than age 5 years when there is violent shaking or abrupt impact with rapid acceleration–deceleration leading to ophthalmic injuries, most readily apparent in the posterior segment.[1,3] Eye findings may manifest in 30% to 40% of child abuse victims.[1]

The Brain Connection

Head trauma and brain trauma are common in cases of NAT with retinal findings and may include epidural, subdural, subarachnoid, intraventricular, and intraparenchymal hemorrhages.[1,2] Skull fractures, cortical contusions, malignant cerebral edema, and diffuse axonal injury may be present.[1,2] The main neurologic manifestations from abusive head trauma include altered consciousness, seizures, and developmental delay.[1,2] In addition, both retinal and neurologic ischemia may occur.[4]

Clinical Features

The most common examination findings include multilayered retinal hemorrhages that occur in the preretinal, intraretinal, and subretinal spaces, occurring in 60% to 85% of nonaccidental head injuries (Fig. 40.1). Hemorrhages in both eyes that extend all the way to the ora serrata especially raise suspicions of abuse. Vitreous hemorrhage and cotton-wool spots may be found; tractional retinal detachment, retinoschisis, retinal folds, macular hole, and retinal ischemia may also occur.

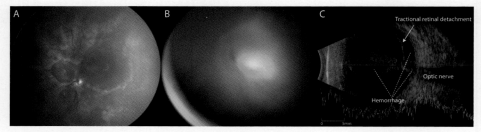

Fig. 40.1 Fundus photographs of the left eye in a 7-week-old infant with (A) numerous preretinal, intraretinal, and subretinal hemorrhages at presentation and (B) evolving vitreous hemorrhage obscuring view of the nerve and macula 3 months later, with a nasal tractional retinal detachment on ocular ultrasonography (C).

OCT Features

Handheld optical coherence tomography (OCT) is often necessary to image young children.[5,6] OCT findings in NAT may include focal separation of the posterior vitreous, as well as subhyaloid/preretinal, intraretinal (e.g., sub–internal limiting membrane [ILM]), and/or subretinal hemorrhages. Moreover, multilayered retinoschisis, disruption of the foveal architecture (including full-thickness macular hole or pseudohole),[6] and subretinal fluid in cases of retinal detachment may be observed (Fig. 40.2). Inner retinal thickening and hyperreflectivity consistent with acute retinal ischemia may also be present (Fig. 40.2). Outer retinal and inner retinal folds have been shown at the site of a pale retinal ring, which is sometimes found encircling the macula.[5] OCT imaging may also be especially helpful in distinguishing retinal pathology (e.g. partial versus full thickness macular hole) immediately after vitrectomy for removal of hemorrhage or associated preretinal tissue.[5,6]

Ancillary Testing

A multidisciplinary approach is necessary in the treatment of suspected child abuse victims. General and focused physical examinations are important. Possible explanations such as accidental trauma, pathologic bone disease, blood dyscrasias, and coagulopathies should be investigated.[1-3] However, because of the devastating consequences of abusive head trauma in children (25%–30% of victims die, and only 15% survive without sequelae of injuries), it is important to evaluate for brain, respiratory, and skeletal injuries.[1,2] When ophthalmic findings are observed, examination findings should be documented with fundus photography.

Treatment

Early recognition and identification of abuse victims is key, with immediate involvement of social services and child protective services. In cases of vitreous hemorrhage and retinal detachment, pars plana vitrectomy may be necessary. Long-term treatment and rehabilitation for visual and neurologic disabilities may be needed in survivors.

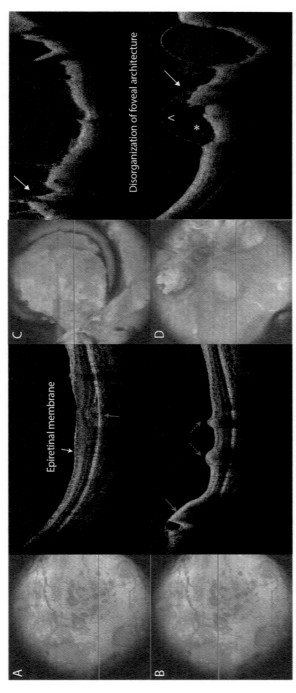

Fig. 40.2 Infrared images and optical coherence tomography (OCT) of the right (A–B) and left (C–D) eyes of an infant with NAT. Hemorrhages appear hyperreflective and are present in multiple layers as noted by the red arrows: pre-retinal or sub-ILM (B), intraretinal (B, dotted arrows), and subretinal (A). OCT reveals multiple areas of traction with retinal elevation (B–D, white arrows) due to the hemorrhagic separation of posterior vitreous and/or internal limiting (ILM) from the retinal surface – both processes that are best seen/distinguished in the left eye (D, ^ vitreous separation, and * ILM separation). In contrast to the distinct retinal layers in the right eye (A–B), in the left eye (C–D), the inner retina is thickened and hyperreflective, with loss of ganglion cell layer distinction, revealing widespread retinal ischemia. Shadowing by the hemorrhage in both eyes and by the inner retina in the left eye, leads to focal or widespread areas where it is difficult to assess the outer retina.

References

1. Paul AR, Adamo MA. Non-accidental trauma in pediatric patients: a review of epidemiology, pathophysiology, diagnosis and treatment. *Transl Pediatr.* 2014;3(3):195–207.
2. Sieswerda-Hoogendoorn T, Boos S, Spivack B, Bilo RA, van Rijn RR. Abusive head trauma. Part I: clinical aspects. *Eur J Pediatr.* 2012;171:415–423.
3. Eliott D, Papakostas TD. Chapter 94: Traumatic chorioretinopathies. In: Schachat AP, ed. *Ryan's Retina.* 6th ed. China: Elsevier; 2018.
4. Caputo G, de Haller R, Metge F, Dureau P. Ischemic retinopathy and neovascular proliferation secondary to shaken baby syndrome. *Retina.* 2008;29(1):127.
5. Scott AW, Farsiu S, Enyedi LB, Wallace DK, Toth CA. Imaging the infant retina with a hand-held spectral-domain optical coherence tomography device. *Am J Ophthalmol.* 2009;147(2):364–373.
6. Seider MI, Tran-Viet D, Toth CA. Macular pseudo-hole in shaken baby syndrome: underscoring the utility of optical coherence tomography under anesthesia. *Retin Cases Brief Rep.* 2016;10(3):283–285.

Ocular Injury

Wenlan Zhang ▪ Lejla Vajzovic

Introduction

Penetrating and nonpenetrating ocular trauma can result in open-globe or closed-globe injuries with a variety of posterior segment pathology. Careful examination of both the globe and the orbit is necessary in these patients.

The Brain Connection

Although head trauma may have occurred in injuries leading to ocular trauma, isolated ocular injuries are not typically associated with neurologic manifestations.

Clinical Features

Open-globe injuries may be associated with vitreous hemorrhage, retinal tears, retinal detachment, or retained intraocular foreign bodies (Fig. 41.1).[1,2] Closed-globe injuries may result in hemorrhage at various levels (Chapter 40), macular holes (Chapter 42), commotio retinae, choroidal ruptures, sclopetaria (Chapter 43), or retinal detachment (Chapter 45).[1,2]

OCT Features

Anterior and posterior segment OCT imaging can help identify various features that are associated with blunt or penetrating trauma. Anterior segment OCT has been shown to help identify angle recession (Fig. 41.2), peripheral anterior synechiae, pupillary block angle closure, iridodialysis, and clyclodialysis.[3] Posterior segment OCT can highlight the presence of subretinal fluid that helps differentiate retinal detachment from retinoschisis (Chapter 45). OCT can be used to identify traumatic macular holes (Chapter 42) and traumatic injuries to the outer retina, such as those seen in choroidal rupture and commotio retinae (Chapter 43). Disruption of outer retinal layers at presentation is often a predictor of poor visual prognosis.[1] Thus OCT can help with patient education and discussion of expectations. OCT can be of little use in the setting of severe anterior segment disruption, cataract, vitreous hemorrhage, or large intraretinal hemorrhage. OCT may, however, help distinguish the location of less severe hemorrhages in the subhyaloid, intraretinal, and subretinal

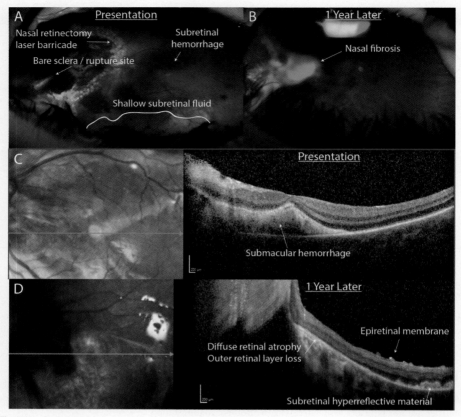

Fig. 41.1 Postretinal detachment repair with nasal retinectomy and laser in a 14-year-old boy who had suffered an open-globe injury (caused by a small metal ball shot from an air rifle, also known as a BB) with inferonasal site of rupture (A) and hyperreflective submacular hemorrhage on optical coherence tomography (OCT) (C). Fundus photo 1 year after surgery shows attached posterior pole with nasal fibrosis and silicone oil fill (B). OCT 1 year after surgery shows extensive loss of outer retinal layers, retinal atrophy, epiretinal membrane, and both preretinal and subretinal hyperreflective material (D) consistent with fibrotic membranes. Elevated nasal tissue shadows the choroid and sclera and has a "flip" artifact on the B-scan.

locations. In particular, eyes following nonaccidental trauma (NAT) often present with blood in all layers; OCT can help document this in these cases (Chapter 40).

Ancillary Testing

Computed tomography (CT) is helpful in cases of suspected open-globe injuries or injuries extending into the orbit. B-scan ultrasonography may additionally help evaluate the posterior globe, especially in the setting of vitreous hemorrhage when the posterior segment cannot be visualized.

Treatment

Regular follow-up care is necessary to monitor for treatable sequelae of posterior traumatic injuries. Prevention of further ocular trauma is equally important. Wearing protective eyewear and polycarbonate spectacles after ocular trauma should be emphasized to patients.

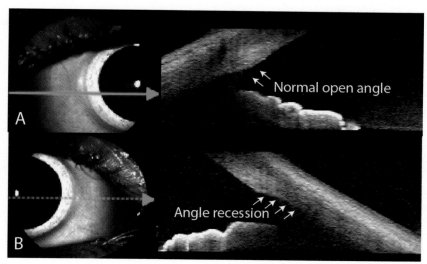

Fig. 41.2 Anterior segment optical coherence tomography (OCT) with nasal angle recession and normal temporal angle in 14-year-old boy who had suffered blunt ocular trauma (A and B). OCT provides documentation of angle configuration to monitor the patient over time. OCT image quality is limited deeper into angle towards location of iris root and ciliary body.

References

1. Puodžiuvienė E, Jokūbauskienė G, Vieversytė M, Asselineau K. A five-year retrospective study of the epidemiological characteristics and visual outcomes of pediatric ocular trauma. *BMC Ophthalmol.* 2018;18 (1):10.
2. Eliott D, Papakostas TD. Chapter 94: Traumatic chorioretinopathies. In: Schachat AP, ed. *Ryan's Retina.* 6th ed. China: Elsevier; 2018.
3. Akil H, Minasyan L, Francis BA, Chopra V. Utility of anterior segment swept-source optical coherence tomography for imaging eyes with antecedent ocular trauma. *Am J Ophthalmol Case Rep.* 2016;3:18–21.

CHAPTER 42

Traumatic Macular Hole

Wenlan Zhang ■ Lejla Vajzovic

Introduction

Full-thickness macular holes may develop after blunt ocular trauma, and the incidence ranges from 1% to 9% following such trauma.[1-3] Blunt force is thought to be transmitted to the macula through sudden globe compression resulting in foveal "rupture," or postcontusion changes, with cystoid degeneration and anteroposterior vitreofoveal traction.[2] Full-thickness and lamellar macular holes have also been reported in nonaccidental trauma.

The Brain Connection

Brain injury is not associated with blunt ocular injury alone and with macular hole, although one should inquire about the extent of head injury. Nonaccidental trauma is associated with brain injury.

Clinical Features

Visual acuity may range from 20/40 to 20/400 with symptomatic metamorphopsia or central scotoma, although vision may be worse if other traumatic findings are present. The lesion appears as a full-thickness, sharply defined hole in the center of the macula. Rarely, full-thickness macular holes may be associated with choroidal rupture, intraretinal and subretinal hemorrhage, and retinal detachment.[3] In nonaccidental trauma, the macular hole may be obscured by hemorrhage of the vitreous, subhyaloid, or sub–internal limiting membrane (ILM) (see Chapter 40).

OCT Features

Optical coherence tomography (OCT) is key to diagnosing and monitoring a traumatic macular hole.[2-4] OCT can distinguish various lamellar holes (rupture of either inner and outer retinal layers) from full-thickness macular holes.[2,3] Traumatic macular holes tend to have a larger basal diameter and to be more eccentric or elliptical and less circular in appearance compared with idiopathic full-thickness macular holes.[2] They may have a surrounding cuff of subretinal fluid, intraretinal cystic changes, or an epiretinal membrane.[2] Associated outer retinal atrophy is often seen. The hyaloid oftentimes remain attached in these eyes (Fig. 42.1).[2]

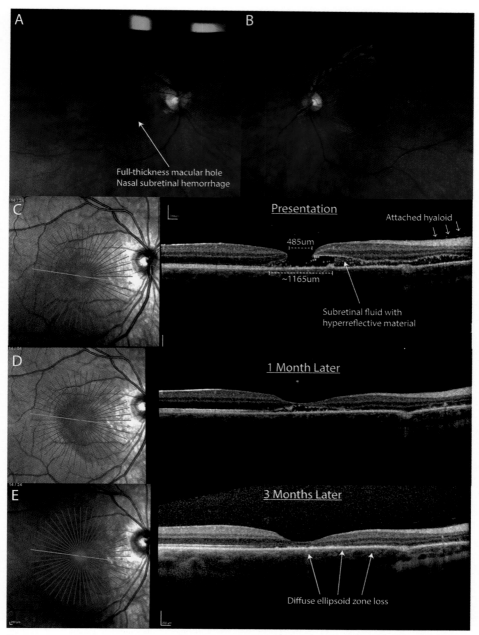

Fig. 42.1 Optos images of 15-year-old male hit in the right eye with a baseball, resulting in a traumatic full-thickness macular hole and adjacent nasal subretinal hemorrhage with 20/320-2 best corrected visual acuity (A) and normal left fundus (B). Optical coherence tomography (OCT) at presentation showed a large full-thickness macular hole with punctate hyperreflective material and nasal hyperreflective subretinal fluid (C). The hole closed spontaneously 1 month after trauma, with bridging retinal tissue, decreasing nasal subretinal fluid, and outer retinal layer disruption (D). At 3 months after injury, the hole remained closed with diffuse ellipsoid zone and interdigitation zone loss in areas of resolved fluid (E). Vision improved to 20/160 level.

OCT evaluation is especially relevant because several of the OCT-determined parameters—smaller diameter holes, eyes with intact posterior hyaloid, and holes with less intraretinal cysts—have been associated with higher rates of spontaneous closure.[4] Spontaneous closure is theorized to result from bridging glial elements, ILM, or formed vitreous gel in younger patients.[2,4-7]

In nonaccidental trauma, OCT is useful to distinguish lamellar hole from full-thickness hole at the time of removal of vitreous and macular hemorrhage (for nonaccidental trauma, see Chapter 40).

Ancillary Testing

Careful dilated examination should also be performed to rule out peripheral retinal pathology in trauma cases.

Treatment

Spontaneous closure in pediatric traumatic macular holes is reported to occur at a high rate in 2 weeks to 12 months after trauma (see Fig. 42.1).[1-3,7] Mitamura et al. reported a spontaneous closure in 6 of 11 such cases.[7] Although there is no consensus on how long to wait for spontaneous closure, 6 months with close follow-up, has been suggested.[1-2,4-8] Although traumatic macular hole closure has been reported after use of topical nonsteroidal antiinflammatory drugs,[2,9] information, to date, is very limited.

For holes that do not close or those that seem to be worsening on follow-up, therapeutic approaches have included vitrectomy.[2,10] Notably, the adherent hyaloid in pediatric patients make vitrectomy more challenging than in adult patients with traumatic macular holes. Adjunctive procedures, such as ILM peeling or ILM flap, autologous plasma-rich plasmin, intraocular gas, or silicone oil tamponade, remain controversial in this setting.

References

1. Gill M, Lou P. Traumatic macular holes. *Int Ophthalmol Clin.* 2002;42:97–106.
2. Liu W, Grzybowski A. Current management of traumatic macular holes. *J Ophthalmol.* 2017;2017:1748135.
3. Eliott D, Papakostas TD. Chapter 94: Traumatic chorioretinopathies. In: Schachat AP, ed. *Ryan's Retina.* 6th ed. China: Elsevier; 2018.
4. Chen H, Chen W, Zheng K, Peng K, Xia H, Zhu L. Prediction of spontaneous closure of traumatic macular hole with spectral domain optical coherence tomography. *Sci Rep.* 2015;5:12343.
5. Pascual-Camps I, Barranco-Gonzalez H, Dolz-Marco R, et al. Spontaneous closure of traumatic macular hole in a pediatric patient. *J AAPOS.* 2017;21(5):414–416.
6. Miller JB, Yonekawa Y, Eliott D, et al. Long-term follow-up and outcomes in traumatic macular holes. *Am J Ophthalmol.* 2015;160(6):1255–1258.
7. Mitamura Y, Saito W, Ishida M, Yamamoto S, Takeuchi S. Spontaneous closure of traumatic macular hole. *Retina.* 2001;21(4):385–389.
8. Azevedo S, Ferreira N, Meireles A. Management of pediatric traumatic macular holes—case report. *Case Rep Ophthalmol.* 2013;4(2):20–27.
9. Li AS, Ferrone PJ. Traumatic macular hole closure and visual improvement after topical nonsteroidal antiinflammatory drug treatment. *Retin Cases Brief Rep.* 2018;.
10. Singh DV, Reddy RR, Kuniyal L, Sharma YR. Excellent visual outcome after vitrectomy for traumatic macular hole associated with choroidal rupture across papillomacular bundle. *Oman J Ophthalmol.* 2018;11(1):90–91.

CHAPTER 43

Commotio Retinae, Choroidal Rupture, and Sclopetaria

Wenlan Zhang ■ Lejla Vajzovic

Introduction

Commotio retinae, choroidal rupture, and sclopetaria are common sequelae from blunt trauma to the globe.[1]

The Brain Connection

None.

Clinical Features

Commotio retinae is characterized by opacification of the deep retina and can range from subtle retinal whitening to widespread retinal opacification. The retinal whitening is hypothesized to occur from sheering of the photoreceptor outer segments.[1,2] This results in intracellular and extracellular edema and loss of retinal transparency. The retinal whitening is transient and resolves over time. Vision is affected when this occurs in the macula but often improves as the retinal whitening resolves.[2] However, in cases of severe commotio, the vision may never be fully recovered because affected areas are replaced by the retinal pigment epithelium (RPE) mottling, or intraretinal pigment deposition.[2]

Choroidal ruptures are tears in the choroid, Bruch membrane, and RPE, whereas the sclera and the retina remain intact.[1] They appear as hypopigmented curvilinear lesions that are concentric to the disc (Fig. 43.1). Acutely, they often occur with subretinal hemorrhage that results from trauma to the choriocapillaris.[3] The choroidal rupture typically develops a gliotic scar within weeks of the initial injury.[3]

In sclopetaria which is a rare consequence of ocular trauma, there is rupture of the choroid and retina, with intact underlying sclera.[1] Clinically, the fundus is characterized by the absence of retina, RPE, Bruch membrane, and choroid; there is often overlying vitreous, intraretinal, and subretinal hemorrhage (Fig. 43.2).[1,4]

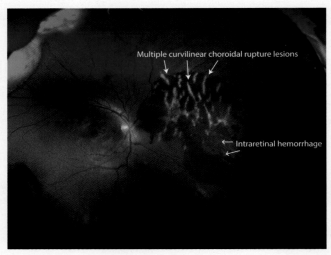

Fig. 43.1   Wide-field fundus photo of the right eye in a 14-year-old boy after closed-globe paintball injury with multiple nasal choroidal ruptures and subretinal hemorrhage.

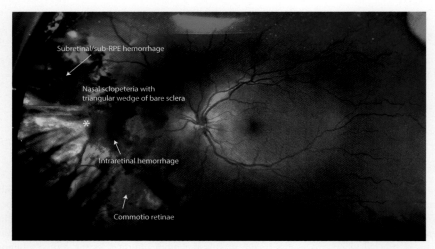

Fig. 43.2   Wide-field fundus photo of the left eye after paintball injury in a 16-year-old boy. There are extensive subretinal, intraretinal, preretinal, and vitreous hemorrhage, with a nasal wedge of bare sclera and adjacent retinal rupture consistent with sclopetaria. Optical coherence tomography (OCT) image capture is often limited by the overlying hemorrhage or the peripheral location out of reach of traditional OCT.

OCT Features

Optical coherence tomography (OCT) is helpful to predict the visual outcome in eyes with commotio retinae, although findings may vary.[2] There may be isolated hyperreflectivity of the ellipsoid zone, or loss of the hyporeflective space occupied by the outer segments of photoreceptors. Changes in adjacent retinal layers may also occur.[2] Other possible OCT changes include hyporeflectivity of the cone outer segment tips, and disruption of the ellipsoid zone and the external limiting membrane (Fig. 43.3).[2] Final visual acuity is worse in eyes that have involvement of multiple retinal layers.[2]

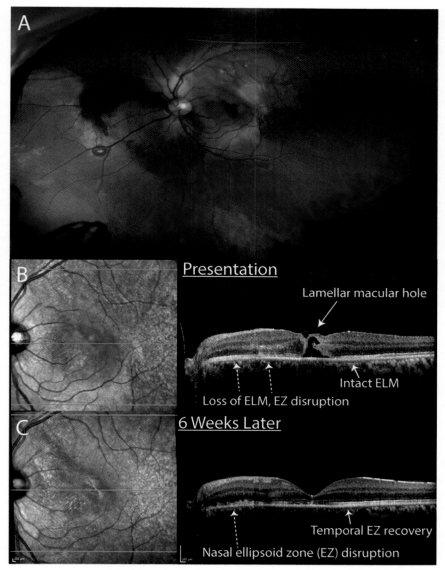

Fig. 43.3 (A) Wide-field fundus photo of the left eye of a 19-year-old female with extensive peripheral and macular commotio retinae after blunt trauma. (B) Initial optical coherence tomography (OCT) image shows a lamellar macular hole, nasal and temporal hyperreflectivity of the ellipsoid zone, and loss of the intervening space between the inner and outer segments. Disruption of the outer retinal layers is more extensive nasally compared with temporally. Nasally, there is ellipsoid zone irregularity and loss of definition of the external limiting membrane. (C) OCT image 6 weeks later shows that the temporal ellipsoid zone is better defined, suggestive of recovery of the temporal photoreceptors *(small solid arrow)*. The nasal outer retina remains disorganized *(dotted arrows)*.

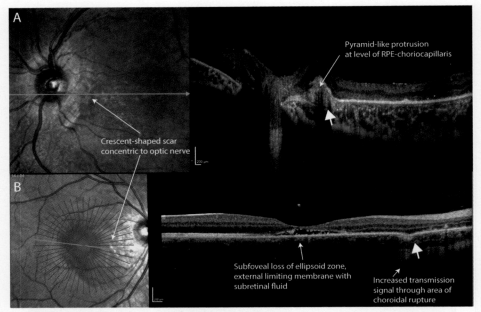

Figure 43.4 (A) Optical coherence tomography (OCT) image of the left eye of a 9-year-old male with a history of blunt trauma from a BB gun injury 2 months earlier. Infrared en face image demonstrates a peripapillary crescent-shaped scar which on the cross-sectional B scan corresponds to a loss of continuity of the retinal pigment epithelium (RPE) with an elevated pyramid-like protrusion (fibrosis versus piled-up RPE) at the level of RPE choriocapillaris through the choroidal rupture (*arrowhead*). (B) OCT of the right eye of a 15-year-old boy after blunt trauma. En face image shows a peripapillary scar concentric to the optic nerve, and this corresponds on the cross-sectional B scan to a loss of continuity of the RPE, resulting in a posteriorly directed concave contour depression. There is also subfoveal fluid with outer retinal atrophy.

In eyes with choroidal rupture, there may also be findings of commotio. Choroidal rupture on OCT may appear as a loss of continuity of the RPE with an elevated pyramid-like or dome-shaped protrusion of the RPE choriocapillaris (Fig. 43.4A).[3] Choroidal rupture may also appear as loss of continuity of the RPE with adjacent disruption of the ellipsoid zone and external limiting membrane, thus resulting in a posteriorly directed concave contour depression (see Fig. 43.4B).[3]

In acute sclopetaria, OCT is of limited use because of the overlying hemorrhage that blocks signal transmission.[4] There are no known published OCT images of acute sclopetaria. OCT of sclopetaria 1 year after ocular injury has been shown to demonstrate full-thickness hyperreflectivity with a transition zone from residual retina into full-thickness chorioretinal hyperreflectivity, which corresponds to a fibrogliotic lesion on clinical examination.[4]

Ancillary Testing

At the site of choroidal rupture, fundus autofluorescence may reveal hypoautofluorescence from loss of RPE. Red-free imaging, as well as the OCT en face image, may also highlight this finding. In eyes with choroidal rupture, there may be a risk of choroidal neovascularization developing at the site of rupture, and fluorescein angiography is useful in identifying late leakage in these eyes.[1,3]

Treatment

There is no treatment for acute commotio retinae or choroidal rupture.[1] Fortunately, extramacular lesions are usually asymptomatic. Commotio retinae affecting the macula may result in a spectrum of visual deficits, depending on the severity and number of retinal layers affected at the time of presentation.[2] It is important to monitor eyes with choroidal ruptures over time as choroidal neovascular membranes may develop and require treatment.[1,3]

References

1. Eliott D, Papakostas TD. Chapter 94: Traumatic chorioretinopathies. In: Schachat AP, ed. *Ryan's Retina*. 6th ed. China: Elsevier; 2018.
2. Ahn SJ, Woo SJ, Kim KE, et al. Optical coherence tomography morphologic grading of macular commotio retinae and its association with anatomic and visual outcomes. *Am J Ophthalmol*. 2013;156(5):994–1001.
3. Nair U, Soman M, Ganekal S, Batmanabane V, Nair K. Morphological patterns of indirect choroidal rupture on spectral domain optical coherence tomography. *Clin Ophthalmol*. 2013;7:1503–1509.
4. Rayess N, Rahimy E, Ho AC. Spectral-domain optical coherence tomography features of bilateral chorioretinitis sclopetaria. *OSLI Retina*. 2015;46(2):253–255.

Retinal Laser Injury

Glenn Yiu

Introduction

Ocular laser injury may result from various types of lasers in industrial, laboratory, or commercial settings, but children are particularly susceptible to injury from recreational lasers which may have been obtained through bypassing consumer safeguards.[1] The refractive structures of the eye focus visible light onto the posterior pole, so the irradiance on the surface of the neurosensory retina is amplified by five to six orders of magnitude. Although natural protective responses, such as blink reflex and pupillary constriction, reduce potential ocular exposure, the primary mode of protection is keeping lasers out of reach of children to prevent misuse.

The Brain Connection

Not applicable.

Clinical Features

The type of retinal injury resulting from lasers depend on the type (continuous versus pulsed emission, power, wavelength, etc.) and conditions of laser exposure (distance, duration, angle of incidence). Lower laser energy that are focused on more superficial layers of the retina may cause vitreous, preretinal (Fig. 44.1A–B), and intraretinal hemorrhages arising from injury to the retinal vessels, whereas higher laser energy applied to the deeper retinal layers may cause choroidal vessel damage that results in subretinal hemorrhages. The median effective dose (energy level necessary to produce a lesion in 50% of cases) measured in threshold studies in nonhuman primates is between 1.7 to 2.3 millijoules (mJ) for choroidal vessel damage and less than 7 microjoules (μJ) for retinal vessel injury. These values serve as a basis for determining laser exposure limits in humans, known as the *maximum permissible exposure (MPE) limits*, as reported in the standards for laser safety established by the American National Standards Institute (ANSI). Therapeutic application of ophthalmic lasers, such as diode or Argon green lasers used for panretinal photocoagulation (PRP) in the treatment of pediatric vitreoretinopathies (e.g., retinopathy of prematurity [ROP] and familial exudative vitreoretinopathy [FEVR]), result in hypopigmented spots or chorioretinal scars.

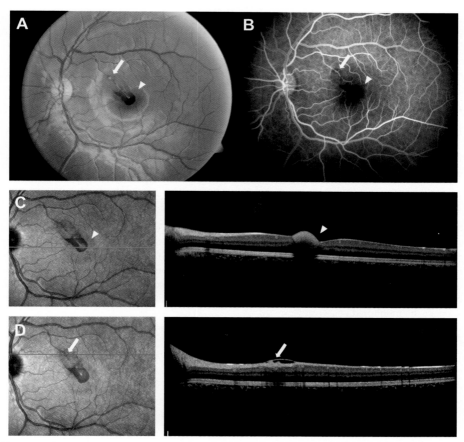

Fig. 44.1 (A) Color fundus photography showing a subhyaloid or sub–internal limiting membrane (ILM) hemorrhage *(arrowhead)* overlying the fovea, resulting from a retinal laser burn site *(arrow)* that damaged a retina vessel branch. (B) Fluorescein angiography (FA) showing blocked fluorescence from the preretinal hemorrhage *(arrowhead)* and no hyperfluorescence or leakage from the laser burn site *(arrow)*. (C) Spectral-domain optical coherence tomography (SD-OCT) image with corresponding infrared retinal image showing a hyperreflective collection on the surface of the retina with posterior shadowing *(arrowhead)* corresponding to the preretinal hemorrhage seen in images A and B. (D) SD-OCT image with corresponding infrared retinal image showing the presumed laser injury site at the retinal vessel *(arrow)* that resulted in the subhyaloid or sub-ILM hemorrhage seen in images A through C.

OCT Features

The features of retinal laser injury depend on the type and setting of the laser injury. Laser energy focused on superficial layers of the retina can result in retinal vessel damage.[2] Subhyaloid or sub–internal limiting membrane (sub-ILM) hemorrhages were caused by retinal vessel damage when a 9-year-old boy was playing with a blue 445 nm high-powered 1250 milliwatt (mW) recreational laser. The hemorrhage appears as a hyperreflective collection on the retinal surface with posterior shadowing (see Fig. 44.1C), even though minimal retinal damage can be detected at the laser injury site (see Fig. 44.1D). Laser energy focused into the deeper layers of the retina and retinal pigment epithelium (RPE) can lead to focally delineated areas of outer retinal damage, with loss of the external limiting membrane (ELM), inner segment ellipsoid zone (EZ), and/or interdigitation zone (IZ), similar to the damage seen in solar retinopathy. Finally, higher laser energy absorbed by the RPE may lead to a break in the Bruch membrane, hemorrhage and choroidal neovascularization (CNV), characterized by the presence of subretinal and/or sub-RPE hyper-reflective material or hyporeflective cystoid spaces if exudation occurs.

Ancillary Testing

Fluorescein angiography (FA) may demonstrate blocked fluorescence in the setting of retinal hemorrhages (see Fig. 44.1B) but may also demonstrate hyperfluorescence from leakage if CNV occurs. Fundus autofluorescence may demonstrate hypoautofluorescence in areas where the RPE is damaged.

Treatment

The treatment of retinal layer injuries depends on the nature of the injury and the degree of visual compromise. If vitreous, preretinal, or intraretinal hemorrhages occur, the patient may be only observed and the hemorrhage left to resolve spontaneously. If a large submacular hemorrhage occurs, pneumatic displacement or submacular surgery with subretinal injection of tissue plasminogen activator (tPA) may be necessary. The presence of CNV may necessitate intravitreal anti–vascular endothelial growth factor (anti-VEGF) therapy. Retinal injuries not involving the macula may generally be monitored conservatively.

References

1. Raoof N, Bradley P, Theodorou M, Moore AT, Michaelides M. The new pretender: a large UK case series of retinal injuries in children secondary to handheld lasers. *Am J Ophthalmol.* 2016;171:88–94.
2. Yiu G, Itty S, Toth CA. Ocular safety of recreational lasers. *JAMA Ophthalmol.* 2014;132(3):245–246.

CHAPTER 45

Retinal Detachment and Proliferative Vitreoretinopathy

Wenlan Zhang ▪ Lejla Vajzovic

Introduction

There are a multitude of etiologies for pediatric retinal detachments. These may be tractional, exudative, hemorrhagic, or rhegmatogenous. Rhegmatogenous retinal detachments may be traumatic in etiology, or be secondary to a preexisting hereditary vitreoretinopathy, such as Stickler syndome.[1,2] Here, we discuss rhegmatogenous retinal detachments.

The Brain Connection

Exudative retinal detachments associated with a morning glory disc anomaly may be associated with abnormalities of the brain (Chapter 61).

Clinical Features

Children often present with chronic retinal detachments with proliferative vitreoretinopathy (preretinal membranes, fixed folds, star folds, subretinal bands).[1,2] Diagnosis is often delayed because children readily compensate with their other eye in the setting of unilateral pathology. Moreover, progression tends to occur slowly as the vitreous is formed in children, and a posterior vitreous detachment is rare.[2]

Retinal dialysis, giant retinal tears, and lattice-associated tears are common etiologies for trauma-related retinal detachment. Vitreous base avulsion may also be a concurrent finding.[1,2]

OCT Features

Optical coherence tomography (OCT) may help distinguish subretinal fluid from retinoschisis. However, OCT utility is often limited by vitreous debris and retinal elevation. In some instances, OCT can help identify preretinal from subretinal membranes (Fig. 45.1). Moreover, in some situations, the status of the posterior hyaloid can be evaluated by using OCT.

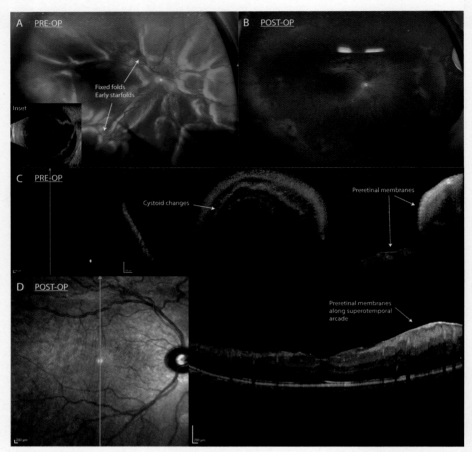

Fig. 45.1 A 19-year-old boy with chronic retinal detachment of the right eye after a basketball injury sustained 6 months earlier. Optos fundus photo shows total retinal detachment with pigment in the vitreous, fixed folds, and early star folds; superior giant retinal tear is not visualized on the photograph. Inset: B-scan shows total retinal detachment and stiff retina and suggests an attached hyaloid (A). Preoperative optical coherence tomography (OCT) image shows elevated thick retinal folds with intraretinal cystoid changes, subretinal fluid, and preretinal membranes (C). After buckle and vitrectomy, the retina is flat with peripheral chorioretinal scarring and pigmentary changes (B). Postoperative OCT shows attached macula with preretinal membranes and retinal thickening along the superotemporal arcade (D).

Ancillary Testing

Ultrasonography is often useful to determine the location and extent of retinal detachment in pediatric patients and may also help determine the status of the hyaloid (Fig. 45.1 A, inset). If there is concern about a predisposition for traumatic retinal detachment (particularly if the fellow eye has significant lattice or vitreous veils), genetic testing for Stickler may be indicated.

Treatment

Retinal detachment repair may be considered in a staged approach in children with traumatic retinal detachments.[2] Scleral buckle with or without cryotherapy is often sufficient in certain situations (especially in treatment of retinal dialysis).[1,2] If vitrectomy is necessary, dilute Triessence may be particularly helpful in visualizing the adherent hyaloid.[2] Occasionally, pars plana lensectomy is necessary for visualization.[2] Tamponade agents, such as gas or oil, are both good options.[2]

References

1. Eliott D, Papakostas TD. Chapter 94: Traumatic chorioretinopathies. In: Schachat AP, ed. *Ryan's Retina.* 6th ed. China: Elsevier; 2018.
2. Read SP, Aziz HA, Kuriyan A, et al. Retinal detachment surgery in a pediatric population: visual and anatomic outcomes. *Retina.* 2018;38:1393–1402.

Tumors and Hamartomas

Retinoblastoma

Prithvi Mruthyunjaya

Introduction

Retinoblastoma (Rb) is the most common primary ocular malignancy in children, with approximately 2300 new cases per year. Mutations in the *Rb1* tumor suppressor gene result in heritable or sporadic forms of Rb, with the former increasing the risk of bilateral disease.

The Brain Connection

Trilateral retinoblastoma is diagnosed when an ectopic tumor is discovered in the pineal gland (pineoblastoma). It is typically found in children with hereditary disease and germline mutations. When uncontrolled, retinoblastoma can spread to the central nervous system (CNS), with poor prognosis for survival.

Clinical Features

Leukocoria and strabismus are common presenting signs. Typically, 50% of children present with unilateral Rb with multifocal tumors. Tumors are typically white, round, and elevated (Fig. 46.1). Intratumoral calcification and engorged vasculature feeding the tumor are also hallmark findings. Associated subretinal fluid, sometimes leading to exudative retinal detachment, and satellite lesions, called *seeds*, can be found in the vitreous cavity or subretinal space. Anterior segment involvement, orbital extension, and metastatic disease are uncommon but serious consequences.

OCT Features

Tumors typically less than 2.5 mm in thickness may be fully imaged by optical coherence tomography (OCT), but visualization of the posterior tumor edge may be limited by shadowing from intratumoral calcium. Early Rb tumors may be seen as almond-shaped, hyperreflective lesions that are presumed to originate from within the inner nuclear layer (Fig. 46.2).[1] Intratumoral calcium may cause microshadowing of the OCT signal (Fig. 46.3). Larger tumors can occupy the full

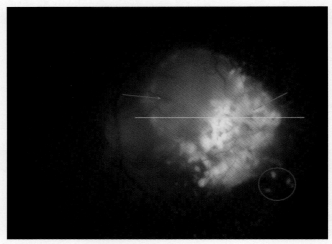

Fig. 46.1 A 3-year-old male child with a large macular retinoblastoma tumor, showing a white domed component *(green arrow)* and a bright white calcific component *(orange arrow)*. Prominent vitreous seeds are seen surrounding the tumor *(blue arrow)*.

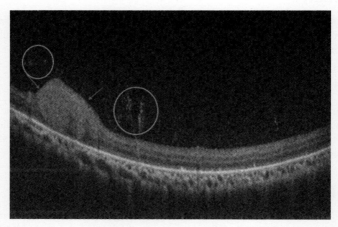

Fig. 46.2 Handheld spectral-domain optical coherence tomography (SD-OCT) images of a retinoblastoma tumor located within the inner nuclear layer and extending to the outer nuclear layer. Dustlike vitreous seeds *(orange circle)* can be seen overlying the tumor mass.

thickness of the retina and the subretinal space. Associated features, such as subretinal fluid or intravitreal seeds, can also be evaluated.[1]

OCT can help monitor for new tumor formation or early tumor relapse during or after systemic or local therapy (Figs. 46.4 through 46.7).[2,3]

Ancillary Testing

Wide-angle fundus photography aids in documenting existing as well as treated lesions. Fluorescein angiography demonstrates dilated vasculature with late leakage. Ultrasonography may reveal highly

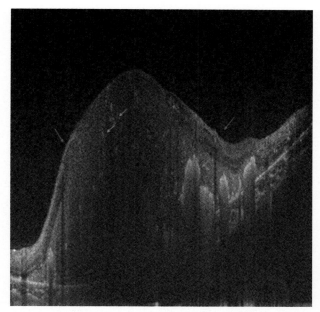

Fig. 46.3 Handheld spectral-domain optical coherence tomography (SD-OCT) images from Fig. 46.1 (*yellow line* indicates scan location). The tumor has infiltrated the inner retina into the subretinal space. There is an abrupt transition *(blue arrow)* from intact neurosensory retina to retina replaced by the tumor mass. Tiny hyperreflective intra-tumoral foci of calcium are seen *(orange arrows)* with streaklike shadowing. Larger hyperreflective calcific foci are seen producing greater shadowing *(green arrows)*.

reflective foci within the tumors suggestive of intratumoral calcification. Orbital and brain imaging with magnetic resonance imaging (MRI) or computed tomography (CT) often reveals intratumoral calcification as well as CNS involvement, including ectopic tumors in the pineal gland.

Treatment

On the basis of accurate tumor size, number, and laterality, treatment is coordinated by a team of ocular oncologists, pediatric oncologists, and, sometimes, radiation oncologists. Advanced-grade unilateral Rb or neovascular glaucoma at presentation may benefit from primary enucleation. Bilateral disease is approached with systemic chemotherapy, with focal consolidation by laser thermotherapy or cryotherapy. Newer chemotherapy delivery via ophthalmic artery or intravitreal routes can be considered in experienced Rb centers. Radiation therapy is used rarely for globe salvage.

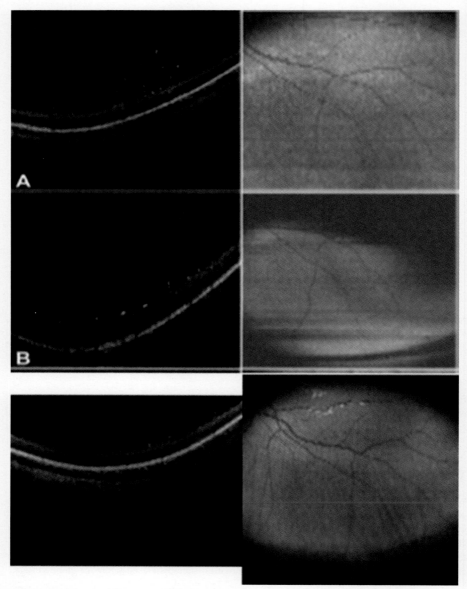

Fig. 46.4   Handheld spectral-domain optical coherence tomography (SD-OCT) peripheral scans demonstrating punctate vitreous seeds (A) not seen on clinical examination. After chemotherapy with intravitreal injection of melphalan, there is reduction in vitreous seeds with hyperreflective seeds on the retinal surface (B). After the third intravitreal melphalan injection, the size and density of the residual seeds continue to decrease. (Reprinted from Seider MI, Grewal DS, Mruthyunjaya P. Portable Optical Coherence Tomography Detection or Confirmation of Ophthalmoscopically Invisible or Indeterminate Active Retinoblastoma. *Ophthalmic Surg Lasers Imaging Retina*. 2016 Oct 1;47(10):965–968. PMID: 27759865.)

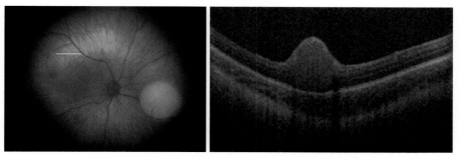

Fig. 46.5 A 2-week-old female infant with a small retinoblastoma lesion and prominent endophytic tumor located nasal to the optic nerve. On clinical examination, no obvious clinical tumor was detected in the macula. By using handheld spectral-domain optical coherence tomography (SD-OCT), a small discrete intraretinal hyper-reflective retinoblastoma tumor involving the inner and outer retinal was identified. This is an example of using OCT to identify clinically "invisible" tumors. (Reprinted from Seider MI, Grewal DS, Mruthyunjaya P. Portable Optical Coherence Tomography Detection or Confirmation of Ophthalmoscopically Invisible or Indeterminate Active Retinoblastoma. *Ophthalmic Surg Lasers Imaging Retina.* 2016 Oct 1;47(10):965–968. PMID: 27759865.)

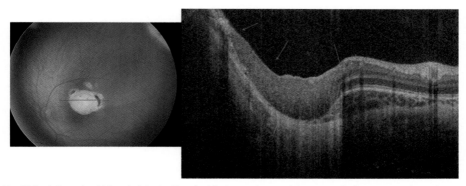

Fig. 46.6 A 2-week-old female infant with retinoblastoma after receiving systemic three-agent chemotherapy and two sessions of 810-nm diode laser thermotherapy to a macular tumor. The resultant inactive tumor is imaged with handheld spectral-domain optical coherence tomography (SD-OCT), which demonstrates a hyper-reflective homogeneous residual tumor mass *(blue arrows)* with loss of retinal layer differentiation. The underlying choriocapillaris is obliterated after laser therapy, with resultant staphyloma formation *(orange arrow).* (Reprinted from Seider MI, Grewal DS, Mruthyunjaya P. Portable Optical Coherence Tomography Detection or Confirmation of Ophthalmoscopically Invisible or Indeterminate Active Retinoblastoma. *Ophthalmic Surg Lasers Imaging Retina.* 2016 Oct 1;47(10):965–968. PMID: 27759865.)

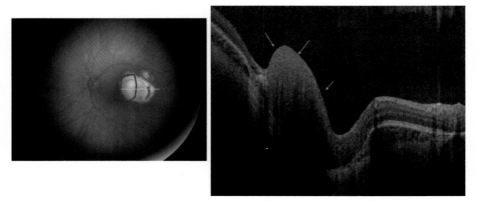

Fig. 46.7 Patient from Fig. 46.6 with clinical evidence of tumor reactivation *(blue outline).* Spectral-domain optical coherence tomography (SD-OCT) image demonstrates elevated reactivated tumor *(green arrow)* with inner retinal hyperreflectivity and shadowing.

References

1. Seider MI, Grewal DS, Mruthyunjaya P. Portable optical coherence tomography detection or confirmation of ophthalmoscopically invisible or indeterminate active retinoblastoma. *Ophthalmic Surg Lasers Imaging Retina.* October 1, 2016;47(10):965–968.
2. Berry JL, Cobrinik D, Kim JW. Detection and intraretinal localization of an 'invisible' retinoblastoma using optical coherence tomography. *Ocul Oncol Pathol.* 2016;2(3):148–152.
3. Soliman S, VandenHoven C, MacKeen L, Héon E, Gallie BL. Optical coherence tomography-guided decisions in retinoblastoma management. *Ophthalmology.* 2017;124(6):859–872.

CHAPTER 47

Diffuse Choroidal Hemangioma

Prithvi Mruthyunjaya

Introduction

Diffuse choroidal hemangioma is seen in nearly half the patients with Sturge-Weber syndrome.

The Brain Connection

Leptomeningeal angiomatosis may result in seizure disorder in young children with Sturge-Weber syndrome, resulting in developmental delay.

Clinical Features

Facial cutaneous hemangioma (nevus flammeus, or "port wine stain") is associated with ipsilateral glaucoma (in up to 70% of cases) and diffuse choroidal hemangioma (Fig. 47.1). The fundus has a characteristic "tomato ketchup" appearance, with associated exudative detachment and optic nerve cupping (Fig. 47.2).[1] Ipsilateral leptomeningeal hemangiomatosis may result in infantile seizures. Most diffuse hemangiomas are asymptomatic, but vision loss may occur from glaucoma or exudative retinal detachment (see Fig. 47.2).

OCT Features

There is engorgement of the choroid with enlarged large-caliber vessels inducing choroidal thickening seen on enhanced depth imaging–optical coherence tomography (EDI-OCT) (Fig. 47.3). Overlying subretinal fluid or intraretinal cystic changes may be seen. After treatment, the choroidal thickness may be reduced but usually is not normalized (Figs. 47.4 and 47.5).[2]

Ancillary Testing

B-scan ultrasonography reveals choroidal thickening, and an exudative retinal detachment may also be present (see Fig. 47.2). Magnetic resonance imaging (MRI) of the brain is used to detect leptomeningeal lesions.

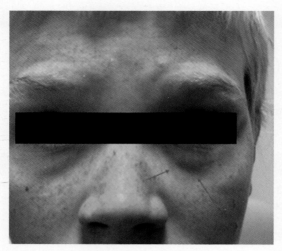

Fig. 47.1   External photograph of an 11-year-old male child with Sturge-Weber syndrome. Periocular cutaneous hemangioma (also called "port wine stain" or "nevus flammeus"), denoted by *arrows*, indicates the ipsilateral involved eye. Glaucoma is also a common finding in these eyes.

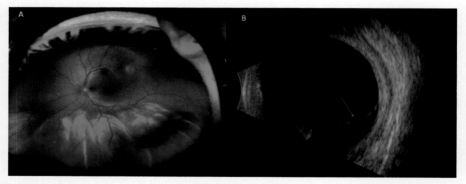

Fig. 47.2   (A) Pretreatment wide-field color photograph demonstrating extensive exudative retinal detachment associated with "tomato ketchup" fundus as a result of a diffuse cavernous choroidal hemangioma. Exudation may be initiated spontaneously or in response to ocular inflammation, after intraocular surgery or sudden intra-ocular pressure lowering. (B) Ultrasonography scan demonstrates diffuse choroidal thickening with exudative retinal detachment *(arrow)*.

Treatment

Intraocular pressure is managed by a pediatric glaucoma specialist. The hemangioma is treated in the setting of symptomatic or progressive retinal detachment or prophylactically prior to intraocular surgery. Low-dose external beam radiotherapy results in reduction in hemangioma thickness and resolution of retinal detachment. Intraocular or external drainage of subretinal fluid may be complicated by choroidal hemorrhage.

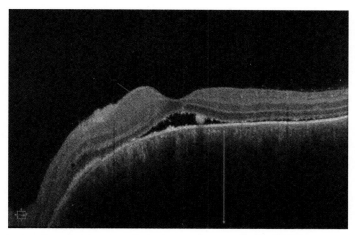

Fig. 47.3 Pretreatment spectral domain–optical coherence tomography (SD-OCT) demonstrates the massive choroidal expansion, with loose compaction of the inner choriocapillaris and shadowing more posteriorly into the choroid. The choroid is massively thickened, as noted where the optic nerve is barely visualized, but not the posterior sclero–choroidal junction. Serial scans failed to clearly identify the sclero–choroidal junction, indicating significant thickness of the choroid (arrow). Subretinal fluid is seen under the fovea with hyperreflective deposits along the retinal pigment epithelium (RPE) and neurosensory retina.

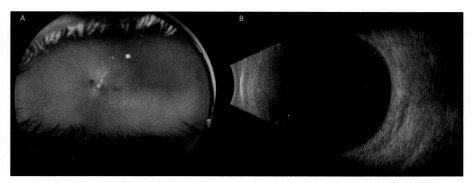

Fig. 47.4 (A) After treatment with external beam radiation therapy at 20 Gy, given over 10 fractions, there is complete resolution of the exudative retinal detachment and early development of retinal pigment epithelium (RPE) pigmentary changes. The "tomato ketchup" fundus appearance is more evident. (B) Ultrasonography scan demonstrates resolution of the exudative retinal detachment and slight decrease in overall choroidal thickening.

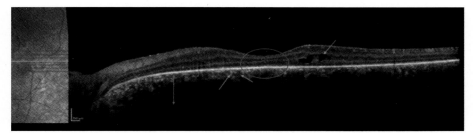

Fig. 47.5 Postradiation treatment optical coherence tomography (OCT) image. The reduction in choroidal thickening is apparent (blue double ended arrow). The inner choriocapillaris has speckled hyper- and hyporeflective areas with small lumen capillaries (orange arrows). The posterior choroidal shadowing is still present. The overlying neurosensory retina has persistent cystic retinal spaces (green arrow). The ellipsoid zone is incomplete with residual external limiting membrane in the subfoveal area (red circle).

References

1. Mantelli F, Bruscolini A, La Cava M, Abdolrahimzadeh S, Lambiase A. Ocular manifestations of Sturge-Weber syndrome: pathogenesis, diagnosis, and management. *Clin Ophthalmol.* 2016;10:871–878. https://doi.org/10.2147/OPTH.S101963. eCollection 2016.
2. Cacciamani A, Scarinci F, Parravano M, Giorno P, Varano M. Choroidal thickness changes with photodynamic therapy for a diffuse choroidal hemangioma in Sturge–Weber syndrome. *Int Ophthalmol.* 2014;34 (5):1131–1135.

CHAPTER 48

Circumscribed Choroidal Hemangioma

Prithvi Mruthyunjaya

Introduction

Circumscribed choroidal hemangioma is a benign vascular lesion associated with vision loss resulting from fluid and lipid exudation. It is uncommon in children but can be seen in association with diffuse chroidal hemangiomas.

The Brain Connection

Vision loss from chronic subretinal fluid in young children may result in amblyopia.

Clinical Features

Circumscribed choroidal hemangioma is a well-delineated and red-orange lesion that, when smaller, may be indistinguishable from the surrounding choroid (Fig. 48.1). Subretinal fluid exudation or cystoid macular edema may result in vision loss. Chronic lesions may have surface retinal pigment epithelium (RPE) hyperpigmentation or fibrosis (Fig. 48.2A).

OCT Features

Circumscribed choroidal hemangioma is an elevated, dome-shaped choroidal lesion with markedly engorged inner choriocapillaris vessels without compression (Fig. 48.3). Choroidal shadowing may be present as a result of increased blood within the hemangioma, often limiting view of the posterior choroidal scleral junction. Secondary overlying subretinal fluid, reflective material (fibrosis), and, in chronic cases, intraretinal cysts may be present (see Fig. 48.3).[1]

Ancillary Testing

B-scan ultrasonography reveals a well-circumscribed hyperreflective choroidal lesion (see Fig. 48.2B). These vascular lesions are visible in the early phases of indocyanine green angiography, with characteristic early washout and late staining in the recirculation phases. Fluorescein

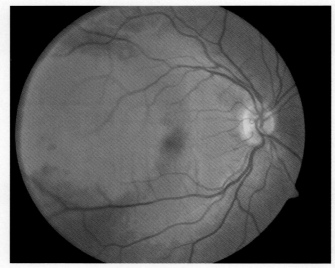

Fig. 48.1 Color fundus photograph of a young adult with elevated, circumscribed, red/orange lesion in temporal macula.

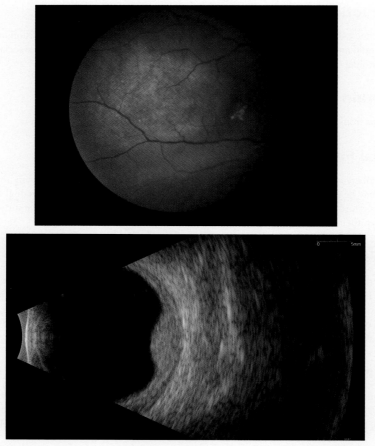

Fig. 48.2 (A) Digital single-lens reflex (SLR) fundus photograph shows the demarcated choroidal lesion with surface fibrosis. (B) Ultrasonography delineates the highly reflective choroidal lesion.

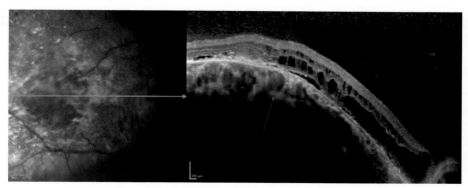

Fig. 48.3   Optical coherence tomography (OCT) reveals an elevated choroidal lesion with large-caliber, enlarged inner choroidal vessels, with shadowing limiting transmission to the outer scleral–choroidal junction. The overlying neurosensory retina shows separation from the subretinal fluid and retinal cystic thickening with irregular loss of the ellipsoid zone.

angiography may outline the image with late hyperfluoresence highlighted by pooling above the lesion from subretinal fluid collections.

Treatment

Asymptomatic lesions without subretinal fluid may be monitored. Actively exuding lesions should be treated with multisession verteporfin photodynamic therapy.[2] Resistant lesions may be treated with thermal ablation or plaque radiation brachytherapy, but there is a risk of collateral vision damage.

References

1. Rojanaporn D, Kaliki S, Ferenczy SR, Shields CL. Enhanced depth imaging optical coherence tomography of circumscribed choroidal hemangioma in 10 consecutive cases. *Middle East Afr J Ophthalmol.* 2015;22 (2):192–197.
2. Liu W, Zhang Y, Xu G, Qian J, Jiang C, Li L. Optical coherence tomography for evaluation of photodynamic therapy in symptomatic circumscribed choroidal hemangioma. *Retina.* 2011;31:336–343.

CHAPTER 49

Choroidal Osteoma

Prithvi Mruthyunjaya

Introduction

These benign lesions are choristomas that have associated intrachoroidal bone deposition.

The Brain Connection

None.

Clinical Features

Typically seen in teenage females, these lesions are asymptomatic unless there is fluid exudation resulting in vision changes. Lesions are unilateral, thin, or only minimally elevated and white-yellow in color. These are usually in the peripapillary location with associated variable retinal pigment epithelium (RPE) hyperpigmentation changes on the surface (Fig. 49.1). Secondary choroidal neovascularization (CNV) may be seen at the margin of the osteoma with subretinal fluid and subretinal hemorrhage (Fig. 49.2).

OCT Features

Lesions produce a minimally expanded choroid with a spongelike appearance (Fig. 49.3).[1,2] Horizontal lamellae, thought to be related to bone lamellae, are common. Secondary RPE deposits and outer retinal atrophy may be detected.[3] Osteoma-associated CNV may result in subretinal fluid and hyperreflective foci, which may represent blood or pigmentary deposits (Fig. 49.4).

Ancillary Testing

B-scan ultrasonography can detect hyperreflective foci, with orbital shadowing consistent with calcium and bone deposition. Fluorescein and/or indocyanine green angiography may detect secondary CNV (see Fig. 49.2).

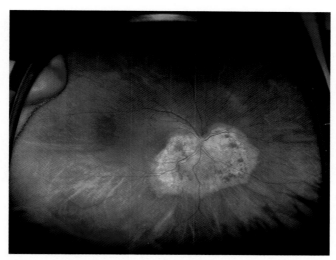

Fig. 49.1 Wide-angle color photo of a choroidal osteoma in a 10-year-old female. The osteoma nearly surrounds the optic nerve. The classic depigmentated lesion is seen with overlying speckled hypertrophy of the
retinal pigment epithelium (RPE). Note the pigmented subretinal choroidal neovascular membrane in the peripapillary region.

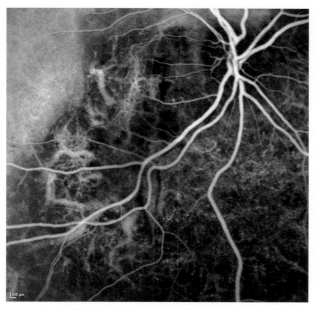

Fig. 49.2 Indocyanine green angiography demonstrates diffuse blockage of the choroidal fluorescence
throughout the osteoma. In the peripapillary region, the choroidal neovascular membrane is highlighted by
large- and small-caliber abnormal choroidal vessels.

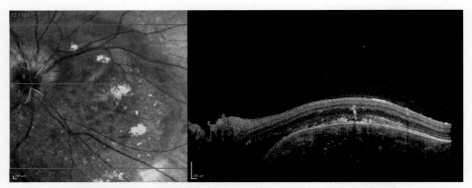

Fig. 49.3 Spectral-domain optical coherence tomography (SD-OCT) in the nasal region of the osteoma demonstrates the expanded choroidal region with horizontal patterns of hyporeflectivity (lamellae). The hyperreflective deposits in the retinal pigment epithelium (RPE) and the focal discontinuity of the ellipsoid zone are seen overlying the osteoma. Subretinal fluid is noted near the optic nerve.

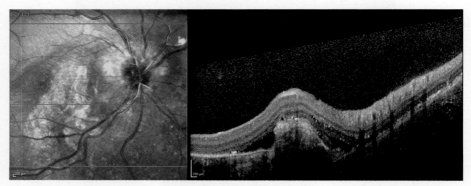

Fig. 49.4 Spectral-domain optical coherence tomography (SD-OCT) in the temporal peripapillary lesion demonstrates osteoma-associated choroidal neovascularization with mounded sub–retinal pigment epithelium (RPE) lesion with irregular reflectivity. Subretinal fluid and fine hyperreflective foci within tiny outer retinal cysts are noted.

Treatment

Several modalities of therapy of been attempted for CNV associated with choroidal osteomas, including argon laser, photodynamic therapy (PDT) with verteporfin, surgical excision, transpupillary thermotherapy (TTT), and anti–vascular endothelial growth factor (anti-VEGF) therapy. Attempts have also been made with decalcify these lesions, particularly if they occur within the fovea and cause vision loss.

References

1. Pellegrini M, Invernizzi A, Giani A, Staurenghi G. Enhanced depth imaging optical coherence tomography features of choroidal osteoma. *Retina.* 2014;34:958–963.
2. Freton A, Finger PT. Spectral domain-optical coherence tomography analysis of choroidal osteoma. *Br J Ophthalmol.* 2012;96:224–228.
3. Shields CL, Arepalli S, Atalay HT, Ferenczy SR, Fulco E, Shields JA. Choroidal osteoma shows bone lamella and vascular channels on enhanced depth imaging optical coherence tomography in 15 cases. *Retina.* 2015;35(4):750–757.

Combined Hamartoma of the Retina and Retinal Pigment Epithelium

Hesham Gabr ▪ Prithvi Mruthyunjaya

Introduction

Combined hamartoma is an uncommon, benign lesion that is caused by focal overgrowth of misarranged sheets of glial tissue, vascular tissue, and pigment epithelial cells. Patients with this lesion typically present during childhood with strabismus and/or reduced visual acuity.[1]

The Brain Connection

Combined hamartomas of the retina and retinal pigment epithelium (RPE), especially bilateral cases, have been strongly associated with and can be the presenting feature of neurofibromatosis type II (NF-II). NF-II manifests as bilateral vestibular schwannomas, which can affect hearing, balance, and trigeminal and facial nerve function when the tumors are small. As the tumors grow larger, they can compress the brainstem and cerebellum. Cases of combined hamartomas of the retina and RPE in NF-I, Gorlin-Goltz syndrome, branchiooculofacial syndrome, and juvenile nasopharyngeal angiofibroma have also been reported.[1] These syndromes can also present with central nervous system (CNS) manifestations.

Clinical Features

The tumor usually presents as a unilateral solitary elevated lesion in the macula (Figs. 50.1 and 50.2), around the optic nerve (Fig. 50.3), or at a peripheral location (Fig. 50.4). It can be dusky brown, green, yellow, gray, or orange in color. The lesion shows characteristic retinal vascular changes, as the distal vessels are straight from traction and intrinsic vessels are tortuous and corkscrewed from contraction. Vitreo–retinal interface changes, traction, fibrosis/gliosis, and epiretinal membrane (ERM) formation are common (see Fig. 50.2). Foveal dragging is seen in 100% of macular tumors and in 42% of extramacular tumors.[1]

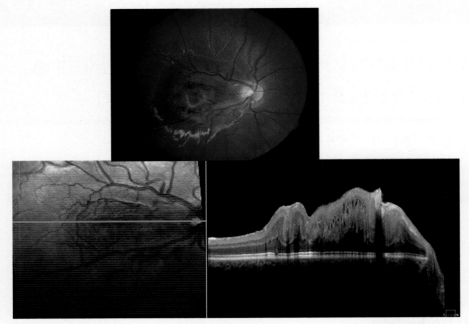

Fig. 50.1 (Top) Color photo of combined hamartoma of the retina and retinal pigment epithelium at the macula with a ring-shaped epiretinal membrane in a 12-year-old boy with grey pigmentation, thickening and an epiretinal membrane. (Lower image) Optical coherence tomography (OCT) image shows disorganized retinal architecture with retinal folds and two sites of more dense epiretinal membrane from the "ring", at the site of lesion and intraretinal hyporeflective spaces in the center of the lesion with normal adjacent retina. The infrared image on the left reveals tortuous mid-sized vessels beneath the epiretinal membrane.

OCT Features

Retinal anatomic disorganization with loss of identifiable retinal layers at the site of the lesion is seen in most cases (see Figs. 50.1 through 50.4). Preretinal fibrosis (see Fig. 50.1), epiretinal membrane (see Fig. 50.2), vitreoretinal interface changes (see Fig. 50.2), and retinal folds/striae (see Figs. 50.1 and 50.4) are prominent features.[2-4] Other features include foveal dragging (see Fig. 50.3), inner retinal hyperreflectivity, outer retinal hyporeflectivity (see Figs. 50.1, 50.2, and 50.4) and optical shadowing[2-4] (see Fig. 50.1). Although the adjacent flat retina appears to be of normal thickness and anatomic configuration (see Figs. 50.1 and 50.4), it gradually thickens into the disorganized retinal tissue at the site of the lesion.

Ancillary Test

Fluorescein angiography (FA) shows corkscrew-shaped blood vessels and early hypofluorescence as a result of blockage in the region of hyperpigmentation (see Fig. 50.2). In the arterial–venous phase, the lesion may show a fine network of abnormal dilated capillaries with leakage[1] (see Fig. 50.4). In the late phase, it may show leakage (see Fig. 50.4) from dilated tortuous vessels.[1] The peripheral lesions (see Fig. 50.4) are characterized on FA by straight blood vessels and relative avascularity.

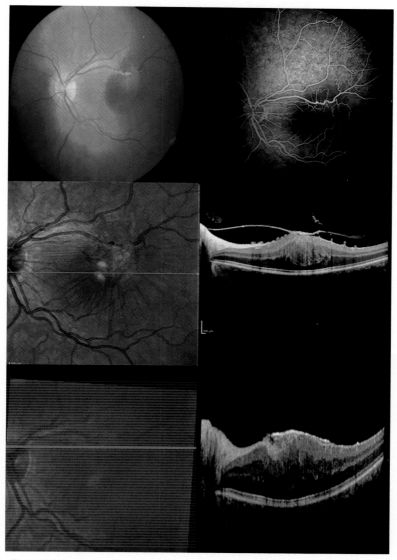

Fig. 50.2 (Top left) Color photo of combined hamartoma of the retina and retinal pigment epithelium in the superotemporal macula in a 13-year-old girl. (Top right) Fluorescein angiography image shows corkscrew-shaped vessels and blocked florescence caused by hyperpigmentation along with subtle hyperfluorescence within the central area of the hamartoma. (Middle row) Optical coherence tomography (OCT) image shows disorganized retinal architecture with partial vitreous separation and vitreoretinal interface changes. (Lower) OCT scan at a different location shows epiretinal membrane *(arrow)*.

Treatment

Management of combined hamartomas of the retina and RPE may often be observation only because they are usually nonprogressive and may have a limited impact on visual acuity. Indications for surgery include retinal traction induced by the ERM or vitreoretinal traction causing loss of

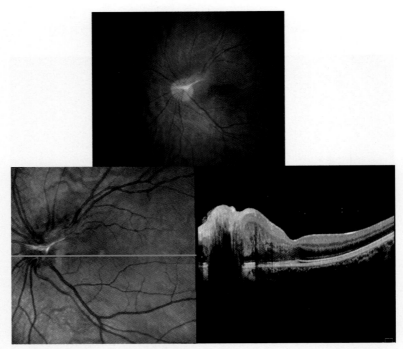

Fig. 50.3 (A) Color photo of peripapillary combined hamartoma of the retina and retinal pigment epithelium *(arrow)* in a 12-year-old girl. (B) Optical coherence tomography (OCT) image shows disorganized retinal architecture *(arrows)* at the optic disc with foveal dragging (*).

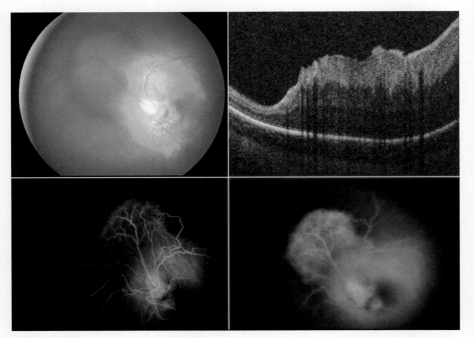

Fig. 50.4 (Top left) Color photo of a peripheral combined hamartoma of the retina and retinal pigment epithelium in a 2-year-old boy. (upper right) Optical coherence tomography (OCT) image within the area of the lesion shows disorganized retinal architecture and retinal folds with outer retinal hyporeflectivity and normal adjacent retina. (Lower left) Arterio–venous phase of fundus fluorescein angiogram (FA) shows straight blood vessels right and leakage from a network of abnormal dilated capillaries. (lower right) Late phase fundus FA shows leakage from the abnormal blood vessels and in areas of traction.

vision. OCT can provide important information regarding vitreo–retinal interface abnormalities caused by this tumor, which can influence surgical decision making. Given the strong association between this condition and NF-II, some authors have recommended screening children with combined hamartomas of the retina and RPE for NF-II.

References

1. Shields CL, Thangappan A, Hartzell K, Valente P, Pirondini C, Shields JA. Combined hamartoma of the retina and retinal pigment epithelium in 77 consecutive patients. *Ophthalmology.* 2008;115(12):2246–2252.
2. Shields CL, Mashayekhi A, Dai VV, Materin MA, Shields JA. Optical coherence tomographic findings of combined hamartoma of the retina and retinal pigment epithelium in 11 patients. *Arch Ophthalmol.* 2005;123 (12):1746–1750.
3. Arepalli S, Pellegrini M, Ferenczy SR, Shields CL. Combined hamartoma of the retina and retinal pigment epithelium: findings on enhanced depth imaging optical coherence tomography in eight eyes. *Retina.* 2014;34(11):2202–2207.
4. Chawla R, Kumar V, Tripathy K, et al. Combined hamartoma of the retina and retinal pigment epithelium: an optical coherence tomography-based reappraisal. *Am J Ophthalmol.* 2017;181:88–96.

CHAPTER 51

Retinal Astrocytic Hamartoma

Prithvi Mruthyunjaya

Introduction

Retinal astrocytic hamartomas (RAHs) as rare, benign tumors of the inner retina associated with the tuberous sclerosis complex.

The Brain Connection

RAHs are associated with the tuberous sclerosis complex. Subependymal nodules can be found in the brain and are associated with seizure disorders and mental retardation.

Clinical Features

These dome-shaped, yellow-white lesions are typically stationary in size (Figs. 51.1 and 51.2). There can be white calcific nodularities on the surface of the lesion (mulberry astrocytic hamartoma), but typically calcific foci are not detected. Lipid exudation and small vitreous seeds may develop. In rare cases, these lesions can grow rapidly with progressive retinal detachment and development of neovascular glaucoma.

RAHs are the most common intraocular manifestation of the tuberous sclerosis complex, occurring in nearly 50% of patients. Bilateral tumors are seen in 25% of patients.

OCT Features

Dome-shaped tumors are seen predominantly within the inner retina and specifically originating within the nerve fiber layer (Fig. 51.3). Outer layers can also be involved with overall full-thickness retinal disorganization in larger tumors (Fig. 51.4). Shadowing from the inner retinal tumors may limit clear identification of deeper involvement. A "moth-eaten" appearance may be seen, with optically empty spaces within the nerve fiber layer correlating with foci of intratumoral calcium.[1]

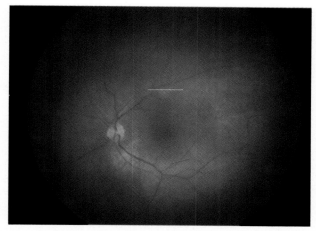

Fig. 51.1   A 13-month-old male child with a history of tuberous sclerosis complex with two *(blue arrows)* small retinal astrocytic hamartomas in the left macula. The superior lesion has a focal bright white calcium inclusion.

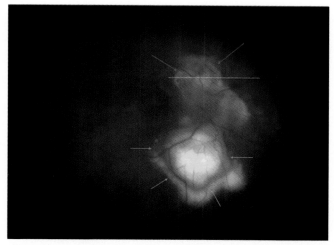

Fig. 51.2   Fellow eye of the patient in Fig. 51.1, with two peripapillary endophytic retinal astrocytic hamartoma *(blue arrow and orange arrows)* with extensive lipid exudation. Superior lesion imaged with handheld spectral-domain optical coherence tomography (SD-OCT), with the view obtained at the *yellow line*.

Ancillary Testing

Fundus photography and B-scan ultrasonography aid in documenting tumor margins to monitor for growth. Fluorescein angiography demonstrates generalized hyperfluoresence, with late leakage within the tumor. Fundus autofluoresence typically shows hypofundus autofluoresence with the exception of the "mulberry" variety, which has interspersed areas of focal bright hyperfundus auto-fluoresence corresponding to areas of calcium.

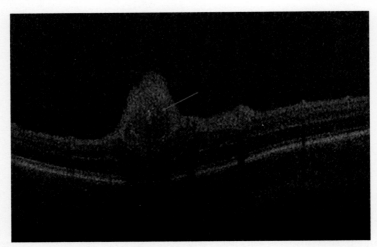

Fig. 51.3 Handheld spectral-domain optical coherence tomography (SD-OCT) image from patient in Fig. 51.1. The hyperreflective inner retinal tumor involves the nerve fiber layer, inner nuclear layer, and inner plexiform layer. There is a focus of bright hyperreflective calcium with a small optically empty space and a minimal variation of the "moth-eaten" appearance seen with extensive intralesional calcium.

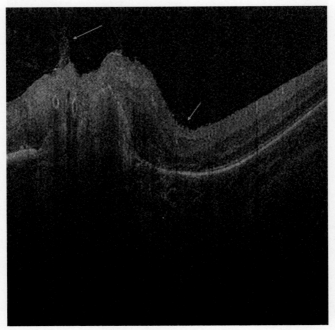

Fig. 51.4 Handheld spectral-domain optical coherence tomography (SD-OCT) image of Fig. 51.3. Bilobular lesion with inner retinal hyperreflectivity and plume of fine retinal seeds *(orange arrow)*. There are round hyperreflective vessel lumens seen within the lesions *(blue arrow)*. A thin epiretinal membrane is noted along the edge of the lesion *(green arrow)*.

Systemic testing, including neuroimaging (central nervous system subependymal nodules) and visceral tumor imaging (for renal and cardiac tumors), is indicated when looking for manifestations of tuberous sclerosis complex.

Treatment

Smaller tumors are monitored closely and typically are stationary and asymptomatic. Tumors developing signs of exudation must be watched closely. Treatment options include 810-nm diode laser thermotherapy, verteporfin photodynamic therapy, plaque brachytherapy, or systemic treatment with mechanistic target of rapamycin (mTOR) inhibitors.[2]

References

1. Shields CL, Benevides R, Materin MA, Shields JA. Optical coherence tomography of retinal astrocytic hamartoma in 15 cases. *Ophthalmology.* 2006;113:1553–1557.
2. Nallisamy N, Seider MI, Gururangan S, Mruthyunjaya P. Everolimus to treat aggressive retinal astrocytic hamartoma in tuberous sclerosis complex. *J AAPOS.* 2017;21(4):328–331.

CHAPTER 52

Retinal Capillary Hemangioblastoma

Prithvi Mruthyunjaya

Introduction

Retinal capillary hemangioblastoma (or hemangioma) (RCH) is a benign vascular proliferative tumor associated with retinal exudation and exudative retinal detachment. These may occur sporadically or as a manifestation of von Hippel Lindau (VHL) disease.

The Brain Connection

RCH is associated with VHL disease, which can manifest as cerebellar and spinal column hemangioblastomas. These can result in increased risk of seizure disorder, increased intracranial pressure and intracranial hemorrhage.

Clinical Features

There are two forms of these pink-red retinal vascular lesions. The endophytic variant is seen a pedunculated vascular tumor associated with dilated feeding arteriole and draining (Fig. 52.1). Located in the retinal periphery, these lesions typically enlarge over time and may produce lipid exudation and extensive exudative retinal detachment. Secondary surface epiretinal membrane proliferation can lead to traction retinal detachment as well. The exophytic variant is seen as a minimally elevated, domed, pink-grey lesion seen near the optic nerve (Fig. 52.2). The lesion is associated with lipid exudation and localized retinal detachment. When sporadic, these lesions may be unifocal, but when they develop as part of VHL disease, they are typically multifocal and bilateral.[1]

OCT Features

Endophytic tumors develop within the inner retina and are seen as hyperreflective, circumscribed lesions with significant posterior shadowing (Fig. 52.3). Rarely intratumoral vascular channels may be detected. Associated surface epiretinal membrane, hyperreflective inner retinal foci corresponding to lipid exudation, and subretinal fluid may be detected around the tumor mass.

242

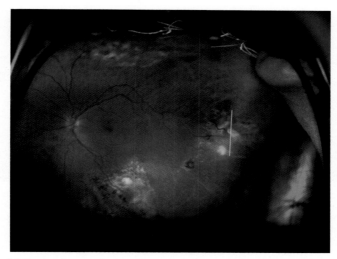

Fig. 52.1 Wide-field fundus photograph of a patient with von Hippel Lindau disease and multiple retinal capillary hemangioblastomas. The temporal lesion *(yellow line)* has classic dilated feeding arteriole and draining venule with surrounding laser scars and surface fibrosis.

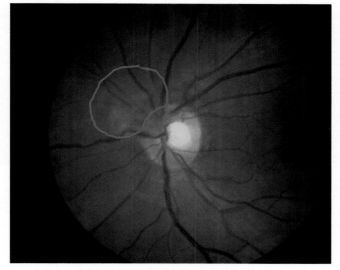

Fig. 52.2 Photograph of an exophytic chronic retinal capillary hemangioblastoma adjacent to the optic nerve. There is no lipid exudation or retinal detachment on clinical examination.

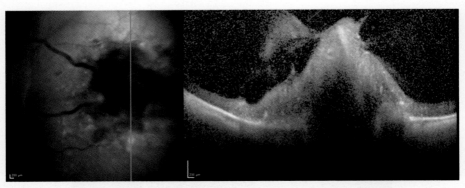

Fig. 52.3 Spectral-domain optical coherence tomography (SD-OCT) image of the lesion in Fig. 52.1 demonstrates an endophytic mounded lesion with preretinal hyperreflective material attached to the lesion apex *(blue arrow)* consistent with organized fibrosis overlying the lesion. The lesion itself is hyperreflective, with loss of clear retinal anatomy and shadowing through the center of the lesion.

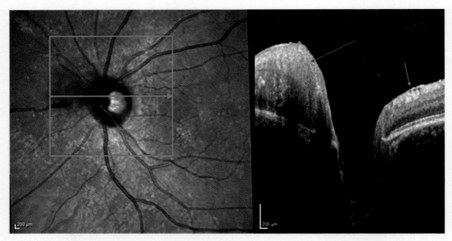

Fig. 52.4 Spectral-domain optical coherence tomography (SD-OCT) image of the lesion in Fig. 52.3 demonstrates a mounded inner retinal hyperreflective domed lesion replacing the inner and middle retinal layers with speckled hyperfluorescent spots and associated shadowing. A very narrow band of ellipsoid zone is noted along the nasal edge that is not obscured by overlying shadowing by the lesion *(red arrow)*. An associated mild epiretinal membrane is seen, along the temporal peripapillary retina *(orange arrow)*.

Exophytic tumors also have a hyperreflective inner retinal component (Fig. 52.4). The posterior shadowing is typically not as extensive as the endophytic variety. Similarly, surface epiretinal membrane, hyperreflective inner retinal foci corresponding to lipid exudation, and subretinal fluid may be detected (Figs. 52.5 and 52.6).

Ancillary Testing

Wide-angle fundus fluorescein angiography is important to detect clinically visible lesions, which demonstrate progressive, bright, circumscribed vascular lesions from the tumors. This technique also can identify subclinical lesions as smaller areas of localized vascular leakage with a typical

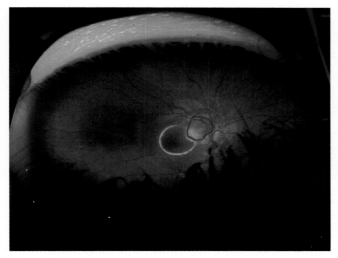

Fig. 52.5 A 2-year-old male with von Hippel Lindau (VHL) disease and an associated exophytic peripapillary retinal capillary hemangioblastoma (or hemangioma) (RCH) *(blue outline)*. There is an associated lipid ring that surrounds the region of the premacular bursa.

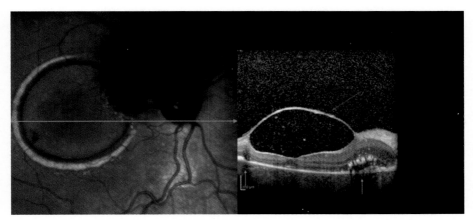

Fig. 52.6 Pretreatment macular spectral-domain optical coherence tomography (SD-OCT) image demonstrates taut elevation of the premacular hyaloid bursa *(blue arrow)* with focal traction to its inner retinal attachment inducing focal deformation of the retina *(orange arrows)*. Nasally, there are outer retinal hyperreflective opacities, consistent with lipid exudation and outer retinal cystoid thickening.

feeding arteriole and draining venule. Ultrasonography aids in documenting tumor size and the extent of coexisting retinal detachment.[2]

Systemic testing for VHL disease includes neuroimaging to screen for brain and spinal cord hemangioblastomas, body scans to look for renal cell carcinoma and pancreatic neuroendocrine tumors, and serologic testing for possible pheochromocytomas. Genetic testing has now critical to establish a diagnosis and to properly counsel the patient on risk of developing further ocular and systemic lesions.

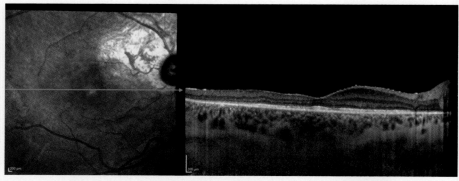

Fig. 52.7 After treatment with two sessions of verteporfin photodynamic therapy (PDT), there is resolution of the lipid exudation, flattening of the peripapillary lesion (now a fibrotic scar). The elevated macular hyaloid bursa is no longer visible, and a fine epiretinal membrane is seen nasal to the foveal depression with associated retinal thickening. The ellipsoid zone and external limiting membrane are intact.

Treatment

Small localized RCH lesions can be managed with direct thermal laser photocoagulation and a yellow dye–based laser system. Diode laser thermotherapy has been used, but it is a risk of increasing fluid leakage immediately after treatment. Verteporfin photodynamic therapy (PDT) can be used to treat tumors near to the optic nerve or even larger tumors in the periphery with repeated treatments (Fig. 52.7). Ablative therapies include external cryotherapy and plaque brachytherapy. The roles of anti–vascular endothelial growth factor (anti-VEGF) therapy and steroid therapy have not been formally studied, but anecdotal experience suggests that fluid exudation and posttreatment inflammation may be partially controlled with these pharmacotherapeutic agents. Surgical resection of large RCHs with vitrectomy and endoresection techniques has been reported. Advanced tumors with extensive retinal detachment may require enucleation in select cases.

References

1. Singh AD, Nouri M, Shields CL, Shields JA, Smith AF. Retinal capillary hemangioma: a comparison of sporadic cases and cases associated with von Hippel Lindau disease. *Ophthalmology.* 2001;108(10): 1907–1911.
2. Heimann H, Jmor F, Damato B. Imaging retinal and choroidal vascular tumors. *Eye (London).* 2013;27 (2):208–216.

Choroidal Nevus and Congenital Hypertrophy of the Retinal Pigment Epithelium

Prithvi Mruthyunjaya

Introduction

These two conditions— choroidal nevus and congenital hypertrophy of the retinal pigment epithelium (CHRPE)—are commonly seen as small circumscribed pigmented lesions, which can be confused for same condition.

A choroidal nevus is an acquired melanocytic choroidal lesion that is usually asymptomatic and detected on routine examination in children. Although these lesions normally grow slowly, in general there is a low risk of malignant transformation to choroidal melanoma. A CHRPE lesion is a congenital benign lesion of the retinal pigment epithelium (RPE) typically discovered on routine examination of the retinal periphery and exhibits very slow growth and extremely low risk of malignant transformation.

The Brain Connection

None.

Clinical Features

A nevus is typically a dark brown lesion with occasional areas of surface depigmentation (Fig. 53.1). The lesion is well circumscribed and generally flat in children but can grow up to 2 mm in thickness. Associated surface features overlying the nevus include subretinal fluid or orange pigment (lipofuscin). Chronic nevi can have overlying degenerative drusen, RPE atrophy, pigment epithelial detachments, or secondary choroidal neovascular membranes.

CHRPE lesions are darkly pigmented, round, flat, and well circumscribed (Fig. 53.2). The margins are more defined and sharper than those of a nevus. Focal areas of depigmentated lacunae can

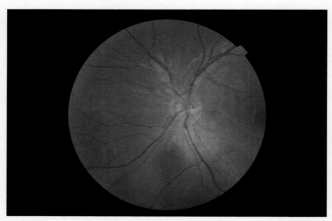

Fig. 53.1   Color fundus photograph of a flat choroidal nevus in the left eye of an 8-year-old male. The lesion is flat on clinical examination, with no overlying subretinal fluid or lipofuscin granules. (Image courtesy of Miguel Materin, MD.)

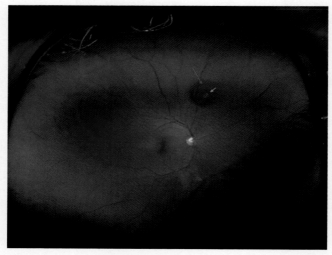

Fig. 53.2   Wide-angle color photo of the right eye of a 15-year-old male with a flat congenital hypertrophy of the retinal pigment epithelium (CHRPE) lesion in the superior periphery posterior to the equator *(blue arrow)*. The lesion is hyperpigmented, oval to round in shape, and has no elevation. The lesion is well circumscribed, with a focal patch of central hypopigmentation representing an area of early lacunae formation *(orange arrow).* - (Image courtesy of Miguel Materin, MD.)

be noted in more chronic lesions. It is not uncommon for these lesions to expand slowly over time. Rarely complete depigmentation may occur.

OCT Features

With a nevus on enhanced-depth imaging (EDI) OCT, expansion of the choroid may be noted. There is hyperreflectivity along the inner choroid with compaction of the choriocapillaris and

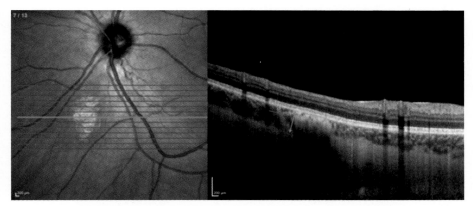

Fig. 53.3 Spectral-domain optical coherence tomography (SD-OCT) with line scan taken through nevus seen in Fig. 53.1. The region of the nevus shows hyperreflective compaction of the choriocapillaris *(blue arrows)* with shadowing. The underlying sclero–choroidal junction can be visualized demonstrating a subtle difference in thickness of the nevus compared with the surrounding normal choroid *(orange arrow)*. There is very subtle upward concave bowing of the neurosensory retina implying that this nevus is nearly flat, but such a subtle degree of elevation cannot be detected clinically. The neurosensory retinal is intact without any subretinal fluid, retinal pigment epithelium (RPE) hyperreflectivity or atrophy, or signs of cystoid macular degeneration.

typical shadowing within the deep choroid (Fig. 53.3).[1] There may be secondary retinal changes overlying the nevus, including subretinal fluid and RPE alterations, but this is less commonly seen in children. Accurate nevus thickness measurements are possible in scans that allow for visualization of the sclerochoroidal junction and can be used to monitor lesion growth.

CHRPE lesions are flat. The RPE in the region of the lesion is typically thickened compared with the normal surrounding RPE, with an abrupt transition; but in some cases, the RPE may be irregular or absent. Lacunae allow signal transmission into the choroid. The overlying retina may demonstrate outer retinal degeneration and retinal thinning (Fig. 53.4).[2]

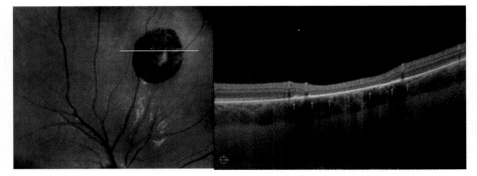

Fig. 53.4 Off-axis long eye scan spectral-domain optical coherence tomography (SD-OCT) through the congenital hypertrophy of the retinal pigment epithelium (CHRPE) lesion *(yellow line)* seen in Fig. 53.2. The surrounding neurosensory retina and retinal pigment epithelium (RPE) is normal. Through the lesion, there is increased thickness and hyperreflectivity of the RPE compared with the surrounding unaffected RPE *(blue arrows)*, with relative signal shadowing in the underlying choroid. There is corresponding loss of the ellipsoid zone and generalized overlying neurosensory retinal thinning over the thickened abnormal RPE, suggesting chronic outer retinal atrophy. No elevation or choroidal expansion of the lesion is noted.

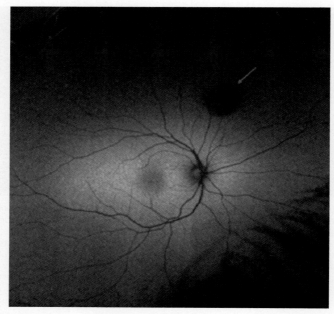

Fig. 53.5 Wide-angle fundus autofluoresence demonstrates the well-circumscribed dark hypofundus autofluoresence from the corresponding lesion in Fig. 53.3 *(blue arrow).*

Ancillary Testing

With both nevi and CHRPE lesions, color fundus photography aids in careful documentation of the lesion borders. B-scan ultrasonography is used to measure lesion thickness, although this method can overestimate the true thickness because both the retinal and choroidal components are typically measured. With a CHRPE lesion, fundus autofluoresence demonstrates well-demarcated, dark hypofundus autofluoresence (Fig. 53.5).

Treatment

Benign nevi are monitored for signs of growth. Malignant transformation into uveal melanoma requires definitive treatment with plaque radiation therapy, although it is rare in the pediatric population. CHRPE lesions are monitored.

References

1. Shah SU, Kaliki S, Shields CL, Ferenczy SR, Harmon SA, Shields JA. Enhanced depth imaging optical coherence tomography of choroidal nevus in 104 cases. *Ophthalmology.* 2012;119:1066–1072.
2. Fung AT, Pellegrini M, Shields CL. Congenital hypertrophy of the retinal pigment epithelium: enhanced-depth imaging optical coherence tomography in 18 cases. *Ophthalmology.* 2014;121:251–256.

Abnormalities of Development

Persistent Fetal Vasculature

Sally S. Ong

Introduction

Persistent fetal vasculature (PFV), previously known as *persistent hyperplastic primary vitreous* (PHPV), is a congenital anomaly that occurs when vessels present during fetal development fail to regress.[1] Fetal vasculature is made up of two vascular meshworks—(1) tunica vasculosa lentis and (2) hyaloid system or primary vitreous. PFV can therefore be subcategorized into anterior or posterior PFV syndrome, depending on whether the persistence of the tunica vasculosa lentis or that of the hyaloid system predominate.[1] In some cases, a combination of both anterior and posterior PFV features can be present. Most cases of PFV are unilateral, idiopathic, and nonheritable.

The Brain Connection

Rarely, PFV can be bilateral and associated with systemic syndromes with neurologic manifestations, such as trisomy 13, Walker-Warburg syndrome, ocular–palatal–cerebral syndrome, and intrauterine herpes simplex virus infection.

Clinical Features

Classically, patients with PFV present with leukocoria, microphthalmia, cataract, and elongated ciliary processes.[1] A stalk from the lens to the optic nerve may also sometimes be visible (Fig. 54.1A). However, clinical presentation can vary because a range of vascular remnants may remain.[1] Specifically, in anterior PFV syndrome, there may also be a shallow anterior chamber with narrow-angle glaucoma, prominent radial vessels or rubeosis iridis (persistent anterior tunica vasculosa lentis vessels), traction on the ciliary body with hypotony, and retrolental fibrovascular membranes causing traction on the peripheral retina.[1] In posterior PFV syndrome, the stalk can exert traction on the retina, causing vitreous hemorrhage and tractional retinal detachment, and there may also be a hypoplastic or dysplastic optic nerve.[1] Of these features, media opacity and retinal changes (traction and dysplasia) are the two determinants of visual outcome. Importantly, the amount of retinal dysplasia has not been found to be associated with the severity of anterior segment pathology, lens involvement, globe size, or vascular appearance.[2]

252

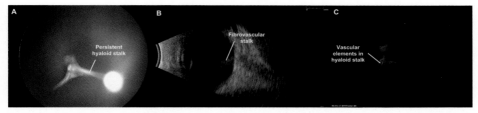

Fig. 54.1   A 3-month-old boy with persistent fetal vasculature of the left eye. (A) On color photograph, the hyaloid stalk is seen extending from the optic nerve to the lens causing a cataract. (B) Ultrasonography shows a fibrovascular stalk and a small globe. (C) Fluorescein angiography demonstrates vascular elements in the hyaloid stalk. (Image courtesy of Laura Enyedi, MD.)

OCT Features

OCT can demonstrate the deformation of the retina and presence of a hyaloid stalk (Fig. 54.2A). It can also show posterior hyaloidal organization, abnormal retinal architecture (see Fig. 54.2B), and diminished foveal contour. Importantly, optical coherence tomography (OCT) can demonstrate the presence of retinal traction, foveal involvement, and retinal dysplasia—morphologic features that may relate to visual outcomes. If significant traction requiring surgery is present, intra- and postoperative OCT can be used to monitor the retinal response after surgery. Given the height of the stalk, it is important to recognize that mirror artifact can occur on OCT (see Fig. 54.2B). The stalk can also cause posterior shadowing, limiting the region of OCT imaging (see Fig. 54.2C).

Ancillary Testing

When there is no view of the fundus, ultrasonography and magnetic resonance imaging (MRI) can be helpful to establish a diagnosis and to rule out other causes of leukocoria, such as retinoblastoma. Each modality can reveal the fibrovascular stalk and small globe in PFV, the absence of calcification, and lack of an intraocular mass (see Fig. 54.1B). When there is a view of the fundus, fluorescein angiography (FA) can help detect abnormal vasculature and perfusion of the retina (see Fig. 54.1C).

Treatment

Cataract with mild PFV is managed surgically with lens removal if the cataract is visually significant and diathermy with stalk division, as well as with refraction and amblyopia therapy to maximize visual potential.[2] When PFV involves the optic nerve and retina (see Figs. 54.1 and 54.2), although the stalk can be removed by using vitreoretinal surgical techniques, visual acuity outcomes are generally poor, depending on the extent of retinal involvement, especially with unilateral disease.[2] Retinal detachment, if present, could also be treated surgically.[2] Visual rehabilitation to address amblyopia and anisometropia after these procedures is important to maximize visual outcomes.

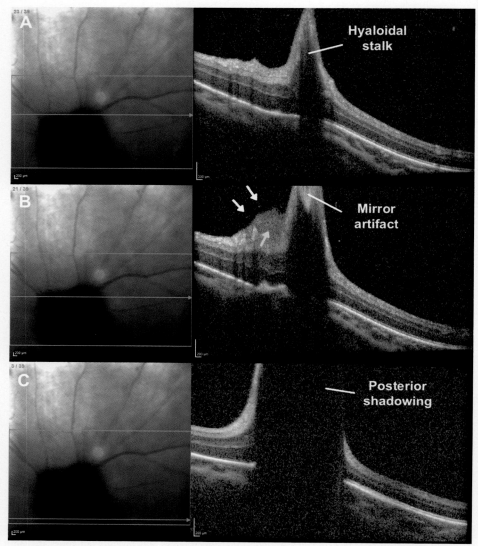

Fig. 54.2 Optical coherence tomography (OCT) image of persistent hyaloidal stalk in the same patient as in Fig. 54.1. (A) Superior edge of the stalk. (B) A more inferior cross section of the stalk demonstrates thickening and disorganization of inner retina *(yellow arrow)*. The hyperreflective flecks represent posterior hyaloidal organization *(white arrows)*. There was also a mirror artifact in an area of elevation. (C) The tall central part of the hyaloidal stalk causes dense posterior shadowing. (Image courtesy of Laura Enyedi, MD.)

References

1. Goldberg MF. Persistent fetal vasculature: an integrated interpretation of signs and symptoms associated with persistent hyperplastic primary vitreous LIV: Edward Jackson Memorial Lecture. *Am J Ophthalmol.* 1997;124(5):587–626.
2. Trese MT, Capone A. Persistent fetal vasculature syndrome (persistent hyperplastic primary vitreous). In: Hartnett ME, Trese MT, Capone A, Keats B, Steidl S, eds. *Pediatric Retina: Medical and Surgical Approaches.* 1st ed. Philadelphia: Lippincott Williams & Wilkins; 2005:437–443.

Chorioretinal Coloboma

Sally S. Ong

Introduction

Chorioretinal coloboma occurs as a result of the failure of the embryonic fissure to close during the sixth and seventh weeks of fetal development.[1,2] It is most common in the inferonasal quadrant and can be associated with iris, ciliary, lens, and optic nerve colobomas.[1] In chorioretinal colobomas, the sclera is staphylomatous, the overlying retina is atrophic, and the retinal pigment epithelium (RPE), Bruch membrane, choriocapillaries, and choroid can be absent and replaced by glial tissue. The atrophic neurosensory retina in the area of coloboma is also known as the *intercalary membrane*.[3]

Some authors have postulated that because the intercalary membrane overlying the choroidal defect is thin and undifferentiated, it is prone to retinal breaks and retinal detachments.[2,3] Hussain et al., however, reported that retinal breaks occurred outside the coloboma in 5 of 15 eyes with colobomatous retinal detachments.[4] These authors hypothesized that there may be an abnormal vitreoretinal interface not limited to the area of the coloboma and its margin in colobomatous eyes. An association has also been demonstrated between chorioretinal colobomas and choroidal neovascularization (CNV) occurrence at the temporal margin of the coloboma through defects in the Bruch membrane.[3,4]

Chorioretinal colobomas can occur in isolation or can be associated with systemic syndromes, such as CHARGE (coloboma, heart abnormalities, anal atresia, renal abnormalities, genitourinary abnormalities, eye abnormalities) syndrome, Goldenhar syndrome, Rubinstein-Taybi syndrome, trisomy 18, 4p syndrome, basal cell nevus syndrome, Aicardi syndrome, congenital rubella, Walker-Warburg syndrome, and Joubert syndrome.[1,2,5]

The Brain Connection

Chorioretinal colobomas can be associated with systemic syndromes with both brain and eye abnormalities. Walker-Warburg syndrome is a severe form of congenital muscular dystrophy associated with anomalies of the brain (lissencephaly, hydrocephalus, cerebellar malformations) and eye (coloboma, microphthlamia, cataracts, persistent fetal vasculature, retinal detachment, optic nerve hypoplasia).[1] In Joubert syndrome, there is underdevelopment of the cerebellar vermis and brainstem, eye abnormalities (coloboma, retinal dystrophy), kidney disease, liver disease, and skeletal and hormone abnormalities.[5]

Clinical Features

If there is no foveal involvement, even if a chorioretinal coloboma is large, the eye may have relatively preserved visual acuity (Fig. 55.1, right eye). Conversely, foveal involvement predicts poor visual acuity (see Fig. 55.1, left eye). Amblyopia and refractive error may further decrease visual acuity in these eyes. Visual field defect is present on testing but may not be noticed by the patient because the defect has been present since birth. Later in life, retinal detachment (Figs. 55.2 and 55.3) and CNV (Fig. 55.4) may occur, resulting in further loss of vision. On clinical examination, chorioretinal colobomas have a glistening yellow-white appearance and distinct hyperpigmented margins.

OCT Features

Optical coherence tomography (OCT) demonstrates staphylomatous sloping of the sclera with an intercalary membrane and absent/atrophic RPE, Bruch membrane, choriocapillaries, and choroid (see Figs. 55.1 through 55.4) in the area of the coloboma. Using OCT, Gopal et al. demonstrated that the transition from normal neurosensory retina to intercalary membrane can be sudden or gradual.[6] These authors hypothesized that the eyes with abrupt transition to a thin intercalary membrane were prone to retinal breaks developing at the margin.[6]

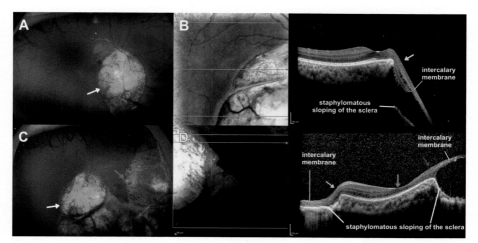

Fig. 55.1 An 8-year-old boy with bilateral optic nerve and chorioretinal colobomas. (A) Wide-field Optos image of the right eye demonstrates the presence of a large inferior chorioretinal coloboma also involving the optic nerve *(white arrow)*. (B) Optical coherence tomography (OCT) of the right eye shows staphylomatous sloping of the sclera with an intercalary membrane in the nasal macula with sparing of the fovea. Transition from the neurosensory retina to the intercalary membrane is gradual *(yellow arrow)* in this eye. (C) Wide-field Optos image of the left eye illustrates presence of a large inferior optic nerve and chorioretinal coloboma *(white arrow)* with extensive macular involvement *(red arrow)*. (D) OCT of the left eye shows staphylomatous sloping of the sclera with intercalary membranes in both the nasal and temporal macula. Transition is gradual nasally *(yellow arrow)* and abrupt temporally *(blue arrow)* between the neurosensory retina and intercalary membranes. Even though there is no coloboma over the fovea, there is generalized retinal thinning in the foveal center *(green arrow)*. Best corrected visual acuity is 20/20 in the right eye and 20/600 in the left eye.

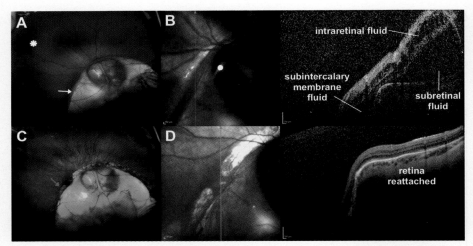

Fig. 55.2 A 10-year-old girl with bilateral chorioretinal colobomas involving the optic nerves presented with total retinal detachment in the right eye. (A) Wide-field Optos image demonstrates the optic nerve and chorioretinal coloboma *(white arrow)* and loss of choroidal markings caused by retinal detachment *(white asterisk)*. (B) Optical coherence tomography (OCT) shows presence of subretinal fluid and subintercalary membrane fluid. There are also intraretinal cystoid spaces. (C) Three months after vitreoretinal surgery with fibrin glue over the break in the intercalary membrane, laser at the coloboma margin but sparing the fovea and temporary silicone oil placement, the retina is attached and pigmentary changes *(red arrow)* from laser along the margin of the coloboma with a skip spot around the fovea are observed. (D) OCT demonstrates the absence of fluid under the neurosensory retina and intercalary membrane. Visual acuity returned to 20/70.

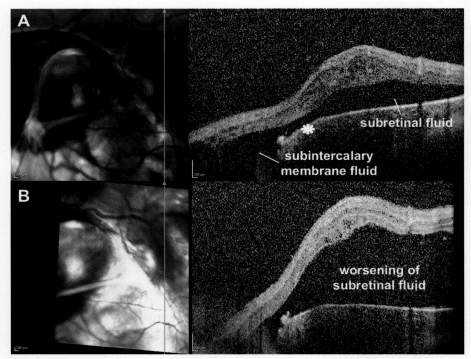

Fig. 55.3 The same patient in Fig. 55.2 subsequently had chronic focal retinal detachment in the left eye. (A) Optical coherence tomography (OCT) shows subretinal fluid communicating with the subintercalary membrane space *(white asterisk)*, suggesting a break within the coloboma. The retinal detachment was initially observed given the limited amount of subretinal fluid and poor visual acuity in this eye. (B) OCT was repeated a few months later and showed interval worsening of the retinal detachment. Retinal detachment repair was then performed.

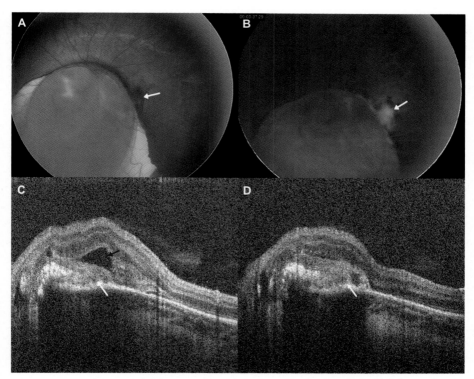

Fig. 55.4   Choroidal neovascular membrane (CNV) in the left eye of a 6-month-old boy with bilateral optic nerve and chorioretinal colobomas. (A) Five months after initial presentation, there is a new CNV with adjacent sub-retinal hemorrhage *(white arrow)* at the temporal border of the coloboma. (B) The lesion has a classic angio-graphic pattern for CNV with early hyperfluorescence and late leakage *(white arrow)*. There are also adjacent areas of blocked fluorescence from subretinal hemorrhage. (C) Optical coherence tomography (OCT) demon-strates a subretinal hyperreflective fibrovascular membrane with surrounding hyperreflective material *(white arrow)*, intraretinal fluid *(green arrow)*, and subretinal fluid *(blue arrow)*. (D) After treatment with anti–vascular endothelial growth factor (anti-VEGF), there was significant decrease in intraretinal and subretinal fluid over a more consolidated-appearing lesion *(white arrow)* on OCT.

Retinal Detachment

(See Figs. 55.2 and 55.3.)

OCT can detect subclinical retinal detachments at the margin. These subclinical detachments could increase future risk of clinical detachments and may be an indication for early treatment along the coloboma margin. If clinical retinal detachment is present, OCT offers cross-sectional imaging of the location and extent of sometimes subtle hyporeflective subretinal fluid. OCT can also show a communication between subretinal fluid and subintercalary membrane fluid. This suggests that the break is within the coloboma, and some authors have reported that focal laser treatment at this area of the margin may suffice. In chronic retinal detachments, intraretinal cystoid spaces may be seen. OCT is also useful to monitor subretinal fluid resolution after retinal detachment repair.

CNV Membrane

(See Fig. 55.4.)

OCT enables cross-sectional visualization of the CNV membrane. The CNV membrane appears on OCT as a fibrovascular pigment epithelial detachment or hyperreflective subretinal material. OCT is also especially useful for monitoring the activity of the neovascular complex. The lesion may be inactive and compact on OCT without associated fluid or hemorrhage, or it may have poorly demarcated borders with associated retinal thickening and intra- and/or subretinal fluid and/or subretinal hemorrhage.[3]

Ancillary Testing

Fluorescein angiography can show late hyperfluorescent leakage when there is a CNV membrane (see Fig. 55.2B). Oral fluorescein angiography may be helpful in monitoring for leakage in some of these young children. As discussed in Chapter 60, visual field testing may also be helpful while looking for any field deficits.

Treatment

Patients with bilateral chorioretinal coloboma or unilateral chorioretinal coloboma plus one other systemic abnormality should be referred for genetic and chromosomal testing for systemic disorders. Treatment of refractive error and amblyopia is important to maximize the visual potential for the affected eye. Monocular precautions are also important with unilateral chorioretinal colobomas. Interval monitoring with a dilated fundus examination, at least annually, is important because of the risk of retinal detachment and CNV in these patients. Colobomatous retinal detachments should be repaired surgically despite a guarded visual prognosis, particularly in children with bilateral chorioretinal colobomas, given the risk of future vision loss in the contralateral eye. Some authors have even suggested prophylactic laser in all patients with chorioretinal colobomas, given the high risk of retinal detachment in this population.[4] CNV in colobomatous eyes can spontaneously resolve or lead to progressive worsening of visual acuity.[4] When associated with worsening vision, CNV can be treated with anti–vascular endothelial growth factor (anti-VEGF), focal laser photocoagulation, or photodynamic therapy.[3]

References

1. Pagon RA. Ocular coloboma. *Surv Ophthalmol.* 1981;25(4):223–236.
2. Daufenbach DR, Ruttum MS, Pulido JS, Keech RV. Chorioretinal colobomas in a pediatric population. *Ophthalmology.* 1998;105(8):1455–1458.
3. Grewal DS, Tran-Viet D, Vajzovic L, Mruthyunjaya P, Toth CA. Association of pediatric choroidal neovascular membranes at the temporal edge of optic nerve and retinochoroidal coloboma. *Am J Ophthalmol.* 2017;174:104–112.
4. Hussain RM, Abbey AM, Shah AR, Drenser KA, Trese MT, Capone Jr A. Chorioretinal coloboma complications: retinal detachment and choroidal neovascular membrane. *J Ophthalmic Vis Res.* 2017;12(1):3–10.
5. Brooks BP, Zein WM, Thompson AH, et al. Joubert syndrome: ophthalmological findings in correlation with genotype and hepatorenal disease in 99 patients prospectively evaluated at a single center. *Ophthalmology.* 2018;125(12):1937–1952.
6. Gopal L, Khan B, Jain S, Prakash VS. A clinical and optical coherence tomography study of the margins of choroidal colobomas. *Ophthalmology.* 2007;114(3):571–580.

CHAPTER 56

Myelinated Nerve Fiber Layer

Sally S. Ong ■ Mays El-Dairi

Introduction

Myelinated nerve fiber layer is a developmental anomaly that results from an abnormal extension of myelination anterior to the lamina cribrosa of the sclera.[1] In normal fetal development, myelination of the optic nerve begins at the lateral geniculate body, progresses toward the eye, and stops posterior to the lamina cribrosa prior to birth. Abnormal myelination that extends anterior to the lamina cribrosa thus occurs along the nerve fiber layers of the optic nerve head and the sensory retina. Although usually congenital and stationary, myelinated nerve fiber layer can also be acquired or progressive in childhood and adolescence.[2]

The Brain Connection

Small case series have reported the presence of myelinated nerve fiber layer in patients with neurofibromatosis type 1 and Goltz-Gorlin syndrome.[3,4] Both syndromes can present with systemic manifestations, including neurological abnormalities. However, association with a systemic syndromic disorder is rare; myelinated nerve fiber layer is usually an idiopathic, isolated developmental anomaly with no neurologic manifestations.[1]

Clinical Features

Myelinated nerve fiber layer has been associated with myopia, amblyopia, and strabismus.[1] Otherwise, the general anatomy and function of the retina are relatively unaffected in this condition. Patients have been reported to have preserved visual fields and, except for obscuration from the opaque myelin sheaths, normal fluorescein angiography findings. Clinically, myelinated nerve fiber layer appears as a cluster of opaque, gray-white patches in the distribution of the retinal nerve fibers (Fig. 56.1). These gray-white patches can obscure the underlying retinal vessels, and have feathered or frayed borders associated with the varying lengths of the myelin sheaths.

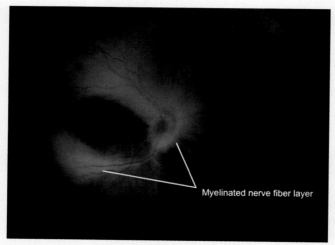

Fig. 56.1 Myelinated nerve fiber layer in the right eye of a 1-year-old girl. Color photography demonstrates the opaque, gray-white patches of abnormal myelination from the optic nerve head to the retina in the distribution of the nerve fibers.

OCT Features

On cross-sectional optical coherence tomography (OCT) imaging, myelinated retinal nerve fiber layer appears uniformly thickened and brightly hyperreflective (Fig. 56.2).[2] There is also backscattering from the thickened nerve fiber layer. Myelin has a high lipid content; thus myelinated nerve fiber layer appears white on the infrared en face image. By revealing the cross-sectional involvement

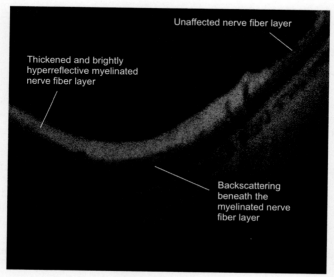

Fig. 56.2 Optical coherence tomography (OCT) from the same eye in Fig. 56.1 shows a thickened and brightly hyperreflective retinal nerve fiber layer in the area of abnormal myelination in comparison with the adjacent unaffected retinal nerve fiber layer. There is also backscattering and shadowing of the outer retina beneath the myelinated nerve fiber layer.

of the nerve fiber layer only, OCT is very helpful in differentiating myelinated nerve fiber layer from more serious conditions. Mimickers that can appear similar on ophthalmoscopy, such as peripapillary epiretinal membrane, retinal pigment epithelium (RPE) detachment, retinal infiltrate, and retinoblastoma,[2] are not localized to the nerve fiber layer. Cotton wool spots can also cause hyperreflective thickening of the nerve fiber layer, but these spots are focal and irregular as opposed to the uniform hyperreflective thickening of the nerve fiber layer seen in myelinated nerve fiber layer. Branch retinal artery occlusion can also cause thickening of the nerve fiber layer in the acute phase but is usually also accompanied by generalized thickening of multiple retinal layers. In myelinated nerve fiber layer, only the nerve fiber layer is affected.

Ancillary Imaging

On color photography, myelinated nerve fiber layer appears as clusters of opaque, gray-white patches in the inner retina with obscuration of the underlying retinal vessels (see Fig. 56.1). The abnormal myelination blocks on fluorescence angiography, appears white on infrared and red-free imaging, and is dark or hypoautofluorescent on autofluorescence imaging.[2]

Treatment

No treatment is required for myelinated nerve fiber layer.

References

1. Straatsma BR, Foos RY, Heckenlively JR, Taylor GN. Myelinated retinal nerve fibers. *Am J Ophthalmol.* 1981;91:25–38.
2. Shelton JB, Digre KB, Gilman J, Warner JE, Katz BJ. Characteristics of myelinated nerve fiber layer in ophthalmic imaging. *JAMA Ophthalmol.* 2013;131(1):107–109.
3. Parulekar MV, Elston JS. Acquired retinal myelination in neurofibromatosis 1. *Arch Ophthalmol.* 2002;120 (5):659–661.
4. De Jong PT, Bistervels B, Cosgrove J, de Grip G, Leys A, Goffin M. Medullated nerve fibers: a sign of multiple basal cell nevi (Gorlin's) syndrome. *Arch Ophthalmol.* 1985;103(12):1833–1836.

CHAPTER 57

Torpedo Maculopathy

Sally S. Ong ■ Akshay S. Thomas

Introduction

Torpedo maculopathy is a congenital lesion that localizes to the temporal macula with a torpedo-like tip pointing to the central macula.[1] The name of the condition is derived from the unique shape of the lesion. Although histopathologic reports on the lesion are lacking, modern imaging techniques of optical coherence tomography (OCT) and autofluorescence have helped provide insight into this entity. This condition has been speculated to represent a persistent defect in retinal pigment epithelium (RPE) development in the fetal temporal bulge that typically occurs at 4 to 6 months gestation.[1]

The Brain Connection

Torpedo maculopathy has been reported in one patient with tuberous sclerosis, a condition that can also present with central nervous system (CNS) lesions.[2] There are otherwise no known associated systemic or neurologic abnormalities in torpedo maculopathy.

Clinical Features

Torpedo maculopathy is asymptomatic and usually found in patients on routine ophthalmologic examination. There may be a scotoma associated with the area of nonfunctional RPE and photoreceptors. Published reports have shown that the condition is stationary and does not progress with time.[1,3] On clinical examination, the lesion appears oval, hypopigmented, and located in the temporal macula with a torpedo-like tip pointing toward the central macula (Fig. 57.1A).[1] The lesion is close to the foveal center but has not been found to affect the foveal center.

Differential diagnoses for torpedo maculopathy include congenital hypertrophy of the RPE (CHRPE) and RPE lesions of Gardner syndrome. Although torpedo maculopathy does not usually have any systemic associations, patients with CHRPE have a rare risk of developing RPE adenoma, and those with Gardner syndrome are at risk of developing colon cancer and other extracolonic tumors.[4] Correct differentiation of torpedo maculopathy from these lesions on clinical examination and OCT is therefore very important. Torpedo maculopathy is usually a single, stationary lesion in

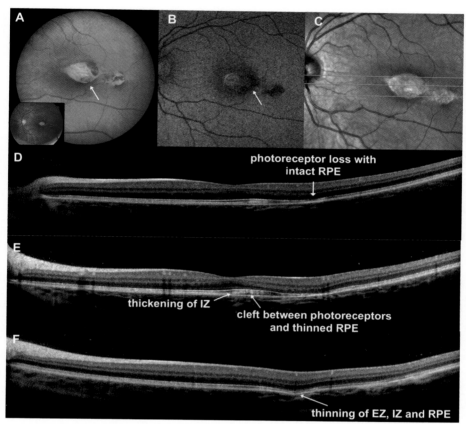

Fig. 57.1 Multimodal imaging in torpedo maculopathy. (A) Color fundus photo showing the characteristic torpedo lesion *(white arrow)* in the temporal macula. (B) Fundus autofluorescence showing relative hypoautofluorescence *(white arrow)* of the lesion with a rim of hyperautofluorescence along the nasal aspect of the lesion. (C) Infrared image with optical coherence tomography (OCT) line scans represented in images D through F. (D) Photoreceptor loss with intact underlying RPE *(arrow)*. (E) Thickening of the interdigitation zone (IZ) with thin hyporeflective cleft formation over thinned RPE *(arrow)*. (F) Thinning of ellipsoid zone (EZ), IZ, and RPE *(arrow)*. (Thomas A, Flaxel C, Pennesi M. Spectral-domain optical coherence tomography and fundus autofluorescence evaluation of torpedo maculopathy. *J Pediatr Ophthalmol Strabismus.* 2015;52: E8-E10. Reprinted with permission from SLACK Incorporated.)

the temporal macula. In contrast, CHRPE, although generally solitary, can occur in clusters, very rarely occurs in the macula, and can grow over time.[4] RPE lesions of Gardner syndrome are usually multiple, small (less than 1mm), bilateral, and occur in the equator and midperiphery.[4]

OCT Features

OCT imaging usually demonstrates normal inner retina and thinned outer retina, with a hyporeflective subretinal cleft between degenerated photoreceptors and thinned RPE in the area of torpedo maculopathy (see Figs. 57.1D-F).[5] These findings, however, are not universal, with some reports of inner retinal thinning and normal RPE architecture.[6] This is in contrast with CHRPE lesions, which, as the name suggests, usually reveal RPE thickening.

Ancillary Testing

In Golchet et al.'s case series of 13 patients with torpedo maculopathy, fluorescein angiography was performed in two patients, and a window defect was demonstrated in the area of the lesion without hyperfluorescence in the area of the cleft.[3] This suggests that the likely fluid in this subretinal hypolucent cleft is not from ongoing vascular leakage, explaining its stability over time. This subretinal hypolucent cleft has been given different names in other reports. Sanabria et al., for example, described the presence of a "serous retinal detachment" in one of two cases with torpedo maculopathy.[7] Without histologic confirmation, what occupies the hyporeflective subretinal cleft in torpedo maculopathy remains unknown. Autofluorescence shows hypoautofluorescence over the area of thinned RPE, occasionally with a rim of stippled hyperautofluorescence (see Fig. 57.1B).

Treatment

Because patients are asymptomatic and the condition does not progress, no treatment is necessary.

References

1. Shields CL, Guzman JM, Shapiro MJ, Fogel LE, Shields JA. Torpedo maculopathy at the site of the fetal "bulge". *Arch Ophthalmology*. 2010;128(4):499–501.
2. Hansen MS, Larsen M, Hove MN. Optical coherence tomography of torpedo maculopathy in a patient with tuberous sclerosis. *Acta Ophthalmol*. 2016;94(7):736–737.
3. Golchet PR, Jampol LM, Mathura JR, Daily MJ. Torpedo maculopathy. *Br J Ophthalmol*. 2010;94(3):302–306.
4. Villegas VM, Schwartz SG, Flynn Jr HW, et al. Distinguishing torpedo maculopathy from similar lesions of the posterior segment. *OSLI Retina*. 2014;45(3):222–226.
5. Thomas AS, Flaxel CJ, Pennesi ME. Spectral-domain optical coherence tomography and fundus autofluorescence evaluation of torpedo maculopathy. *J Pediatr Ophthalmol Strabismus*. 2015;13(52):e8–e10.
6. Tsang T, Messner LV, Pilon A, Lombardi L. Torpedo maculopathy: in-vivo histology using optical coherence tomography. *Optom Vis Sci*. 2009;86:E1380–E1385.
7. Sanabria MR, Coco RM, Sanchidrian M. OCT findings in torpedo maculopathy. *Retin Cases Brief Rep*. 2008;2:109–111.

Pathologic Myopia

Sally S. Ong

Introduction

Pathologic myopia was originally described as high myopia (defined as an eye with a refractive error of greater than −6.0 diopters) that is accompanied by characteristic degenerative changes in the sclera, choroid, and retinal pigment epithelium (RPE) associated with decreased vision.[1] Pathologic myopia is usually an isolated condition with no systemic associations. However, it can also be associated with systemic conditions, such as Stickler syndrome, Marfan syndrome, and homocystinuria.[1] Pathologic myopia is becoming an emerging public health issue, especially in East Asia, because of its increasing prevalence in the past few decades and because of the potential sight threatening complications associated with the condition. A reported 10% to 20% of those completing secondary schooling in urban East Asian cities now have pathologic signs associated with high myopia.[1]

The Brain Connection

Myopia has been found to be associated with higher intelligence quotients (IQs), but the relationship is poorly understood.[2] Some have hypothesized that children with myopia, with their cumbersome glasses, are more likely to devote time to studying indoors, which helps increase their educational achievements,[3] although others think that the relationship may result from highly intelligent children spending more time studying indoors and less time outdoors, which increases their risk of myopia.[2] Separately, some have suggested that shared genetic factors influence the development of both myopia and intelligence,[4] and there is now some evidence supporting this postulation. Using a powerful twin data set, Williams et al. demonstrated that genetic factors were responsible for 78% of the phenotypic correlation between IQ and refractive error.[2]

Clinical Features

Axial elongation of the eye in pathologic myopia leads to stretching of ocular tissue and progressive thinning of the sclera, choroid, and RPE. On clinical examination, the fundus in these eyes can appear tessellated as a result of the irregular distribution of RPE atrophy (Figs. 58.1A and

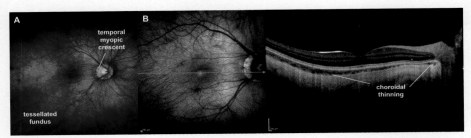

Fig. 58.1 A 5-year-old boy with −12 diopters myopia in his right eye. (A) Color photograph demonstrates a tessellated fundus and a temporal myopic crescent by the optic nerve. (B) On optical coherence tomography (OCT), diffuse choroidal thinning is observed and particularly also surrounding the optic nerve.

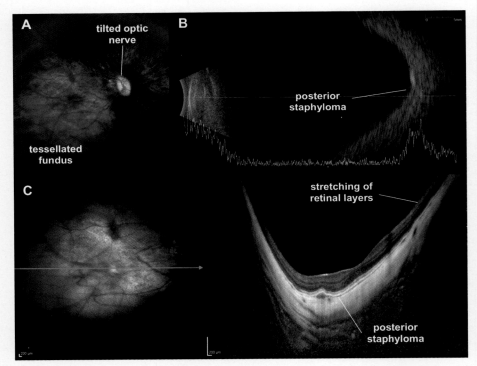

Fig. 58.2 A 13-year-old boy with Stickler syndrome has an axial length of 38 mm and −24 diopters myopia in his right eye. (A) Color photograph shows a tessellated fundus, visible choroidal vessels, and a tilted optic nerve. (B) Ultrasonography illustrates the posterior bowing of the sclera and presence of a posterior staphyloma. (C) Optical coherence tomography (OCT) demonstrates the presence of a posterior staphyloma and stretching of the retinal layers.

58.2A). The optic disc can appear tilted in these eyes as the optic nerve inserts into the elongated globe at an angle. When RPE atrophy surrounds the optic nerve, this is known as *peripapillary atrophy*. A hypopigmented myopic crescent characterized by temporal flattening of the optic disc can be observed. The choroidal vessels beneath atrophic RPE may also be visible. Posterior staphyloma occurs when there is outpouching of scleral tissue typically involving the optic nerve or macula.

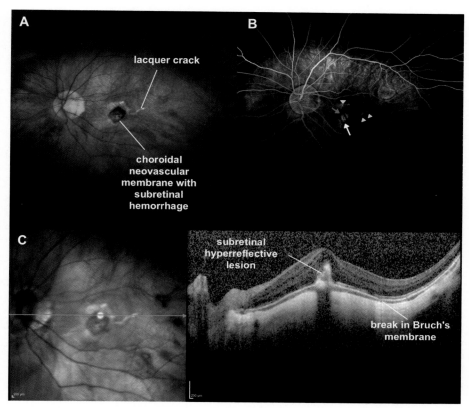

Fig. 58.3 A 16-year-old female patient with −17 diopters myopia in the left eye presented with lacquer cracks associated with a choroidal neovascular membrane and subretinal hemorrhage. (A) Color photograph shows linear hypopigmented lacquer cracks with a choroidal neovascular membrane and adjacent subretinal hemorrhage. (B) Fluorescein angiography demonstrates blockage from subretinal hemorrhage *(red arrow)*, late leakage from the choroidal neovascular membrane *(white arrow)* and staining of the lacquer cracks *(yellow arrowheads)*. C. Optical coherence tomography (OCT) illustrates a hyperreflective lesion consistent with choroidal neovascularization (CNV) and breaks in the Bruch membrane consistent with lacquer cracks. The more intensely hyperreflective areas on the choroidal neovascular membrane likely represents subretinal hemorrhage.

Lacquer cracks are irregular yellow-appearing bands representing breaks in the Bruch membrane (Fig. 58.3A). Myopic choroidal neovascularization (CNV) (see Fig. 58.3A), Forster-Fuchs spots (areas of RPE hyperplasia suspected to be RPE response to previously regressed CNV), macular or foveal schisis, and epiretinal membrane may also occur.[5] Eyes with pathologic myopia are also at increased risk for retinal detachment (Fig. 58.4A).

OCT Features

Axial length is an important variable that can affect the qualitative and quantitative measurements in optical coherence tomography (OCT) imaging. Manual focus adjustments based on refractive error are important to optimize image quality. Particularly in handheld OCT systems, adjustments to the reference arm are also essential to prevent image clipping.[6] In axial myopia (axial length ≥26 mm), the OCT image spans a larger lateral area than in an eye with normal axial length.[6]

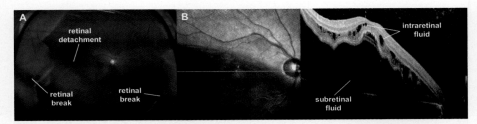

Fig. 58.4 A 17-year-old male patient with −10 diopters myopia in the right eye presented with rhegmatogenous retinal detachment. A wide-field photograph of the right eye shows a macula-off inferior retinal detachment with two retinal breaks at the 8 o'clock and 4 o'clock positions. (B) Optical coherence tomography (OCT) of the right eye reveals the presence of intraretinal fluid and subretinal fluid involving the fovea.

To correct for the lateral magnification, it is important to adjust the scan length on the retina accordingly.[6] The larger area imaged in a longer eye also decreases scan density, causing undersampling of the eye. To correct this, it is necessary to adjust the A-scan/B-scan parameter under scan settings to standardize the number of A-scans and B-scans per millimeter of eye.[6] See Chapter 3 for more information on optimizing OCT capture for an elongated eye.

Various myopia related pathologies are well visualized on OCT. OCT can demonstrate choroidal thinning, peripapillary atrophy, and thinning and disruption of the RPE. (see Fig. 58.1B). OCT can show posterior bowing of the sclera in posterior staphyloma (see Fig. 58.2C). Lacquer cracks appear on OCT as a break/discontinuity in the Bruch membrane. Complications associated with lacquer cracks, such as subretinal hemorrhage, can appear as subretinal hyperreflective material, whereas myopic CNV can appear as a hyperreflective lesion associated with subretinal fluid, intraretinal fluid, or pigment epithelial detachment (see Fig. 58.3C). The cross-sectional view provided by OCT allows for identification and differentiation of the epiretinal membrane, retinal detachment (see Fig. 58.4B), and macular retinoschisis.

Ancillary Testing

Fluorescein angiography demonstrates atrophic hyperfluorescent staining in RPE atrophy and late hyperfluorescent leakage in myopic CNV (see Fig. 58.3B). B-scan ultrasonography can also show the posterior scleral bowing of a posterior staphyloma (see Fig. 58.2B).

Treatment

In pathologic myopia, myopic CNV can be treated with anti–vascular endothelial growth factor (anti-VEGF) injections, and OCT may be used to monitor resolution of fluid. Retinal detachment and vision threatening macular schisis and epiretinal membrane are often treated with vitreoretinal surgical techniques.[5] Substantial research focus is now placed on the prevention of progression to high myopia and pathologic myopia through topical therapy or environmental modifications.[1]

References

1. Morgan IG, Ohno-Matsui K, Saw SM. Myopia. *Lancet.* 2012;379(9827):1739–1748.
2. Williams KM, Hysi PG, Yonova-Doing E, Mahroo OA, Snieder H, Hammond CJ. Phenotypic and genotypic correlation between myopia and intelligence. *Scientific Reports.* 2017;7:45977.
3. French AN, Ashby RS, Morgan IG, Rose KA. Time outdoors and the prevention of myopia. *Exp Eye Res.* 2013;114:58–68.
4. Cohn SJ, Cohn CM, Jensen AR. Myopia and intelligence: a pleiotropic relationship? *Hum Genet.* 1988;80 (1):53–58.

5. Ohno-Matsui K, Lay TYY, Lai CC, Cheung CMG. Updates of pathologic myopia. *Prog Retin Eye Res.* 2016;52:156–187.

6. Maldonado RS, Izatt JA, Sarin N, et al. Optimizing hand-held spectral domain optical coherence tomography imaging for neonates, infants and children. *Invest Ophthalmol Vis Sci.* 2010;51(5):2678–2685.

Optic Nerve Abnormalities and Diseases

Optic Nerve Pit

Mays El-Dairi

Introduction

An optic nerve pit is usually a unilateral excavation of the optic nerve head rim (most common location is inferotemporal). The majority of the time they are asymptomatic (identified incidentally on a routine examination), but they can also be associated with visual field defects or even intraretinal or subretinal fluid.

The Brain Connection

Optic nerve pits are usually isolated and are not associated with intracranial anomalies.[1] Some authorities argue that the optic nerve head pit may be connecting the vitreous cavity to cerebrospinal fluid (CSF) as has been suggested by reports of silicone oil or gas seen in the subarachnoid space after repair of a retinal detachment.[2,3] However, subretinal silicone oil or air have also been reported after vitrectomies in the presence of pits.[4] Ehlers et al. reported that after posterior hyaloid removal, direct aspiration over the optic nerve pit results in collapse of intraretinal cystoid spaces, suggesting a connection between the vitreous cavity and intraretinal fluid.[5] Another theory suggests that the source of subretinal fluid in optic nerve head pit associated maculopathy is actually CSF[1]; however, in the absence of cytologic analysis, this theory remains unproven. A few rare cases of optic nerve head pit associated with encephalocele have been described,[6,7] but in the absence of midline abnormalities, neuroimaging is not recommended.

Clinical Features

The pit is usually seen at the border of the optic nerve on a routine eye examination and may be associated with a gray-dark color (Fig. 59.1). If the pit location is in the papillomacular bundle, central visual acuity can be affected. Peripheral pits may be associated with arcuate scotomas.[8]

OCT Features

Optical coherence tomography (OCT) of the optic nerve may show a triangular slit posterior to the lamina cribrosa. The nerve fiber layer is shifted opposite to the pit, and some of the retina can

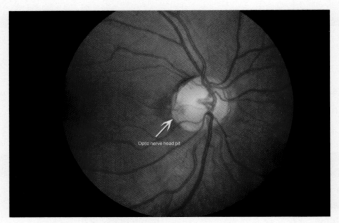

Fig. 59.1   Color fundus photo showing a gray optic nerve pit.

herniate into the pit (Fig. 59.2). Reflective strands or sheets may be found over the retinal surface, or the pit may also appear empty.[9] There may be associated retinal detachment and/or cystoid intraretinal fluid, which may be found in multiple layers. OCT is useful to monitor the volume extent and growth or decrease in fluid, as well as photoreceptor changes (reflectivity or thickness) over the subretinal fluid (Figs. 59.3 and 59.4). OCT can also be used intraoperatively to evaluate for intraoperative changes in vitreous strands, flaps, or intra- or subretinal fluid.[5]

Ancillary Testing

Visual fields can help determine the presence of a scotoma.

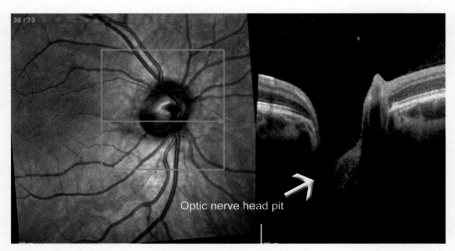

Fig. 59.2   Enhanced-depth imaging (EDI) scan of the right optic nerve from a 13-year-old boy demonstrates deep excavation of the inferotemporal optic nerve head (pit border).

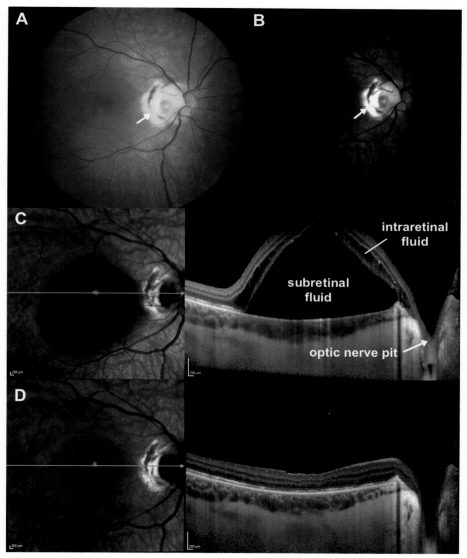

Fig. 59.3 (A) Color and (B) red-free photographs of an optic nerve pit *(arrow)* with serous retinal detachment in an 18-year-old female. (C) Optical coherence tomography (OCT) through the fovea and optic nerve demonstrates presence of the optic nerve pit with subretinal fluid and intraretinal fluid. The patient underwent vitrectomy with internal limiting membrane peel, endolaser, platelet-rich plasma to plug the pit, and intraocular gas tamponade. (D) Two months after surgery, OCT demonstrates resolution of retinal detachment and intraretinal fluid. (Adapted from Todorich B, Sharma S, Vajzovic L. Successful repair of recurrent optic disk PIT maculopathy with autologous platelet rich plasma: report of a surgical technique. *Retin Cases Brief Rep.* 2017 Winter;11(1):15–17.)

Treatment

Rarely, a pit can be associated with a serous retinal detachment or cystoid intraretinal fluid, which may be observed if mild and minimally affecting vision and may be treated, especially if progressive

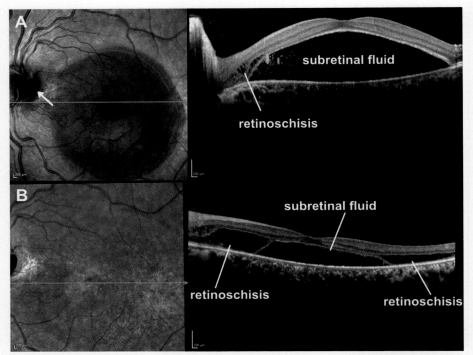

Fig. 59.4   Optic pit maculopathy in a 7-year-old girl. (A) Optical coherence tomography (OCT) at presentation demonstrates peripapillary retinoschisis and subretinal fluid extending into the fovea. The optic nerve pit can be visualized on the en face infrared image *(white arrow)*. (B) OCT taken 5 years later reveals improved retinal detachment and an increase in extrafoveal cystoid cavities. Visual acuity remained stable at 20/30 over the 5-year period. (Courtesy of Cynthia Toth, MD.)

and associated with decrease in visual acuity (see Figs. 59.3 and 59.4). However, controversy remains regarding the optimal techniques to treat the maculopathy. Laser along the pit margin and vitrectomy with use of various adjuncts (internal limiting membrane peel and sometimes placement of laser, gas exchange, fibrin, or platelet-rich plasma glue within the pit) have been suggested. Vitrectomy with posterior hyaloid separation alone has been shown to be a useful treatment, and during surgery, direct aspiration over the optic nerve pit with use of OCT was shown to partially drain intra- and subretinal fluid—arguing that there is a vitreous connection via the optic pit in some eyes.[5]

References

1. Gowdar JP, Rajesh B, Giridhar A, Gopalakrishnan M, Hussain R, Thachil T. An insight into the pathogenesis of optic disc pit-associated maculopathy with enhanced depth imaging. *JAMA Ophthalmol.* 2015;133 (4):466–469.
2. Kuhn F, Kover F, Szabo I, Mester V. Intracranial migration of silicone oil from an eye with optic pit. *Graefes Arch Clin Exp Ophthalmol.* 2006;244(10):1360–1362.
3. Johnson TM, Johnson MW. Pathogenic implications of subretinal gas migration through pits and atypical colobomas of the optic nerve. *Arch Ophthalmol.* 2004;122(12):1793–1800.
4. Grzybowski A, Pieczynski J, Ascaso FJ. Neuronal complications of intravitreal silicone oil: an updated review. *Acta Ophthalmol.* 2014;92(3):201–204.

5. Ehlers JP, Kernstine K, Farsiu S, Sarin N, Maldonado R, Toth CA. Analysis of pars plana vitrectomy for optic pit related maculopathy with intraoperative optical coherence tomography. *Arch Ophthalmol.* 2011;129 (11):1483–1486.
6. Seth A, Gupta R, Gupta A, Raina UK, Ghos B. Bilateral optic disc pit with maculopathy in a patient with cleft lip and cleft palate. *Indian J Ophthalmol.* 2015;63(4):346–348.
7. Goldhammer Y, Smith JL. Optic nerve anomalies in basal encephalocele. *Arch Ophthalmol.* 1975;93 (2):115–118.
8. Aboobakar IF, Mettu P, El-Dairi MA. Optic nerve head pit with sectoral inner retinal hypoplasia: a bottomless pit. *JAMA Ophthalmol.* 2015;133(6):e1572.
9. Ohno-Matsui K, Hirakata A, Inoue M, Akiba M, Ishibashi T. Evaluation of congenital optic disc pits and optic disc colobomas by swept-source optical coherence tomography. *Invest Ophthalmol Vis Sci.* 2013;54 (12):7769–7778.

Optic Nerve Coloboma

Mays El-Dairi

Introduction

An optic nerve coloboma is a congenital malformation marked by a defect in the optic nerve. It is caused by an incomplete closure of the embryonic fissure (optic fissure or choroidal fissure) during the first trimester of pregnancy. It can be unilateral or bilateral.

The Brain Connection

Colobomas can be isolated or part of a syndrome with other congenital brain malformations (see Chapter 55). The presence of a coloboma does not, however, necessarily correlate with a brain abnormality.

Clinical Features

It usually involves the inferonasal part of the optic disc and frequently involves the retina as well. It is frequently associated with ocular abnormalities, such as microphthalmos and colobomas in other parts of the eye: iris, ciliary, lens, and retina. As discussed in Chapter 55, although the cause is sporadic most of the time, it can also be associated with systemic abnormalities, such as CHARGE (coloboma, heart defects, atresia choanae, growth retardation, genital abnormalities, and ear abnormalities) syndrome, Aicardi syndrome, Goldenhar sequence, and Walker-Warburg renal coloboma syndrome.[1,2]

OCT Features

The coloboma manifests as a deep excavation next to or in part of the optic nerve area (Fig. 60.1A and B). The optical coherence tomography (OCT) signal deep to the area of thinned tissue is brighter than that of the normal Bruch membrane opening. An intercalary membrane or sometimes herniated retina can be found in the colobomatous area (see Fig. 60.1B and Fig. 60.2A).[3] Intraretinal cystoid spaces, retinal detachment, or fluid connection to deeper optic nerve and retrobulbar structures may also be found on OCT imaging; the deeper structures may be best visualized with swept-source OCT imaging.[3]

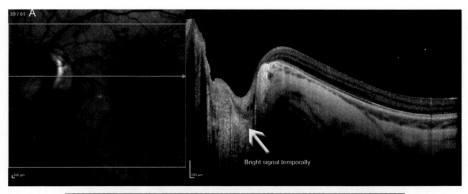

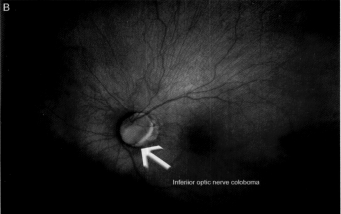

Fig. 60.1   (A) Infrared scanning laser ophthalmoscopic image and enhanced-depth imaging (EDI) spectral-domain optical coherence tomography (SD-OCT) scan of the left optic nerve head of a 5-year-old female with an optic nerve coloboma, showing deep excavation of the inferior aspect of the optic nerve. The signal temporally is brighter than the normal Bruch membrane opening. (B) Color fundus photo of the same 5-year-old female showing the optic nerve coloboma.

Ancillary Testing

As discussed in Chapter 55, it is usually recommended to screen for associated systemic abnormalities in patients with bilateral optic nerve colobomas or unilateral coloboma with one other systemic abnormality. If the child can cooperate for a visual field, this can be useful to demonstrate field deficits associated with the optic nerve coloboma (see Fig. 60.2C).

Treatment

There is no treatment for optic nerve coloboma. However, these patients need to be observed because of the high risk of choroidal neovascularization (CNV) and retinal detachment that would need treatment (see Chapter 55 for more information).

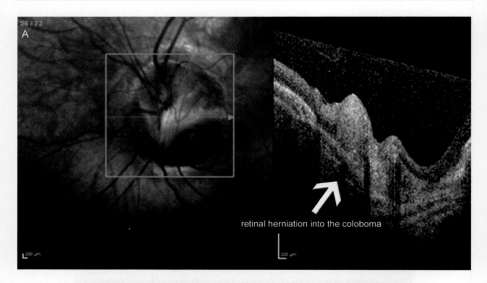

retinal herniation into the coloboma

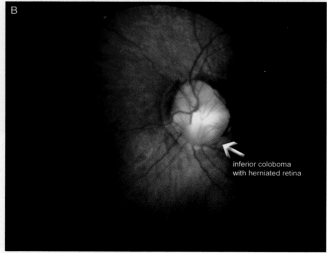

inferior coloboma
with herniated retina

Fig. 60.2   A 15-year-old female patient presenting with an optic nerve coloboma of the left eye; associated retinal herniation is demonstrated on OCT images (A) and color fundus photo (B).

(Continued)

Fixation Monitor: Blind Spot
Fixation Target: Central
Fixation Losses: 2/13
False POS Errors: 0%
False NEG Errors: 0%
Test Duration: 04:52

Stimulus: III. White
Background: 31.5 ASB
Strategy: SITA-Fast

Pupil Diameter:
Visual Acuity:
RX: +0.00 DS +2.25 DC X 115

Date: 12-12-2018
Time: 3:37 PM
Age: 17

Fovea: 28 dB ■

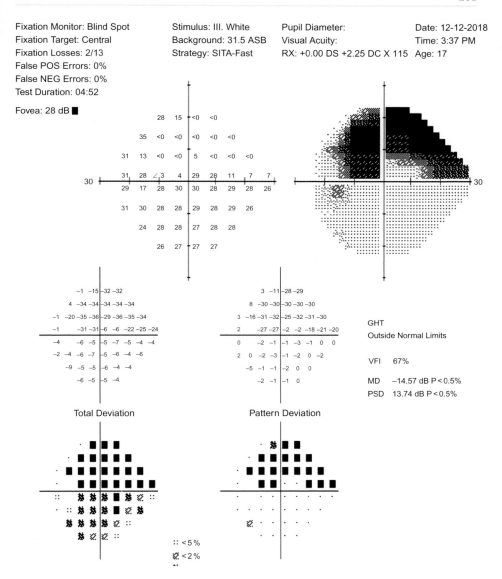

GHT
Outside Normal Limits

VFI   67%

MD   −14.57 dB P < 0.5%
PSD   13.74 dB P < 0.5%

Total Deviation

Pattern Deviation

:: < 5 %
※ < 2 %

Fig. 60.2—cont'd   (C) Visual field of the left eye, demonstrated by using a size 5 Humphrey stimulus (same patient).

References

1. Amador-Patarroyo MJ, Pérez-Rueda MA, Tellez CH. Congenital anomalies of the optic nerve. *Saudi J Ophthalmol.* 2015;29(1):32–38.
2. Nicholson B, Ahmad B, Sears JE. Congenital optic nerve malformations. *Int Ophthalmol Clin.* 2011; 51(1):49–76.
3. Ohno-Matsui K, Hirakata A, Inoue M, Akiba M, Ishibashi T. Evaluation of congenital optic disc pits and optic disc colobomas by swept-source optical coherence tomography. *Invest Ophthalmol Vis Sci.* 2013; 54(12):7769–7778.

Morning Glory

Mays El-Dairi ▪ James Tian

Introduction

The morning glory disc anomaly is a unilateral congenital malformation of the optic disc and surrounding retina, occurring in approximately 2.6 per 100,000 patients.[1] The anomaly is thought to be caused by either abnormal development of the distal optic stalk or abnormal closure of the choroidal fissure.[2]

The Brain Connection

Morning glory anomaly has been associated with basal encephalocele, pituitary dysfunction, and disorders of intracranial vascular development, such as PHACE (posterior fossa anomalies, hemangioma, arterial anomalies, cardiac anomalies, and eye anomalies) syndrome, Moyamoya disease, and other cerebrovascular malformations.[2]

Clinical Features

The morning glory disc appears as a funnel-shaped excavation of the optic disc with surrounding retinal disturbance (Fig. 61.1). Visual acuity is usually anywhere from 20/100 to 20/200 but can range from 20/20 to NLP ("no light perception"). Choroidal neovascular membranes or retinal detachment can occur in approximately one-third of affected patients.[3] Rarely, the nerve can be seen to exhibit contractile movements.[4]

OCT Features

Optical coherence tomography (OCT) usually shows a peripapillary staphyloma with glial tissue overlying the center of the optic disc. If an associated retinal detachment or choroidal neovascularization (CNV) are present, these can be visualized on OCT.[5]

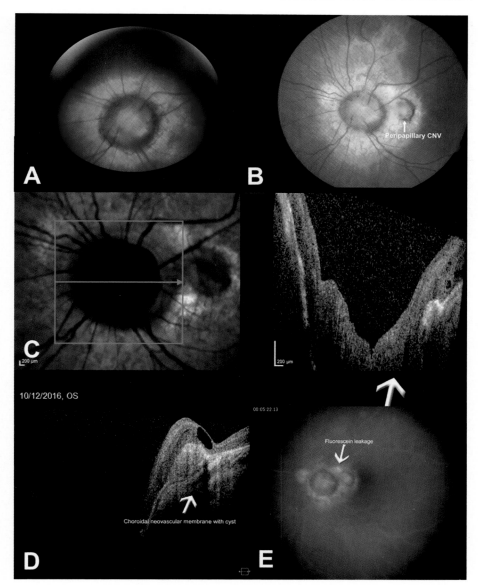

Fig. 61.1   Color fundus photo (A) of the left optic nerve in a 6-month-old girl demonstrates an optic nerve that is excavated in a funnel shape with a central tuft of gliosis and associated peripapillary changes. Left eye fundus photo (B) of the same patient at age 2 years after developing a temporal peripapillary neovascular membrane. At this follow-up appointment, optical coherence tomography (OCT) shows a peripapillary staphyloma (C) and peripapillary choroidal neovascularization (CNV) with an adjacent cyst (D). Late-frame of fluorescein angiography (E) shows leakage from the CNV, which was treated with intravitreal avastin.

Ancillary Testing

Given the high association with intracranial and vascular malformations, patients with morning glory optic nerves should undergo magnetic resonance imaging (MRI) of the brain and orbits with contrast as well as magnetic resonance angiography (MRA) of the head and neck. In the setting of an associated CNV or retinal detachment, fluorescein angiography may be needed.

Treatment

Reparative surgery may be required if a basal encephalocele is present. Intracranial vascular malformation usually needs serial monitoring or prophylactic treatment with aspirin. The presence of CNV or retinal detachment may be treated with surgery, laser, or intravitreal avastin injections. OCT may demonstrate vitreoretinal traction, which may be a consideration in surgical planning.[6]

References

1. Ceynowa DJ, Wickstrom R, Olsson M, et al. Morning glory disc anomaly in childhood—a population-based study. *Acta Ophthalmol.* 2015;93(7):626–634.
2. Lee BJ, Traboulsi EI. Update on the morning glory disc anomaly. *Ophthalmic Genet.* 2008;29(2):47–52.
3. Akiyama K, Azuma N, Hida T, Uemura Y. Retinal detachment in Morning Glory syndrome. *Ophthalmic Surg.* 1984;15(10):841–843.
4. Lee JE, Kim KH, Park HJ, Lee SJ, Jea SY. Morning glory disk anomaly: a computerized analysis of contractile movements with implications for pathogenesis. *J AAPOS.* 2009;13(4):403–405.
5. Cennamo G, de Crecchio G, Iaccarino G, Forte R, Cennamo G. Evaluation of morning glory syndrome with spectral optical coherence tomography and echography. *Ophthalmology.* 2010;117(6):1269–1273.
6. Chang S, Gregory-Roberts E, Chen R. Retinal detachment associated with optic disc colobomas and morning glory syndrome. *Eye (Lond).* 2012;26(4):494–500.

CHAPTER 62

Optic Nerve Hypoplasia

Mays El-Dairi ▪ Robert James House

Introduction

Optic nerve hypoplasia (ONH) is a developmental abnormality presenting with small optic nerves associated with a loss of the ganglion cell layer (GCL) and retinal nerve fiber layer (RNFL). ONH is one of the most common causes of visual impairment and blindness in children in the United States and Europe. It is a congenital anomaly of the optic nerve, rarely isolated and often part of other functional and anatomic abnormalities of the central nervous system.[1,2] Potential risk factors include prenatal exposures, genetic abnormalities, and maternal factors (e.g., young maternal age and primiparity).[2] Although most commonly bilateral, ONH can also occur in one eye only.

The Brain Connection

Corpus callosum abnormalities, hypothalamic dysfunction, pituitary abnormalities, and other neurologic conditions are commonly associated with ONH, as outlined in the other sections of this chapter.[2]

Clinical Features

ONH can present with a range of severity, vision loss, and associated conditions. Clinical findings include low vision, blindness, nystagmus, and strabismus; refractive errors also may be present. Systemic associations include hypothalamic dysfunction, pituitary dysfunction/panhypopituitarism, seizure disorders, autism spectrum disorders, infectious causes (e.g., Zika virus infection),[3] and other neurodevelopmental disorders. ONH is diagnosed by using ophthalmoscopic examination of the optic disc. The examination reveals small optic nerves; a "double ring" sign may be present (Fig. 62.1) and appears as a peripapillary yellow or white ring (often termed "halo") around the small nerve. Through clinical examination or fundus photography, nerve size is measured by determining the ratio of disc–diameter (DD) distance to disc–macula (DM) distance, and ONH is often diagnosed when this ratio is less than 0.35, although some patients with a DD/DM ratio of 0.30:0.35 have been described as still having normal vision.[2,4]

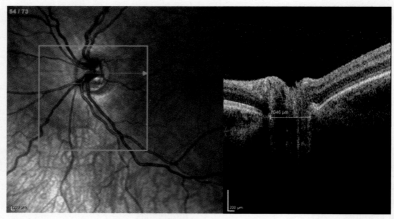

Fig. 62.1 Optical coherence tomography (OCT) demonstrating a small nerve and the Bruch membrane opening, measured at 1046 microns, in a 12-year-old girl with unilateral left optic nerve hypoplasia. The infrared image demonstrates the classic "double ring" sign.

OCT Features

OCT findings correlate with the general lack of GCL and RNFL layers.[5] These include a thinning of the RNFL (Fig. 62.2), a small Bruch membrane opening (Fig. 62.3), and a correlation with foveal hypoplasia. Although many features of ONH are seen on a clinical fundus examination, OCT allows for quantification of the RNFL and has been shown to demonstrate high sensitivity and high specificity for detecting the disease.[5]

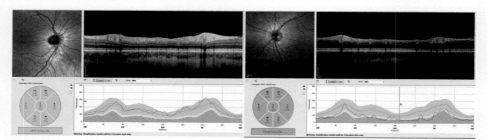

Fig. 62.2 A 10-year-old boy with unilateral optic nerve hypoplasia of the left eye. Optical coherence tomography (OCT) of the retinal nerve fiber layer (RNFL) demonstrated a normal RNFL of the right eye and global thinning in the left eye.

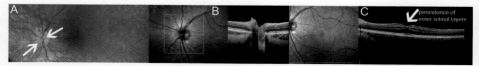

Fig. 62.3 The left eye of a 5-year-old patient with bilateral optic nerve hypoplasia and growth hormone deficiency. Optos color fundus photo (A) demonstrates a small optic nerve and a "double ring" sign *(arrows)*. Optic nerve head scan demonstrates a small Bruch membrane opening (B), measured at 912 microns. Single-line macular scan (C) through the fovea demonstrates persistence of the inner retina layer over the fovea center *(arrows)*, consistent with grade 1 foveal hypoplasia (fovea plana).

Ancillary Imaging

Magnetic resonance imaging (MRI) may help identify the presence of associated brain abnormalities. Fundus photography can also be useful.

Treatment

Patients diagnosed with ONH should be referred to a pediatric neurologist and/or endocrinologist to investigate for neuroendocrine disorders, including panhypopituitarism. Manifestations secondary to ONH, including refractive errors, strabismus, amblyopia, and nystagmus, should be managed accordingly. Children with unilateral ONH may benefit from patching to lessen the effect of amblyopia.

References

1. Dutton GN. Congenital disorders of the optic nerve: excavations and hypoplasia. *Eye (Lond).* 2004;18(11):1038–1048.
2. Garcia-Filion P, Borchert M. Optic nerve hypoplasia syndrome: a review of the epidemiology and clinical associations. *Curr Treat Options Neurol.* 2013;15(1):78–89.
3. Ventura LO, Ventura CV, Lawrence L, et al. Visual impairment in children with congenital Zika syndrome. *J AAPOS.* 2017;21(4):295–299. e292.
4. Borchert M, Garcia-Filion P. The syndrome of optic nerve hypoplasia. *Curr Neurol Neurosci Rep.* 2008;8(5):395–403.
5. Pilat A, Sibley D, McLean RJ, Proudlock FA, Gottlob I. High-resolution imaging of the optic nerve and retina in optic nerve hypoplasia. *Ophthalmology.* 2015;122(7):1330–1339.

CHAPTER 63

Tilting of the Disc and Megalopapilla

Mays El-Dairi ■ Robert James House

Introduction

Tilting of the optic disc is an anomaly sometimes discovered on routine childhood clinical examinations and can be caused by congenital[1] or acquired[2] processes. The congenital form, tilted disc syndrome (TDS), is thought to be caused by an oblique insertion of the optic nerve as it enters the eye, causing rotation of the nerve and an oval shape.[3] An acquired form in pediatric patients can also occur secondary to a myopic shift, in which an increase in axial length causes scleral stretching and peripapillary atrophy (PPA).

Megalopapilla is a congenital anomaly of the optic nerve, in which the size of the optic disc is larger than 2500 μm.

The Brain Connection

Tilted disc and megalopapilla are generally isolated findings and are not associated with any specific neurologic findings.

Clinical Features

Tilted discs are most commonly seen bilaterally. Clinical examination of the nerve typically shows temporal PPA with visible sclera in a crescent formation (Fig. 63.1). As the sclera is stretched, the temporal margin flattens, and the optic nerve is pulled temporally, leading to a protrusion of the Bruch membrane and choroid on the nasal/inferonasal side. This causes the classic elevation of the nasal margin and the horizontally tilted appearance of the nerve. Patients tend to present with moderate[4] to severe myopia, myopic astigmatism, and can have situs inversus of the retinal vessels. Bitemporal superior visual field defects not respecting the vertical midline can occur. These are often refractive scotomas and can be corrected with myopic correction. Visual prognosis is generally good.

Megalopapilla usually presents as an incidental finding, with preserved vision and normal visual fields. However, central vision can be mildly decreased. It can be a mimicker for glaucoma (Fig. 63.2). Refer to Chapter 70 for more information on how to differentiate glaucoma from its mimickers.

288

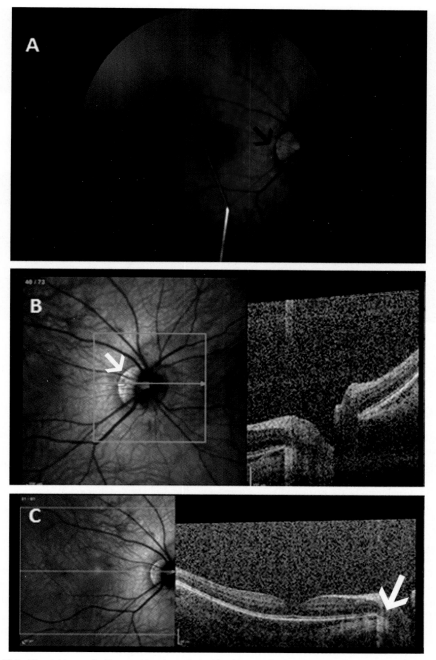

Fig. 63.1   The right eye of a 5-year-old male patient with a history of axial myopia with a prescription of −9.00 diopters (D) and an axial length of 26.62 mm. Color fundus photography (A) and infrared images (B and C) demonstrate thinning of the temporal margin. Bilateral tilting of the nerve is outlined on an optical coherence tomography (OCT) optic nerve head scan (B) along with peripapillary atrophy (*arrows in images A–C*). OCT image of the macula (C) shows the thinning of the Bruch membrane in the peripapillary area.

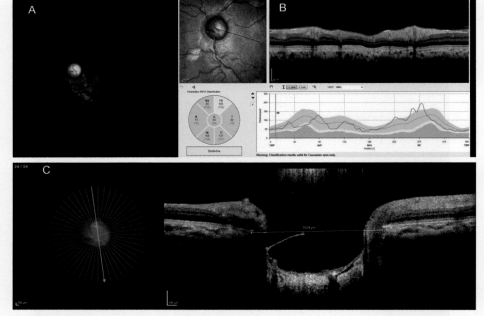

Fig. 63.2 Left optic nerve of a 15-year-old boy with megalopapilla. Color fundus photo (A) of a patient with megalopapilla, demonstrating what appears to be a large cup-to-disc ratio. Retinal nerve fiber layer (RNFL) scan (B) of a patient with megalopapilla shows that the peripapillary RNFL thickness is grossly normal despite the abnormal clinical appearance of the nerve. Optic nerve head scan (C) shows the Bruch membrane opening measuring 2529 microns.

OCT Features

In tilting of the disc, OCT cross-sectional scans of the disc demonstrate a protrusion of the Bruch membrane and choroid with concurrent thinning at the nasal margin of the optic disc, causing sloping of the lamina cribosa (see Fig. 63.1). The same scan also demonstrates nasal elevation in comparison with the temporal margin of the disc.

In megalopapilla, the nerve will have a large optic disc diameter (see Fig. 63.2), disc, and cup-to-disc ratio; however, the peripapillary retinal nerve fiber layer (pRNFL) is normal.[5]

Ancillary Imaging

In the case of a tilted disc, color fundus photography demonstrates the previously mentioned temporal PPA leading to the crescent shape of the visible sclera, along with an oblique, misshapen disc. For megalopapilla, visual fields, intraocular pressure (IOP), and central corneal thickness may be used to rule out glaucoma.

Treatment

Treatment is generally not required for a tilted disc unless associated with other clinical diagnoses, such as degenerative myopia and glaucoma. These conditions should be managed accordingly. No treatment is required for megalopapilla.

References

1. Pichi F, Romano S, Villani E, et al. Spectral-domain optical coherence tomography findings in pediatric tilted disc syndrome. *Graefes Arch Clin Exp Ophthalmol.* 2014;252(10):1661–1667.
2. Kim TW, Kim M, Weinreb RN, Woo SJ, Park KH, Hwang JM. Optic disc change with incipient myopia of childhood. *Ophthalmology.* 2012;119(1):21–26. e1–3.
3. Shinohara K, Moriyama M, Shimada N, et al. Analyses of shape of eyes and structure of optic nerves in eyes with tilted disc syndrome by swept-source optical coherence tomography and three-dimensional magnetic resonance imaging. *Eye (Lond).* 2013;27(11):1233–1242.
4. Maruko I, Iida T, Sugano Y, Oyamada H, Sekiryu T. Morphologic choroidal and scleral changes at the macula in tilted disc syndrome with staphyloma using optical coherence tomography. *Invest Ophthalmol Vis Sci.* 2011;52(12):8763–8768.
5. Lee HS, Park SW, Heo H. Megalopapilla in children: a spectral domain optical coherence tomography analysis. *Acta Ophthalmol.* 2015;93(4):e301–e305.

Optic Atrophy

Mays El-Dairi

Introduction

Optic atrophy is the result of damage to some (partial) or all (complete) the ganglion cells that form the optic nerve. It is a nonspecific end-stage process and is usually not seen before 3 to 4 weeks of the disease process. Causes can be varied, and include, but are not limited to, compressive lesions, papilledema, inflammation, vascular events, trauma, nutritional (vitamin B_{12} or folate deficiency), genetic, toxic (from certain medications, such as ethambutol), or secondary to certain chronic retinopathies.

The Brain Connection

When optic atrophy results from an isolated ocular cause (genetic, traumatic vascular event to the eye, or secondary to optic neuropathy), it would not necessarily be indicative of a central nervous system (CNS) problem. When the optic atrophy is a manifestation of a systemic or neurologic/neurodegenerative disease, the degree of optic atrophy (or measured retinal nerve fiber layer [RNFL] thinning) may correlate with the severity of the disease. This relationship has been established in adults with multiple sclerosis[1] and in premature babies with periventricular leukomalacia.[2] Optic atrophy may also be indicative of a brain lesion or injury causing compression or chronic papilledema.

Clinical Features

Funduscopic examination usually reveals optic nerve head pallor. Depending on the cause and severity, vision, color vision, or visual fields may be affected.

Mild optic nerve pallor may be harder to recognize in children compared with adults, and optical coherence tomography (OCT) plays a very important role in helping diagnose and follow up optic atrophy in children (Figs. 64.1 through 64.3), especially when they cannot perform reliably on automated perimetry.

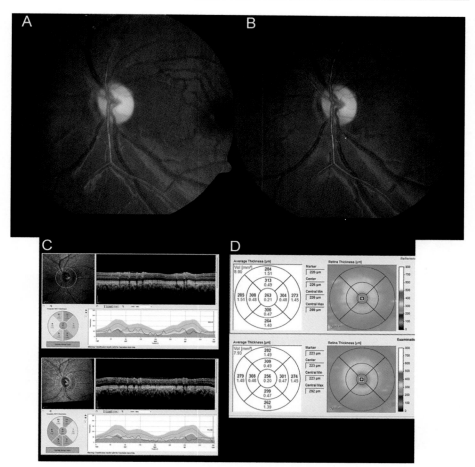

Fig. 64.1 Progression of optic atrophy in the left optic nerve of a female patient with Wolfram (DIDMOAD) syndrome from ages 8 to 15 years. Color fundus photos of the patient at age 8 years (A, *left pane*) and age 15 years (B, *right pane*) show worsening pallor. Retinal nerve fiber layer (RNFL) optical coherence tomography (OCT) at age 8 years (C) demonstrated an average RNFL of 61. At age 15 years, average RNFL (D) was 49. Note that there are some uncorrectable segmentation errors. Macular maps of the ganglion cell layer (E) could not be segmented until macular volume decreased from 8 mm³ cubed to 7.93 mm³.

OCT Features

Optic atrophy will manifest as thinning on the RNFL scan and the macular map (the inner retinal layers: nerve fiber layer [NFL], ganglion cell layer [GCL], and inner plexiform layer [IPL] are thinned) (see Figs. 64.1 through 64.3). The location of RNFL thinning may narrow down the potential location of the causative lesion (see Fig. 64.2). Sometimes cystoid spaces in the inner nuclear layer can be seen on the macular scan (see Fig. 64.3). The cystoid spaces may result from schisis, occur at the level of the inner nuclear layer, and be more common with nonglaucomatous optic atrophy than in pediatric glaucoma.[3] When optic atrophy is superimposed on active optic disc edema, it may be difficult to decipher resolution of edema from superimposed atrophy in the acute phase, and sometimes the RNFL may appear falsely reassuring when the there is a combination of

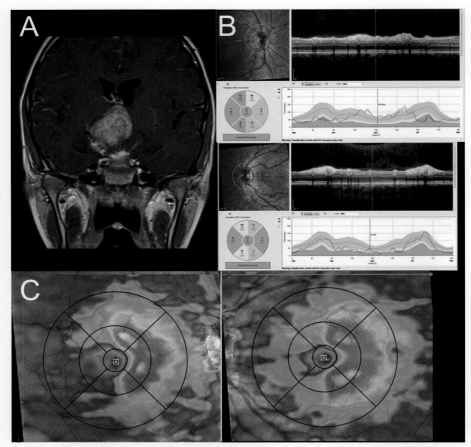

Fig. 64.2 A 5-year-old boy with bowtie optic atrophy caused by a large third ventricular mass crossing the floor of the third ventricle and pressing on the right optic tract. Contrast magnetic resonance imaging (MRI) (A) shows a large brain mass. Retinal nerve fiber layer (RNFL) optical coherence tomography (OCT) (B) of the right eye *(top)* and left eye *(bottom)* showing partial optic atrophy with a RNFL thickness of 74 and 67, respectively. Macular ganglion cell layer map (C) showing homonymous thinning of the ganglion cell layer on the right side, suggestive of injury producing a left homonymous hemianopia.

both pallor and atrophy in the same nerve. Therefore relying purely on the RNFL OCT to rule out partial optic atrophy can yield misleading results, so we recommend looking at the macular GCL as well[4] (Chapter 14; and see Fig. 64.3).

Ancillary Testing

It is very important to identify the cause of optic atrophy. A pale optic nerve is assumed to be caused by a compressive lesion until proven otherwise. The workup in a child with optic atrophy should include magnetic resonance imaging (MRI) of the brain and orbits with contrast, vitamin levels for B_{12} and folate. If negative and the pattern of optic atrophy is consistent with a possible genetic cause, genetic testing can be performed for Leber hereditary optic neuropathy (LHON), dominant

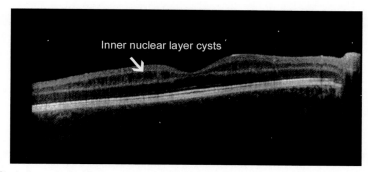

Fig. 64.3 Single-line optical coherence tomography (OCT) of the macula in the right eye of a 6-year-old boy with optic atrophy in the setting of acute demyelinating encephalomyelopathy optic neuritis. The ganglion cell layer is thin, and there are cystic changes in the inner nuclear layer *(arrow)*.

optic atrophy, Wolfram syndrome (see Fig. 64.1), and other genetic optic neuropathies (depending on the clinical history and associated manifestations).

Treatment

Once optic atrophy has occurred, it cannot be reversed. Treatment is aimed at identifying the cause and addressing it, if possible, to prevent progression.

References

1. Lange AP, Zhu F, Sayao AL, et al. Retinal nerve fiber layer thickness in benign multiple sclerosis. *Mult Scler.* 2013;19(10):1275–1281.
2. Rothman AL, Sevilla MB, Mangalesh S, et al. Thinner retinal nerve fiber layer in very preterm versus term infants and relationship to brain anatomy and neurodevelopment. *Am J Ophthalmol.* 2015;160 (6):1296–1308.
3. Jiramongkolchai K, Freedman SF, El-Dairi MA. Retinal changes in pediatric glaucoma and nonglaucoma-tous optic atrophy. *Am J Ophthalmol.* 2016;161:188–195.
4. Goldhagen BE1, Bhatti MT, Srinivasan PP, Chiu SJ, Farsiu S, El-Dairi MA. Retinal atrophy in eyes with resolved papilledema detected by optical coherence tomography. *J Neuroophthalmol.* 2015;35(2):122–126.

CHAPTER 65

Optic Nerve Glioma

Mays El-Dairi

CHAPTER OUTLINE

Introduction

Optic pathway glioma (OPG) is the most common intraconal tumor in children and is classified as juvenile pilocytic astrocytoma. These tumors are usually benign and slow growing and therefore can be asymptomatic for years.[1,2] It is estimated that about 50% of patients with OPG will have neurofibromatosis type I (NF-I).[3] However, the incidence of OPG in individuals with NF1 is about 15% to 30%; of those, only 50% of them will experience visual consequences. Mean age of diagnosis is around 5 years.[4,5]

The Brain Connection

Optic pathway gliomas are usually retrobulbar. In children with NF-I, gliomas are most common in the optic pathway (retrobulbar is most common, but these may be found in the chiasmatic–hypothalamic region or the posterior optic pathway) and may also occur in the brainstem. The detection of optic atrophy or retinal nerve fiber layer (RNFL) thinning on optical coherence tomography (OCT) may help diagnose a visually significant optic pathway glioma in when accurate assessment of visual function in a child is limited.[6]

Clinical Features

The presentation can vary from asymptomatic optic atrophy on a routine ophthalmic examination to findings of vision or visual field loss, optic disc edema or atrophy, relative afferent papillary defect, nystagmus, proptosis, and strabismus.

OCT Features

The most common OCT finding is optic atrophy (similar to a compressive lesion), although if discovered very early, mild optic disc edema may be present. Because most experts currently agree that the need to treat an OPG is based on whether or not there is vision loss, the use of OCT has become important to make this decision, especially in children who may not be cooperative during eye

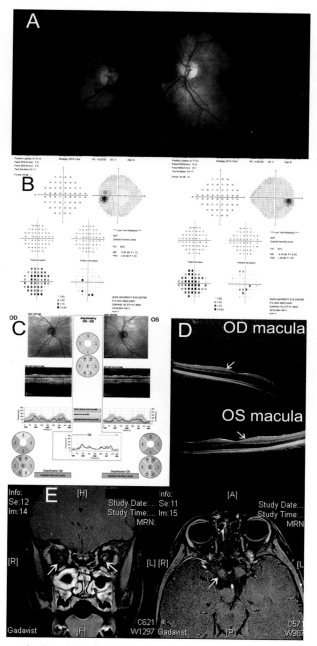

Fig. 65.1 Assessment of optic pathway glioma in an 8-year-old boy with neurofibromatosis type I (NF-I) and with visual acuity of 20/30 OD and 20/40 OS. (A) Color fundus photographs showed mild pallor (if any) of the left optic nerve, whereas the right optic nerve appeared normal. (B) The 24-2 Humphrey visual fields showed mild decreased sensitivity and nonspecific defects in both eyes. (C, D) Optical coherence tomography (OCT) of the optic nerve head (C) showed thinning of the peripapillary retinal nerve fiber layer (RNFL) more temporally than nasally in both eyes. Although a complete macular map could not be obtained because of lack of patient cooperation, a single-line macular OCT (D) showed significant thinning of the ganglion cell layer in both eyes *(arrows)*. In this case, OCT was more sensitive for detection of optic atrophy compared with fundus photography and clinical examination. (E) Magnetic resonance imaging (MRI) of the brain and orbits with contrast showed bilateral optic nerve gliomas with active enhancement in the left optic nerve and a nonenhancing chiasmal glioma *(arrows)*.

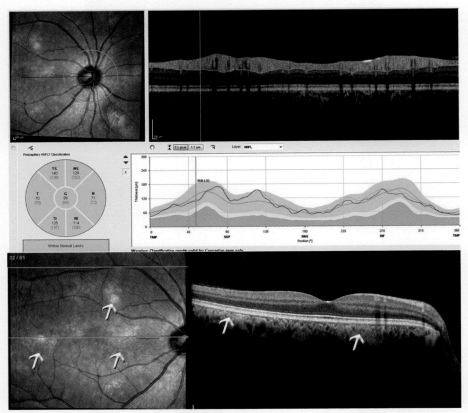

Fig. 65.2 Neurofibromatosis type I (NF-I) without optic pathway glioma. A 13-year-old boy with NF-I and a visual acuity of 20/20 OU and normal visual fields underwent magnetic resonance imaging (MRI), which demonstrated no evidence of glioma. Although the retinal nerve fiber layer (RNFL) thickness was normal, the infrared scanning laser ophthalmoscopic image (A) and macular optical coherence tomography (OCT) (B) showed multiple choroidal neurofibromas *(arrows)*.

examination. It has been shown that the peripapillary RNFL thickness correlates with vision loss and can help differentiate patients who may have a visual decline as a result of an OPG (Fig. 65.1A–E).

Independent of the presence of an optic pathway glioma, choroidal neurofibromas in individuals with NF-I (Fig. 65.2) may be demonstrated by macular OCT. These tumors are usually visually insignificant, very much like Lisch nodules.

Ancillary Testing

If an optic pathway glioma is suspected, brain MRI of the orbits with contrast is recommended to confirm the diagnosis. Endocrine workup is also recommended in case the pituitary gland is also involved.

Treatment

Treatment with chemotherapy is reserved only for patients with vision loss. If the glioma is not associated with vision changes, the recommendation is observation only.

References

1. King A, Listernick R, Charrow J, Piersall L, Gutmann DH. Optic pathway gliomas in neurofibromatosis type 1: the effect of presenting symptoms on outcome. *Am J Med Genet A.* 2003;122a(2):95–99.
2. Louis DN, Ohgaki H, Wiestler OD, et al. The 2007 WHO classification of tumours of the central nervous system. *Acta Neuropathol.* 2007;114(2):97–109.
3. Miller NR. Primary tumours of the optic nerve and its sheath. *Eye (Lond).* 2004;18(11):1026–1037.
4. Thiagalingam S, Flaherty M, Billson F, North K. Neurofibromatosis type 1 and optic pathway gliomas: follow-up of 54 patients. *Ophthalmology.* 2004;111(3):568–577.
5. Czyzyk E, Jóźwiak S, Roszkowski M, Schwartz RA. Optic pathway gliomas in children with and without neurofibromatosis 1. *J Child Neurol.* 2003;18(7):471–478.
6. Avery RA, Liu GT, Fisher MJ, et al. Retinal nerve fiber layer thickness in children with optic pathway gliomas. *Am J Ophthalmol.* 2011;151(3):542–549. e542.

CHAPTER 66

Papilledema and Disc Swelling Versus Traction Elevation

Mays El-Dairi

Introduction

Papilledema is swelling of the optic nerve caused by high intracranial pressure (ICP) and is usually bilateral. Causes include compressive intracranial lesions (congenital or acquired) that cause cerebral spinal fluid (CSF) flow obstruction, venous sinus thrombosis, malignant hypertension, meningitis, or certain medications, or it may be idiopathic.

The Brain Connection

Increased ICP is often associated with swelling of the optic nerves. The term *papilledema* is reserved to describe swelling of the optic nerve caused by high ICP. Although the grade of papilledema has not been shown to correlate with the measurement of the ICP, it has been correlated with risk of vision loss.[1,2]

Clinical Features

The clinical presentation varies and may include complaints of positional headaches, intracranial noise, transient vision obscuration, vision changes, and diplopia caused by sixth cranial nerve palsy. The optic nerves are swollen (usually it is bilateral, and the severity of the papilledema is graded from 0 to 5 according to the Frisén scale (based on fundus photographs) of blurring of disc margins and major vessels.[3]

OCT Features

Optical coherence tomography (OCT) can help diagnose and grade papilledema. In papilledema, the RNFL is thickened (average retinal nerve fiber layer [RNFL] >131 μm); the Bruch membrane opening is enlarged (average >1718 μm).[4] Depending on the severity of the papilledema, peripapillary retinal changes, such as schisis, subretinal fluid, and loss of photoreceptor ellipsoid zone, can also be seen (Fig. 66.1).[2] The grading of papilledema via OCT (based on RNFL or even total retinal thickness) has been shown to be more reliable than a masked expert panel—especially for mild and moderate papilledema.[5] OCT can also be used to monitor the changes in RNFL after treatment (see Fig. 66.1; Fig. 66.2) or the development of optic atrophy. While looking at the Bruch

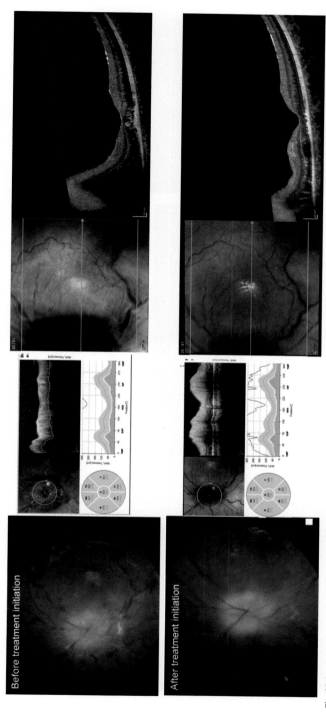

Fig. 66.1 A 14-year-old female with idiopathic intracranial hypertension. Top panel: Before treatment, Color fundus photo (A) of the left eye shows severe papilledema grade 5. Optical coherence tomography (OCT) of the retinal nerve fiber layer (RNFL) (B) demonstrates severely thickened RNFL (segmentation had to be manually corrected). Single-line macular OCT image (C) shows subretinal fluid, schisis of the outer nuclear layer, and photoreceptor changes. Bottom panel: After treatment, color fundus photo (D) shows decrease in the papilledema, now grade 3/4. Peripapillary RNFL (E) shows decrease in the elevation of RNFL thickening. Single-line macular OCT image (F) shows resolution of the subretinal fluid and of the outer nuclear layer schisis, with partial recovery of the photoreceptors.

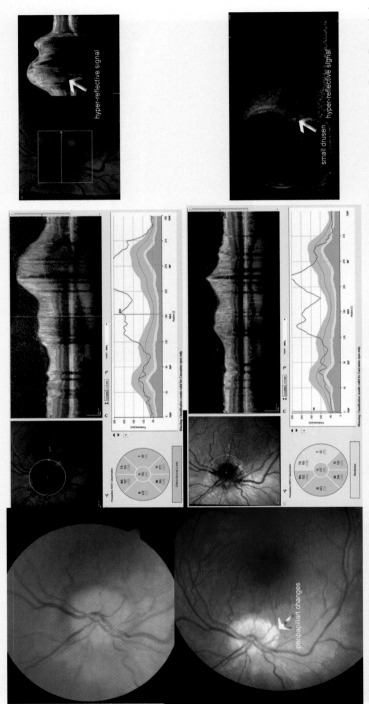

Fig. 66.2 A 6-year-old boy with papilledema secondary to hydrocephalus. Top panel: Before treatment, color fundus photo (A) shows grade 2 papilledema. Peripapillary optical coherence tomography (OCT) of the retinal nerve fiber layer (RNFL) image (B) shows moderate thickening with average RNFL at 186 microns. Enhanced depth imaging (EDI) OCT (C) shows a hyperreflective signal under the optic nerve, suggestive of an optic nerve head drusen. Bottom panel: After treatment, color fundus photo (D) does not demonstrate any edema, but peripapillary changes are now seen (arrow). OCT RNFL scan (E) shows mildly thickened RNFL with an average of 137 microns. EDI OCT showed no change in the disc drusen, which was also demonstrated on ultrasonography (F). The coexistence of optic nerve head drusen and papilledema is not uncommon.

membrane opening on the optic nerve head (ONH) map or scan, an upward angle is suggestive of increased intracranial pressure (ICP); however, this finding is not sensitive or specific.[6] Changes in the outer retina (ellipsoid absence or discontinuation) on a macular scan can be predictive of a worse final visual outcome[2,7] (see Fig. 66.1). In a cohort of 31 children with papilledema caused by idiopathic intracranial hypertension, optic disc drusen were noted in 48% of study eyes by enhanced depth imaging (EDI) OCT (see Fig. 66.2C) and confirmed by ultrasonography (see Fig. 66.2F).[2]

Ancillary Testing

The cause of the high ICP should be investigated. Depending on the clinical suspicion, workup should include blood pressure check, imaging of the brain and orbits, and venous sinus imaging (magnetic resonance imaging/magnetic resonance venography [MRI/MRV] or computed tomography/computed tomography venography [CT/CTV], followed by lumbar puncture if the neuroimaging results are normal.

Treatment

The treatment is to reduce the ICP, either medically or surgically. In the cases of idiopathic intracranial hypertension, in particular, surgical treatment is reserved for patients who fail maximal medical therapy. Optic nerve sheath fenestration is indicated in cases of severe or impending vision loss without significant headaches. A CSF diversion procedure is reserved for those in whom maximal medical therapy fails to control headaches.

References

1. Wall M, Falardeau J, Fletcher WA, et al. Risk factors for poor visual outcome in patients with idiopathic intracranial hypertension. *Neurology.* 2015;85(9):799–805.
2. Gospe 3rd SM, Bhatti MT, El-Dairi MA. Anatomic and visual function outcomes in paediatric idiopathic intracranial hypertension. *Br J Ophthalmol.* 2016;100(4):505–509.
3. Frisén L. Swelling of the optic nerve head: a staging scheme. *J Neurol Neurosurg Psychiatry.* 1982;45 (1):13–18.
4. Thompson AC, Bhatti MT, El-Dairi MA. Bruch's membrane opening on optical coherence tomography in pediatric papilledema and pseudopapilledema. *J AAPOS.* 2018;22(1):38–43. e33.
5. Scott CJ, Kardon RH, Lee AG, Frisén L, Wall M. Diagnosis and grading of papilledema in patients with raised intracranial pressure using optical coherence tomography vs clinical expert assessment using a clinical staging scale. *Arch Ophthalmol.* 2010;128(6):705–711.
6. Kupersmith MJ, Mandel G, Anderson S, Meltzer DE, Kardon R. Baseline, one and three month changes in the peripapillary retinal nerve fiber layer in acute optic neuritis: relation to baseline vision and MRI. *J Neurol Sci.* 2011;308(1-2):117–123.
7. Tawse KL, Hedges 3rd TR, Gobuty M, Mendoza-Santiesteban C. Optical coherence tomography shows retinal abnormalities associated with optic nerve disease. *Br J Ophthalmol.* 2014;98(suppl 2):ii30–33.

CHAPTER 67

Optic Neuritis and Multiple Sclerosis

Mays El-Dairi

Introduction

Optic neuritis is inflammation of the optic nerve. It is rare in children. It may be an isolated event or a manifestation of a systemic recurrent of chronic demyelinating diseases such as acute demyelinating optic neuropathy, neuromyelitis optica, and multiple sclerosis.

The Brain Connection

It has been shown in adult subjects with multiple sclerosis that the retinal nerve fiber layer (RNFL) measurement reflects disease activity. This finding allows for the use of the RNFL as a biomarker for disease activity and efficacy of treatment in clinical trials.[1-5]

Clinical Features

Patients usually present with acute vision loss (usually unilateral in adults; in children, it is either unilateral or bilateral), with eye pain that is exacerbated by eye movements. In unilateral or asymmetric cases, there should be a relative afferent pupillary defect. Fundus examination may be normal (which is the usual scenario in adults because the process is retrobulbar) or can show optic nerve edema (in up to 66% of children).

OCT Features

In the acute phase of optic neuritis, optical coherence tomography (OCT) usually shows thickening of the RNFL even if no edema is seen on funduscopic examination (Fig. 67.1).[6,7] In the later stage, as optic atrophy develops, the RNFL becomes thin (Fig. 67.2).[6-11]

Imaging of the retina in optic neuritis–induced optic atrophy may reveal cystic lesions in the inner nuclear layer.[12] These are seen in other types of optic atrophy and are thought to be caused by microschisis at the level of the inner nuclear layer.

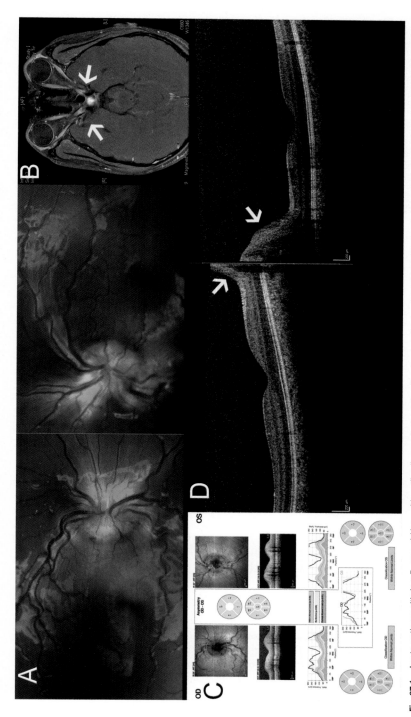

Fig. 67.1 Acute optic neuritis in a 5-year-old boy with antibodies against myelin oligodendrocyte glycoprotein (MOG). Optos color fundus photos (A) demonstrate bilateral optic nerve head swelling. Magnetic resonance imaging (MRI) scan (B) shows enhancement of the optic nerves bilaterally *(arrows)*. Optical coherence tomography (OCT) image (C) shows the retinal nerve fiber layer (RNFL) being bilaterally thickened, with an average RNFL of 207 (OD) and 232 (OS). Single-line macular OCT image (D) shows normal inner and outer retinal architecture. The nasal macula is elevated in both eyes *(arrows)*.

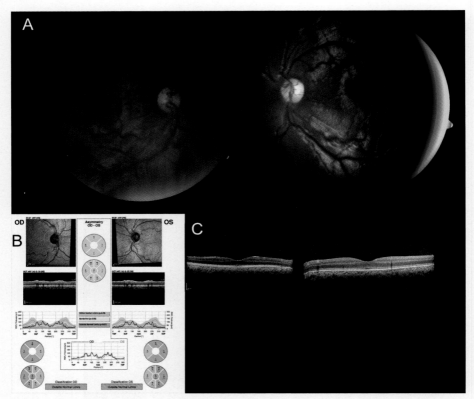

Fig. 67.2 The same patient from Fig. 67.1 a month later. Color fundus photos (A) show bilateral optic nerve head pallor. Optical coherence tomography (OCT) retinal nerve fiber layer (RNFL) image (B) shows bilateral RNFL thinning, with an average RNFL of 59 (OD) and 57 (OS). Single-line macular OCT image (C) shows severe thinning of the ganglion cell layer.

Ancillary Testing

Contrast magnetic resonance imaging (MRI) of the orbits shows enhancement of the retrobulbar optic nerve (see Fig. 67.1B). Brain MRI and spine MRI are essential to look for white-matter lesions that may suggest the diagnosis of multiple sclerosis or neuromyelitis optica. Lumbar puncture may be indicated to rule out infectious, malignant, or inflammatory conditions that may have long-term neurologic sequelae. Laboratory testing for aquaporin V antibodies is done to rule out neuromyelitis optica and myelin oligodendrocyte glycoprotein (MOG) antibodies.

Treatment

High-dose intravenous solumedrol has been shown to shorten the course of optic neuritis in adults, but it has not been shown to alter the final visual outcome. Data on children are still being collected as part of the pediatric optic neuritis treatment trial. If neuromyelitis optica is suspected, treatment may include high-dose solumedrol for 3 to 5 days, intravenous immunoglobulin (IVIG), or even plasmapheresis. If the diagnosis of multiple sclerosis or neuromyelitis optica is suspected, long-term treatment would be required to prevent complications and early disability.

References

1. Sergott RC. Optical coherence tomography: measuring in-vivo axonal survival and neuroprotection in multiple sclerosis and optic neuritis. *Curr Opin Ophthalmol.* 2005;16(6):346–350.
2. Zimmermann H, Freing A, Kaufhold F, et al. Optic neuritis interferes with optical coherence tomography and magnetic resonance imaging correlations. *Mult Scler.* 2012;19(4):443–450.
3. Costello F, Coupland S, Hodge W, et al. Quantifying axonal loss after optic neuritis with optical coherence tomography. *Ann Neurol.* 2006;59(6):963–969.
4. Costello F, Hodge W, Pan Y, Eggenberger E, Coupland S, Kardon R. Tracking retinal nerve fiber layer loss after optic neuritis: a prospective study using optical coherence tomography. *Mult Scler.* 2008;14(7):893–905.
5. Kallenbach K, Frederiksen J. Optical coherence tomography in optic neuritis and multiple sclerosis: a review. *Eur J Neurol.* 2007;14(8):841–849.
6. Pro MJ, Pons ME, Liebmann JM, et al. Imaging of the optic disc and retinal nerve fiber layer in acute optic neuritis. *J Neurol Sci.* 2006;250(1-2):114–119.
7. Kupersmith MJ, Mandel G, Anderson S, Meltzer DE, Kardon R. Baseline, one and three month changes in the peripapillary retinal nerve fiber layer in acute optic neuritis: relation to baseline vision and MRI. *J Neurol Sci.* 2011;308(1-2):117–123.
8. Noval S, Contreras I, Rebolleda G, Muñoz-Negrete FJ. Optical coherence tomography in optic neuritis. *Ophthalmology.* 2007;114(1):200.
9. Syc SB, Saidha S, Newsome SD, et al. Optical coherence tomography segmentation reveals ganglion cell layer pathology after optic neuritis. *Brain.* 2012;135:521–533.
10. Trip SA, Schlottmann PG, Jones SJ, et al. Retinal nerve fiber layer axonal loss and visual dysfunction in optic neuritis. *Ann Neurol.* 2005;58(3):383–391.
11. Trip SA, Schlottmann PG, Jones SJ, et al. Optic nerve atrophy and retinal nerve fibre layer thinning following optic neuritis: evidence that axonal loss is a substrate of MRI-detected atrophy. *Neuroimage.* 2006;31(1):286–293.
12. Kaufhold F, Zimmermann H, Schneider E, et al. Optic neuritis is associated with inner nuclear layer thickening and microcystic macular edema independently of multiple sclerosis. *PLoS One.* 2013;8(8):e71145.

Neuroretinitis

Mays El-Dairi

Introduction

Neuroretinitis is inflammation of both the optic nerve and the macula. Causes can be infectious, inflammatory, or infiltrative. The most common cause in children is *Bartonella henselae*, or cat scratch disease.

The Brain Connection

The typical neuroretinitis is usually isolated. In rare scenarios (e.g., syphilis, leukemia, sarcoid, other rare infections, or even *Bartonella* infection in certain individuals[1,2]), neuroretinitis may be indicative of (or concurrent with) brain involvement (encephalitis).[1,3]

Clinical Features

Patients usually present with acute unilateral vision loss and a relative afferent pupillary defect (RAPD). The optic nerve is swollen with exudative fluid in the peripapillary area (Fig. 68.1A). The accumulation of exudates in the outer plexiform layer gives the classic macular star pattern. The macular star may not be visible acutely and appears about 5 to 7 days later.

OCT Features

RNFL thickening is seen acutely. Despite the possible absence of a frank macular star on examination, macular optical coherence tomography (OCT) shows foveal contour changes, hyperreflective foci within the retina and especially in outer plexiform, Henle and photoreceptor layers. These may be thicker in association with macular star. Further findings include loss of distinct photoreceptor outer bands (external limiting membrane, ellipsoid zone and interdigitation zone), thickening, and subretinal fluid and exudates[4] (see Fig. 68.1B). OCT helps differentiate neuroretinitis from isolated optic neuritis (the macular star may not be seen in the early stages of neuroretinitis on clinical examination, but OCT will show edema and subretinal fluid), or other causes of optic nerve edema.

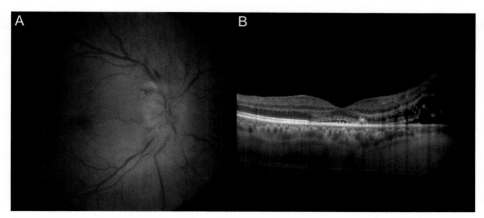

Fig. 68.1   Color fundus photo (A) of the right eye of a 13-year-old Hispanic girl with *Bartonella* infection–related neuroretinitis, showing swollen right optic nerve with peripapillary hemorrhages and a right hemi-macular star *(arrow)*. Single-line macular optical coherence tomography (OCT) scan (B) showing subretinal fluid, many hyperreflective foci on the foveal RPE surface and in the outer retina, a larger hyperreflective focus in the nasal fovea in the location of the hemi-macular star, and photoreceptor changes which include disruption of the photoreceptor outer layers (ellipsoid zone and interdigitation zone).

Ancillary Testing

In classic isolated neuroretinitis, orbital magnetic resonance imaging (MRI) shows enhancement that is isolated to the intraocular portion of the optic nerve. Laboratory work should include screening for *B. henselae* titers, rapid plasma reagin (RPR), fluorescent treponemal antibody absorption (FTA-ABS), Lyme titers, angiotensin-converting enzyme (ACE), Rocky Mountain Spotted Fever (RMSF) titers, and purified protein derivative (PPD) test. Chest imaging (radiography or computed tomography [CT], depending on suspicion) are obtained to rule out tuberculosis or sarcoidosis.

Treatment

Treatment is dependent on the etiology. Consultation with infectious disease specialist or rheumatologist should be sought if infections, such as syphilis or tuberculosis, are found. In cat scratch neuroretinitis, in particular, visual outcome has not been shown to be influenced by systemic treatment with antibiotics.[5]

References

1. Rondet B, Sarret C, Lacombe P, et al. [Neurological symptoms with Bartonella henselae infection: report on 2 pediatric cases]. *Arch Pediatr.* 2012;19(8):823–826.
2. Marra CM. Neurologic complications of Bartonella henselae infection. *Curr Opin Neurol.* 1995;8(3):164–169.
3. Sivakumar RR, Prajna L, Arya LK, et al. Molecular diagnosis and ocular imaging of West Nile virus retinitis and neuroretinitis. *Ophthalmology.* 2013;120(9):1820–1826.
4. Habot-Wilner Z, Zur D, Goldstein M, et al. Macular findings on optical coherence tomography in cat-scratch disease neuroretinitis. *Eye (Lond).* 2011;25(8):1064–1068.
5. Bhatti MT, Lee MS. Should patients with *Bartonella* neuroretinitis receive treatment? *J Neuroophthalmol.* 2014;34(4):412–416.

Optic Nerve Head Drusen

Mays El-Dairi

Introduction

Optic nerve head drusen are deposits of protein and calcium salts that accumulate in the optic nerve head. They are usually buried in the patient's first decade of life and become visible around the teenage years.

The Brain Connection

Optic nerve head drusen is usually isolated to the eye and not indicative of a neurologic condition.

Clinical Features

In teenagers, optic nerve head drusen are usually asymptomatic and are incidentally found on a routine funduscopic examination. They may cause arcuate peripheral visual field defects (usually later in life). Although usually asymptomatic, optic nerve head drusen can mimic papilledema and thus calls for a complex workup.

OCT Features

Imaging the optic nerve head can be accomplished with spectral-domain optical coherence tomography (SD-OCT); however, enhanced-depth imaging (EDI) is preferred. The EDI protocol can reveal the buried drusen, appearing as a hyperreflective body underneath the nerve (Fig. 69.1). Sometimes the angle formed by the edge of the RPE can be deflected inward in high intracranial pressure (ICP) and normally deflected in an optic nerve head drusen (poor sensitivity and specificity).[1-3] The presence of drusen may cause peripapillary choroidal neovascular membrane (CNVMs) that can be easily detected by OCT (see Fig. 69.1). Nasal drusen do not require treatment, and temporal ones may need treatment if central vision is affected.[4,5]

A decreased average RNFL in the setting of an optic nerve heard drusen is suggestive of partial optic atrophy and the presence of a visual field defect.[6]

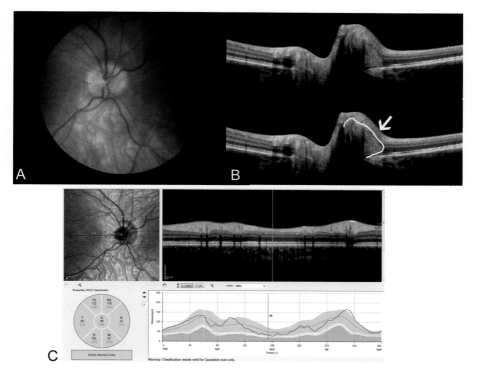

Fig. 69.1 Color fundus photo (A) of the right optic nerve of a 13-year-old white girl. The nerve is nasally elevated, but there is no obscuration of the vessels. Enhanced-depth optical coherence tomography (EDI OCT) (B, *top*) shows hyperreflective material underneath the nerve fiber layer. The drusen has been outlined and labeled with an arrow (B, *bottom*). Peripapillary retinal nerve fiber layer (C) is normal with an average RNFL thickness of 98 microns.

Ancillary Testing

Ocular ultrasonography can show the hyperreflective calcification (so would computed tomography [CT]; however, we would not advise CT for the purpose of differentiating optic nerve head drusen from papilledema). However, the sensitivity of ultrasonography can be low because some of the wave signals can be dampened by the intraocular lens. Fundus autofluorescence will only show hyperautofluorescence if the drusen is superficial and visible. In some cases, fluorescein angiography (FA) can help distinguish an optic nerve head drusen from true optic disc edema (the swollen nerve would show late leakage, but the optic nerve head drusen would not). An optic disc drusen surrounded by CNVM will also leak on FA, thus giving a false-positive result.

Treatment

No treatment is required for optic nerve head drusen unless there is temporal CNVM affecting the central vision.

References

1. Kulkarni KM, Pasol J, Rosa PR, Lam BL. Differentiating mild papilledema and buried optic nerve head drusen using spectral domain optical coherence tomography. *Ophthalmology*. 2014;121(4):959–963.

2. Silverman AL, Tatham AJ, Medeiros FA, Weinreb RN. Assessment of optic nerve head drusen using enhanced depth imaging and swept source optical coherence tomography. *J Neuroophthalmol.* 2014;34 (2):198–205.
3. Sibony P, Kupersmith MJ, Rohlf FJ. Shape analysis of the peripapillary RPE layer in papilledema and ischemic optic neuropathy. Invest *Ophthalmol Vis Sci.* 2011;52(11):7987–7995.
4. Knape RM, Zavaleta EM, Clark 3rd CL. Intravitreal bevacizumab treatment of bilateral peripapillary choroidal neovascularization from optic nerve head drusen. *J AAPOS.* 2011;15(1):87–90.
5. Duncan JE, Freedman SF, El-Dairi MA. The incidence of neovascular membranes and visual field defects from optic nerve head drusen in a large cohort of pediatric patients. *J AAPOS.* 2016;20(1):44-48.
6. Noval S, Visa J, Contreras I. Visual field defects due to optic disk drusen in children. *Graefes Arch Clin Exp Ophthalmol.* 2013;251(10):2445–2450.

CHAPTER 70

Childhood Glaucoma

Sharon Freedman ■ Amanda Ely

Introduction

Childhood glaucoma represents a heterogeneous group of disorders that share the common features of elevated intraocular pressure (IOP) and resultant secondary ocular changes/damage. Onset can occur anytime from birth to age less than 18 years. Recently, international consensus has helped unify the definitions of "glaucoma" and "glaucoma suspect" in children and offers a simple classification system for both primary and secondary childhood glaucomas. These are listed in Tables 70.1 and 70.2, respectively.[1]

Clinical Features

Before the introduction of optical coherence tomography (OCT), baseline optic nerve status documentation was limited to photography and very often to subjective documentation of optic nerve head cupping, which varied according to the method of viewing (e.g., slit-lamp biomicroscopy versus indirect ophthalmoscopy) as well as from one clinician to another. These methods are still used when OCT imaging is not feasible.

GLAUCOMA SUSPECT

Typically, the pediatric glaucoma suspect presents with either elevated IOP with a healthy-appearing optic nerve or an unusual optic nerve configuration with or without elevated IOP. At other times, the "glaucoma suspect" is a child with other ocular or systemic features that herald a high risk for the development of glaucoma (e.g., eyes with "port wine stain" on one or both sides of the upper face, Axenfeld-Rieger syndrome, or aniridia; childhood cataract removal, uveitis, or trauma) (see Table 70.2).

CHILDHOOD GLAUCOMA

The clinical features of childhood glaucoma vary widely, depending on the type and underlying cause, as well as age of onset and severity of disease. As mentioned earlier, common features usually

TABLE 70.1 ■ Definitions of Glaucoma and Glaucoma Suspect in Children

Term	Features
Glaucoma (≥2 features required)	IOP >21 mm Hg (discretion if examination under anesthesia data alone), Optic disc cupping: a progressive increase in cup-to-disc ratio, cup-to-disc asymmetry of ≥0.2 when the optic discs are similar size, or focal rim thinning Corneal findings: Haab striae or diameter ≥11mm in newborn, >12 mm in child <1 year of age, >13 mm any age Progressive myopia or myopic shift coupled with an increase in ocular dimensions out of keeping with normal growth Reproducible visual field defect consistent with glaucomatous optic neuropathy with no other observable reason for the visual field defect
Glaucoma suspect (at least one feature required)	IOP >21 mm Hg on two separate occasions Or suspicious optic disc appearance for glaucoma (i.e., increased cup-to-disc ratio for size of optic disc) Or suspicious visual field for glaucoma Or increased corneal diameter or axial length in setting of normal IOP

IOP, Intraocular pressure.
Adapted from Beck A, Chang TCP, Freedman S. Definition, classification, differential diagnosis. In *Childhood Glaucoma. The 9th Consensus Report of the World Glaucoma Association.* Amsterdam, The Netherlands: Kugler Publications; 2013.

TABLE 70.2 ■ Classification of Childhood Glaucoma

Broad Category	Subtypes and Examples
Primary childhood glaucoma	Primary congenital glaucoma (PCG) Juvenile open-angle glaucoma (JOAG)
Secondary childhood glaucoma	Glaucoma associated with nonacquired ocular anomalies—includes conditions of predominantly ocular anomalies present at birth which may or may not have associated systemic signs (e.g., Axenfeld-Rieger, Peters, and Aniridia syndromes] Glaucoma associated with non-acquired systemic disease or syndrome—includes conditions predominantly of systemic disease present at birth which may have associated ocular signs (e.g., Trisomy 21/other chromosomal abnormalities, Marfan syndrome/other connective tissue disorders, Lowe syndrome/other metabolic disorders, Sturge-Weber syndrome/other phacomatoses) Glaucoma associated with acquired condition—(e.g., secondary to uveitis, trauma, steroid, tumors, retinopathy of prematurity, postsurgical other than cataract removal) Glaucoma following cataract surgery—after removal of congenital idiopathic cataract, congenital cataract associated with ocular/systemic anomalies (but no previous glaucoma), acquired cataract (but no previous glaucoma)

Adapted from Beck A, Chang TCP, Freedman S. Definition, classification, differential diagnosis. In *Childhood Glaucoma. The 9th Consensus Report of the World Glaucoma Association.* Amsterdam, The Netherlands: Kugler Publications; 2013.

include elevated IOP, which—in infants and young children with ocular tissues susceptible to stretching—causes one or more of the classic clinical triad of tearing, photophobia, and blepharospasm, in response to corneal enlargement with Descemet tears (Haab striae) and resultant corneal edema and scarring. Other, sometimes less clinically obvious, ocular changes include axial elongation with progressive myopia, and optic nerve damage, which occur in affected children of all ages and may lead to mild or profound vision loss. Multifactorial causes of blindness include corneal scarring, high refractive errors, optic nerve damage (cupping and loss of ganglion cells and axons), amblyopia in asymmetric cases, cataract, and even retinal detachment.

OCT Features

OCT has revolutionized the evaluation and management of glaucoma in cooperative children with a sufficiently clear visual axis, enough visual function to allow fixation, and absent or mild nystagmus by providing detailed quantifiable measurement of the peripapillary retinal nerve fiber layer (RNFL) as well as macular thickness.[2,3] There are important considerations and limitations to the use of OCT in the diagnosis and monitoring of children at risk for or with glaucoma. Relative obstacles to using OCT to definitively differentiate between normal and glaucomatous optic nerves in children include the wide range of normal values for optic nerve parameters on OCT for children of different ages and ethnicities and the limited normative data for various time-domain OCT (TD-OCT) and spectral-domain OCT (SD-OCT) imaging devices. Nonetheless, this noninvasive imaging modality has proven to be tremendously useful for establishing an objective baseline for a given child.

THREE MAIN PARAMETERS FOR THE DETECTION OF GLAUCOMATOUS LOSS

These include measures of the circumperipapillary retinal nerve fiber layer (cpRNFL) (parameters available on the Cirrus and Spectralis), the optic nerve head (parameters, such as rim area, disc area, average cup-to-disc ratio, cup volume available on the Cirrus), and the perimacular "ganglion cell complex" (parameters available on the Cirrus and Spectralis).[4] An OCT baseline for the RNFL and macular thickness can now be longitudinally monitored for change, in both a pediatric glaucoma suspect without treatment and in a known and treated pediatric glaucoma case for verification of optic nerve head stability (or deterioration) over time.[5] To directly measure and quantify RNFL thickness, OCT calculates the area between the internal limiting membrane (ILM) and the RNFL border; however, the RNFL edge determination varies among machines. These determination algorithms are not interchangeable among machines, and thus one cannot compare RNFL measurements among different types of OCT devices. More recently, segmentation of the ganglion cell complex has also become available, although its use in children is still in its infancy.[6]

ACQUISITION TIME AND EYE TRACKING

The advancement from TD-OCT to SD-OCT has revolutionized RNFL imaging in children by allowing for faster imaging acquisition from an average 400 A-scans per second in the standard Stratus TD-OCT (Carl Zeiss Meditec, Jena, Germany) to 18,000 to 50,000 A-scans per second in SD/Fourier-domain OCT devices, such as Cirrus HD-OCT (Carl Zeiss Meditec) and Spectralis SD-OCT (Heidelberg Engineering, Heidelberg, Germany).[7,8] For children, the Spectralis SD-OCT device may be preferred over the Cirrus HD-OCT device because Spectralis has a dual-beam eye-tracking system that allows for more accurate reproducibility of scan location between images and an eye tracker that averages multiple B-scan images to help eliminate motion artifact, thus increasing the potential for a quality image in a wiggly child.[9]

LACK OF A COMPLETE NORMATIVE DATABASE FOR CHILDREN AND VARIATION IN NORMAL PARAMETERS AMONG CHILDREN OF DIFFERENT AGES AND RACES/ETHNICITIES

Like most ophthalmologic imaging analysis software products, the built-in comparison algorithm in OCT is based on a normative database for adults. For example, the Spectralis unit includes only white adults ages 18 to 78 years, mean age 48.2 +/− 14.5 years (Spectralis HRA + OCT 510(k) Summary 2012, FDA). Various studies have attempted to establish normative values for peripapillary RNFL and macular thickness in the pediatric population; however, an analysis software package for these age groups has yet to be designed for any OCT machine. El-Dairi et al. published a normative pediatric RNFL database obtained by using measurements from the Stratus TD-OCT device.[10] These authors examined 286 healthy children, ages 3 to 17 years, with a near-equal proportion of black (114) and white (154) participants. Their data showed that in the older age group (11-17 years), black children had a larger optic nerve head cup-to-disc ratio and average cup area. Black children were also found to have a higher superior peripapillary RNFL thickness across all age groups compared with white children. Yanni et al. published a more recent study of 83 healthy, mostly non-Hispanic white, North American children ages 5 to 15 years, by using the Spectralis SD-OCT device.[11] They reported mean peripapillary RNFL thickness of 107.6 +/− 1.2 μm, thicker than previously reported in adults (97.2 +/− 9.7 μm), which, they concluded, resulted from a known negative correlation of peripapillary RNFL thickness with advancing age.[11,12] Average macular thickness was reported as 271.2 +/− 2.0 μm, similar to adult data.[12] Without a built-in pediatric normative database for these commercial OCT units, peripapillary RNFL measurements in children are best studied for longitudinal change as opposed to a one-time initial measurement. Table 70.3 provides a quick reference for the previous studys' peripapillary RNFL data on normal pediatric subjects.

Childhood Glaucoma Assessment with OCT

In evaluating the SD-OCT images of the eyes of a child with possible glaucoma, it is important to consider global parameters, such as the average RNFL, as well as the pattern of both peripapillary

TABLE 70.3 ■ **Variability of Pediatric Peripapillary RNFL Thickness (microns) in Normal Children per OCT Device**

	Spectralis OCT (SEM)[11]	Stratus OCT[10]
Global	107.6 (1.2)	108
S		143
NS	116.2 (2.8)	
N	84.5 (1.9)	83
NI	125.4 (3)	
I		129
TI	147.0 (2.1)	
T	76.5 (1.9)	78
TS	145.1 (2.2)	

Note: Numbers given in table are mean peripapillary RNFL in microns across the entire study population, with SEM given when available from both the Spectralis OCT (Heidelberg Engineering) and Stratus OCT (OCT-3, Carl Zeiss Meditec) studies by Yanni et al.[11] and El-Dairi et al.[10]

G, Global average; I, inferior; N, nasal; NI, nasal–inferior; NS, nasal–superior; OCT, optical coherence tomography; RNFL, retinal nerve fiber layer; S, superior; SEM, standard error of the mean; T, temporal; TI, temporal–inferior; TS, temporal–superior.

Adapted from: Yanni SE, Wang J, Cheng CS, et al. Normative reference ranges for the retinal nerve fiber layer, macula, and retinal layer thicknesses in children. Am J Ophthalmol. 2013;155(2):354-360.e351; El-Dairi MA, Asrani SG, Enyedi LB, Freedman SF. Optical coherence tomography in the eyes of normal children. Arch Ophthalmol. 2009;127(1):50-58.

RNFL and macular thickness. For example, uniformity within one eye and symmetry of both eyes can confirm that a child with large optic nerve cups and a normal/average RNFL has physiologic cupping and can, therefore, be safely monitored for progression without treatment (assuming normal IOP and otherwise normal ocular findings) (Fig. 70.1).

The RNFL is thinned with glaucomatous optic nerve damage (Fig. 70.2). Sometimes the damage is focal, but at other times, it is global. The average RNFL is a good overall measure of optic nerve health in a pediatric patient with glaucoma, with changes of approximately 6 to 10 microns considered significant enough to warrant concern in a quality scan.[13,14] Spectralis OCT also provides a change report, whereby it shows graphically the location and amount of significant loss in RNFL thickness from a preselected baseline measurement of peripapillary RNFL, shown as a red area (see Fig. 70.2A juvenile open-angle glaucoma [JOAG]) Additionally, comparison of the macular thickness map within one eye and between both eyes can be a confirmatory sign of health (see Fig. 70.1B) or glaucomatous damage (see Fig. 70.2B JOAG) although nonglaucomatous causes of macular thickness increase has to be ruled out (see following section).

Pitfalls in Childhood Glaucoma Assessment with OCT

RNFL TOO THIN FOR ACCURATE GLAUCOMA ASSESSMENT

Segmentation of RNFL thickness in both adult and pediatric populations can be more difficult in the late stages of glaucoma. A study by Chan et al. showed that the RNFL level in patients with end-stage glaucomatous optic atrophy and no light perception vision did not fall below 30 μm.[15] This so-called floor effect is believed to be a fault of segmentation algorithms that cannot differentiate RNFL from glial tissue.[16] This effect may limit the ability to monitor RNFL loss in advanced cases of glaucomatous optic atrophy. In these cases, other parameters, such as visual field status, are more sensitive and reliable for monitoring stability or progression over time (Fig. 70.3A and B). Ganglion cell layer (GCL) segmentation analysis may be useful in monitoring progression when the RNFL has reached a plateau, but this modality is still limited by the fact that the segmentation software can generate significant error in the setting of a very thin GCL layer.

BAD TRACING

OCT images of poor quality can result from numerous causes when imaging children. Among them are motion artifact (especially in cases of poor vision and nystagmus) (Fig. 70.4A and B); impediments to a clear visual axis, including corneal or lens opacities; and poorly dilating pupils. Additionally, eyes with a very thin RNFL are difficult to segment accurately (see Fig. 70.3B).

Segmentation errors can also occur as a result of poor automated tracing around the retinal blood vessels embedded within the RNFL, making it difficult to delineate the RNFL boundaries in these areas. Recently Ye et al. demonstrated that in advanced glaucoma cases (defined by Humphrey visual field mean deviation criteria of ≤12 dB and found to have average mean cpRNFL 51.9 +/− 11.65 μm by Spectralis SD-OCT), there was a 15% chance of segmentation error believed to be secondary to the increased proportion of retinal blood vessels of up to 24.9% in these cases of severe RNFL thinning.[16] Thus careful inspection of automated RNFL tracing in comparison with the examiner's assessment of RNFL reflectivity, averaged on the OCT B-scan, should be performed especially in those cases of advanced glaucomatous optic atrophy to avoid the RNFL assessment showing falsely elevated values (see Fig. 70.3A and B)

CUPPING REVERSAL

Optic nerve head cupping reversal after marked IOP reduction in pediatric glaucoma is widely known. OCT has been used to investigate RNFL thickness as it relates to this phenomenon.

For many years, it was believed that cupping reversal indicated an improvement of glaucomatous optic nerve damage with successful treatment of childhood glaucoma; however, recent work has suggested that initial cupping of the optic nerve on pediatric glaucoma presentation likely reflects true damage to the RNFL and not just compliance of the optic nerve head tissues themselves.[17] In the case of cupping reversal, OCT, rather than optic nerve clinical appearance, may more accurately represent the optic nerve health after successful glaucoma surgery (see Fig. 70.3C)

Nonglaucomatous OCT Abnormalities that Can Be Mistaken for Glaucomatous Change

In general, any other coexisting abnormalities on OCT imaging, including the presence of inner nuclear layer cysts, cystoid macular edema, outer retinal and photoreceptor loss, total retinal atrophy, pigment epithelial detachment with associated subretinal fluid, choroidal folds, or inner segment ellipsoid (ISE) disruption, should raise suspicion for *nonglaucomatous atrophy* and the need for further workup.[18] When glaucoma is secondary, other retinal pathology, such as retinal cysts or macular edema, can actually artefactually thicken the RNFL and macula, masking glaucomatous optic nerve damage (Fig. 70.5A and B).

1. Congenital optic nerve abnormality (see also Chapter 10)
   - Optic nerve hypoplasia may be focal and subtle and represent either a unilateral or bilateral loss in RNFL (Fig. 70.6). If the Bruch membrane opening is imaged with OCT in these cases, one would expect to see this opening smaller in optic nerve hypoplasia (see Chapter 10).
   - An optic nerve pit will show unilateral loss of the RNFL, typically in the temporal location. SD-OCT in the location of an optic pit may show a schisis-like separation between the outer and inner retinal layers, with or without subretinal fluid accumulation in this area.
   - An optic nerve coloboma may also be focal and subtle and typically represents a unilateral versus bilateral asymmetric RNFL loss, usually in the inferonasal quadrant.
   - Megalopapillae, or a congenitally anomalous large disc (area >2.5 mm^2), often is mistaken for a glaucomatous optic nerve because of its increased cup area, shape, and volume. As shown in Fig. 70.7, however, despite their abnormal appearance, these optic nerves contain normal RNFL thickness. If the OCT were to show the Bruch membrane opening, one would expect to see a wider opening in megalopapillae (see Fig. 70.7).

2. CNS pathology (see also Chapter 14)
   - A history of prematurity may include significant CNS disease, such as cerebral palsy, periventricular leukomalacia, history of intraventricular hemorrhage, hydrocephalus, and so on. These children may present with an enlarged cup-to-disc ratio secondary to postsynaptic degeneration of the optic pathways. In the premature child who fits this scenario and who is able to sit for a tabletop SD-OCT, the OCT may show worrisome thinning of both the RNFL and macular thickness.[19] Serial SD-OCT examination is warranted, but this thinning may remain stable over time and is unlikely to represent true glaucoma (Fig. 70.8).
   - Optic nerve gliomas, most of them secondary to NF-I in this age group, can present with optic cupping or atrophy that shows typically unilateral or asymmetric RNFL thinning. In this setting, one needs to obtain a thorough history for first-degree relatives with an NF-I diagnosis, multiple café au lait spots and to perform an ophthalmic examination as thoroughly as possible, looking for any signs of low vision, decreased color vision, afferent pupillary defects, presence of Lisch nodules, IOP, and eyelid abnormalities. There should be a low threshold for neuroimaging in any case of significant asymmetric or unilateral RNFL thinning with a positive history as listed previously or other signs of NF-I.

CNS pathology of any kind that affects the optic pathways enough to cause significant visual field loss may also show up as RNFL thinning on OCT. One should beware findings that suggest a homonymous hemianopia or bitemporal loss (Chapter 67).

Ancillary Testing

Although OCT is very useful as a tool for diagnosis and monitoring of children with known and suspected glaucoma, there is no substitute for the clinical examination. In the case of children, this includes not only other features of the eye examination but also examination of the entire child to identify features that may either reassure or cause additional worry to the clinician.

Automated visual field testing is helpful in older cooperative children with adequate vision to perform reliable testing. This is useful, particularly for monitoring children who have advanced cupping and thinning of the RNFL on OCT and who may show progression on the visual field even after the RNFL has hit "bottom"(see Fig. 70.3A–C).

Many younger children can be successfully coaxed to allow tabletop SD-OCT imaging, even when visual field testing is completely unreliable because of poor fixation and concentration.

Photography can also be helpful for baseline optic nerve documentation in children with glaucoma, but reversal of optic nerve cupping, although it indicates control of IOP, may not represent true recovery of damaged optic nerve axons or lost visual field (see above section on "Cupping Reversal", and Fig. 70.3C).

Axial length measurement can be very useful in young children, even more so than corneal diameter measurement, in monitoring for adequate IOP control.

Simple cycloplegic refraction, in itself, can serve as a good surrogate for ocular enlargement and should be monitored regularly in children with glaucoma.

Treatment

The treatment of childhood glaucoma usually includes surgical and medical interventions aimed at reducing IOP and then managing other related problems, such as refractive error, amblyopia, strabismus, cataract, and low vision.

Future Advances in OCT for Pediatric Glaucoma

HANDHELD SD-OCT

Although handheld OCT imaging (Envisu C-2300; Leica Microsystems, Wetzlar, Germany) has shown promise for identifying optic atrophy in preterm infants[15] and for identifying and monitoring progression of optic atrophy secondary to optic nerve gliomas in patients with NF-I, data on its use are limited to allow for monitoring the progression of optic atrophy secondary to glaucoma. Currently, there is no available algorithm for purchase to analyze the RNFL thickness automatically.

SPECTRALIS FLEX MODULE

The Spectralis Flex Module (Heidelberg Engineering, Heidelberg, Germany) was designed for use in patients in the supine position. The Spectralis device is affixed to a flexible arm that is adjustable with respect to height and tilt. The Spectralis Flex module, not yet commercially available, should allow use of all Spectralis functions, including the same analysis software available for the tabletop version and is useful for imaging children who are unable to cooperate during tabletop imaging (see Fig. 70.4B).

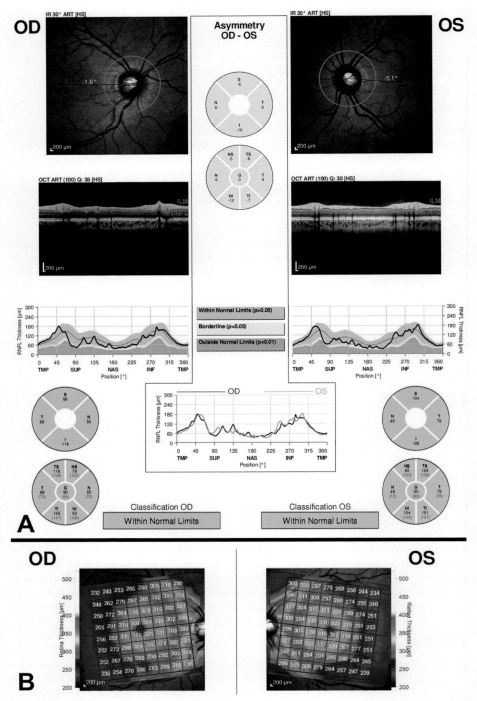

Fig. 70.1 (A,B) Physiologic cupping. This 12-year-old girl was referred for large optic nerve cups; she had intra-ocular pressure (IOP) values in the mid-teens and mild myopia but was otherwise healthy, with a negative family history. Heidelberg Spectralis spectral-domain optical coherence tomography (SD-OCT) imaging showed normal peripapillary retinal nerve fiber layer (RNFL) (average 90 µm OD and OS) (A) and macular segmentation mapping (B) in both eyes. She was followed over 2 years and continued to have stable IOP, RNFL measurements, and normal Humphrey visual field examinations.

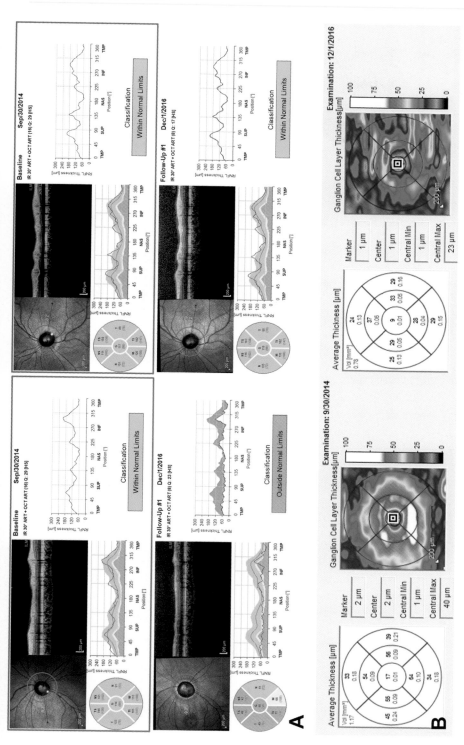

Fig. 70.2, cont'd (A-C) Glaucoma suspect turned juvenile open-angle glaucoma (JOAG) over a 2-year interval.

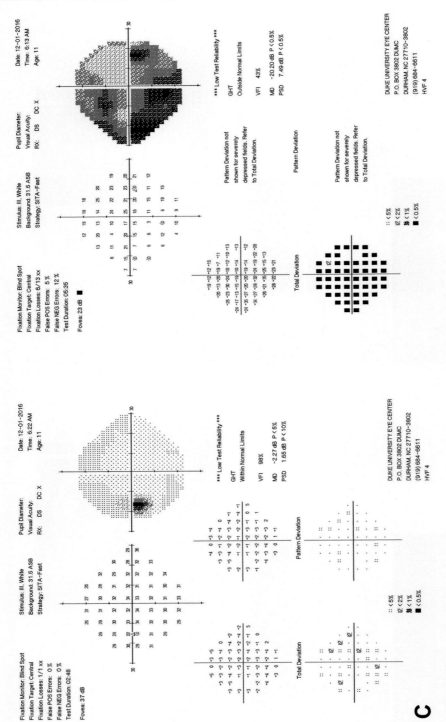

Fig. 70.2, cont'd (A–C) Glaucoma suspect turned juvenile open-angle glaucoma (JOAG) over a 2-year interval.

Fig. 70.2, cont'd (A–C) Glaucoma suspect turned juvenile open-angle glaucoma (JOAG) over a 2-year interval. This 11-year old boy was seen with mild myopia, healthy "phys-iologic" optic nerve cups and intraocular pressure (IOP) in the low 20s with central corneal thickness (CCT) in the high 500s, and a negative family history. Heidelberg Spectralis spectral-domain optical coherence tomography (SD-OCT) imaging showed normal retinal nerve fiber layer (RNFL) in both eyes (average OD 114 μm, OS 112 μm) (top of figure A).

He was recommended to have a diurnal curve and follow-up in 6 months with his own eye care provider. He was lost to follow-up for 2 years, returning to his eye doctor with IOP in the low 30s and treated with travoprost. Upon return to Duke University, he had IOP (Goldmann applanation tonometry [GAT]) OD 26 mm Hg, OS 24 mm Hg, with progression of his myopia, and dramatic increase in cupping OD with loss of RNFL OD, but stable RNFL OS. SD-OCT RNFL scan showed huge asymmetry of cupping, as well as a decline in OD RNFL average (from 114 to 70) but not OS (112 versus 113) (bottom of figure A).

Segmentation of the macular OCT scans demonstrated thinning of the ganglion cell layer from initial presentation to the follow-up 2 years later, correlating well with loss of the RNFL and overall macular thickness in the right eye (B).

Humphrey visual field (HVF) showed glaucomatous loss OD, not OS (C). Magnetic resonance imaging (MRI) was done to rule out central nervous system (CNS) pathology, given the asymmetry and the rapidity of loss OD (normal brain and orbits). The boy required surgical as well as medical therapy to control his glaucoma.

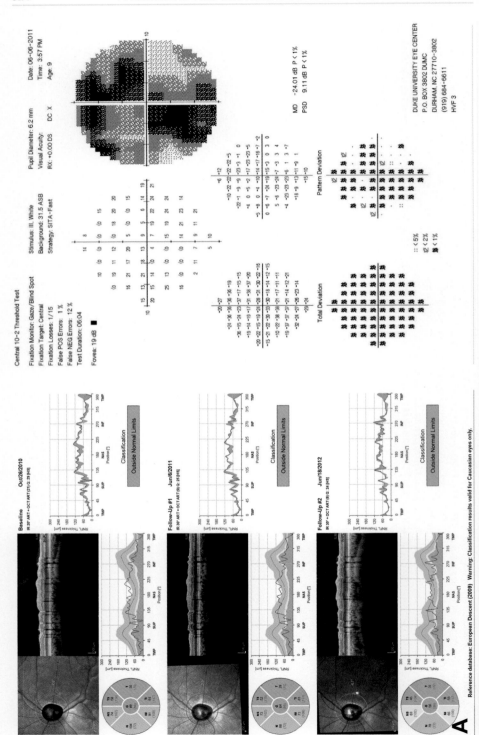

Fig. 70.3, cont'd (A–C) Severe juvenile open-angle glaucoma (JOAG) with very thin retinal nerve fiber layer (RNFL), demonstrating difficulty with accurate autosegmentation tracing and need to monitor visual fields rather than the extremely thin RNFL by using OCT alone.

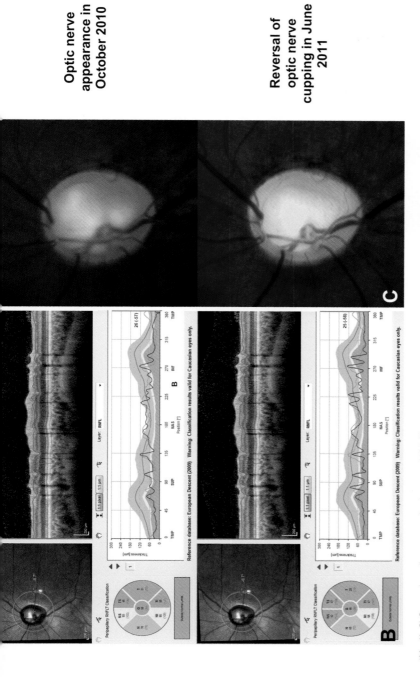

Optic nerve appearance in October 2010

Reversal of optic nerve cupping in June 2011

Fig. 70.3, cont'd (A–C) Severe juvenile open-angle glaucoma (JOAG) with very thin retinal nerve fiber layer (RNFL), demonstrating difficulty with accurate autosegmentation tracing and need to monitor visual fields rather than the extremely thin RNFL by using OCT alone. This 9-year-old boy presented with a failed vision screen and had corrected vision 20/200 OS with intraocular pressure (IOP) 43 mm Hg, total cup, and very thin RNFL. Although 360-degree trabeculotomy and medication controlled the IOP in the range of 10 mm Hg, monitoring the very thin RNFL over time was problematic, making visual field testing more reliable as a method to demonstrate stability (A). His very thin RNFL also made accurate segmentation of the remaining RNFL difficult (B). The top spectral domain optical coherence tomography (SD-OCT) image demonstrates the uncorrected scan, with average RNFL 63 μm, which, when corrected for faulty segmentation caused by the very thin RNFL (bottom image), was actually even lower (about 48). The very cupped left optic nerve did demonstrate mild cupping reversal (C) but the RNFL, macular thickness, and visual fields showed no recovery (not shown).

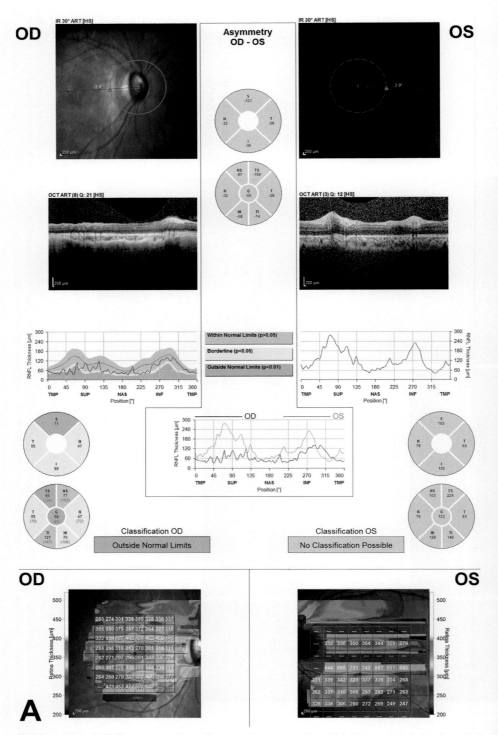

Fig. 70.4, cont'd (A,B) Glaucoma suspect with poor patient cooperation with tabletop spectral-domain optical coherence tomography (SD-OCT); there was improved imaging possible with FLEX scanning under anesthesia during strabismus surgery.

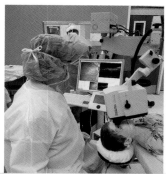

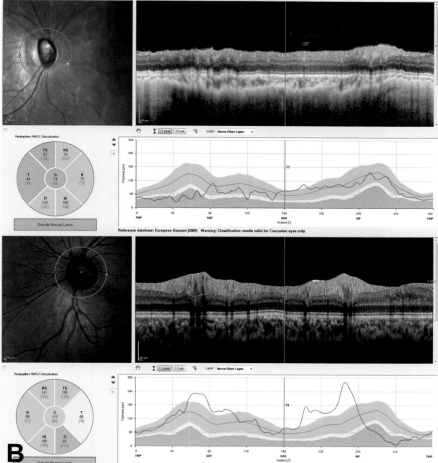

Fig. 70.4, cont'd (A,B) Glaucoma suspect with poor patient cooperation with tabletop spectral-domain optical coherence tomography (SD-OCT); there was improved imaging possible with FLEX scanning under anesthesia during strabismus surgery.

This 11-year-old girl born at 34 weeks' gestation, had a controlled seizure disorder, unilateral high myopia in the right eye, exotropia of the right eye, and enlarged optic nerve cups in both eyes with high normal intraocular pressure (IOP); she underwent baseline tabletop SD-OCT (Spectralis), attempted for determining baseline retinal nerve fiber layer (RNFL) and macular thickness (A). Although tabletop scanning was of limited value because of poor patient cooperation, the FLEX arm provided the opportunity for better-quality baseline RNFL scanning during anesthesia at planned strabismus surgery for her exotropia (B).

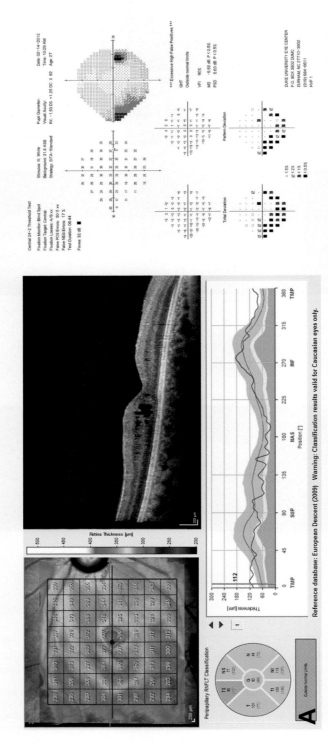

Fig. 70.5, cont'd (A,B) Uveitic glaucoma with cystic changes of the macular retina superimposed on glaucomatous thinning of the retinal nerve fiber layer (RNFL), and macula in the right eye.

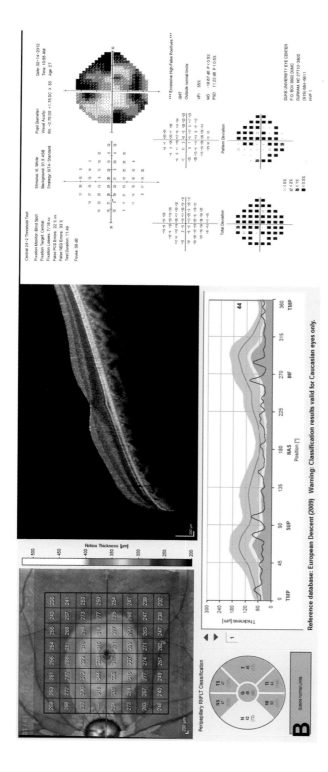

Fig. 70.5, cont'd (A,B) Uveitic glaucoma with cystic changes of the macular retina superimposed on glaucomatous thinning of the retinal nerve fiber layer (RNFL) and macula in the right eye. Severe uveitic glaucoma (juvenile idiopathic arthritis and uveitis) in a patient with persistent retinal thickening after severe cystoid macular edema (CME) prompted by secondary intraocular lens (IOL) OD; best vision is OD 20/125, OS 20/20, with intraocular pressure (IOP) in the low teens after multiple glaucoma surgeries. Heidelberg spectral-domain optical coherence tomography (SD-OCT) showed RNFL with mild thinning (overall 92 μm) OD versus very severe thinning (46 μm) OS (A right eye, B left eye). Macular SD-OCT showed artifactual thickening of the macula caused by persistent cystic changes and TD-OCT showed frank CME, which first occurred 9 years earlier OD. (A, left image). By contrast, the OS showed expected thinning throughout from glaucoma (B, left image). Note that despite the rather "preserved" RNFL OD, there is a visual field defect suggesting that the retinal thickening may extend to affect the RNFL measurement OD as well (A, right image).

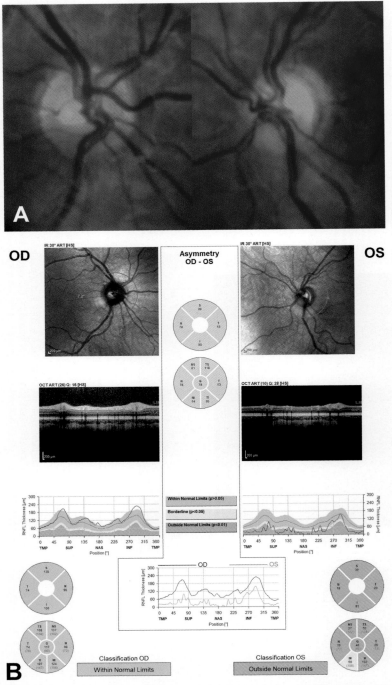

Fig. 70.6 (A,B) Optic nerve hypoplasia presenting as amblyopia left eye, discovered on pediatric vision screening. This 7-year-old girl presented for evaluation and treatment of poor vision caused by amblyopia OS. Past ocular, medical, and family histories were unremarkable. Examination revealed best corrected vision OD 20/20, OS 20/200, possible trace left afferent pupillary defect, intraocular pressure (IOP) OD 15 mm Hg, OS 16 mm Hg (by rebound tonometry), minimal refractive error, no strabismus, fundus showing optic nerve hypoplasia (A). Heidelberg Spectralis spectral-domain optical coherence tomography (SD-OCT) showed normal retinal nerve fiber layer (RNFL) OD, very thin OS (OD 117 μm, OS 40 μm) (B), macular scan artefact (not shown).

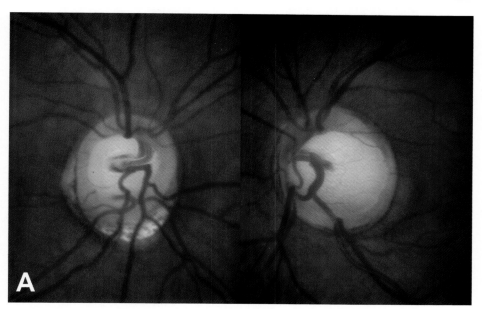

Fig. 70.7, cont'd (A-C) Megalopapilla.

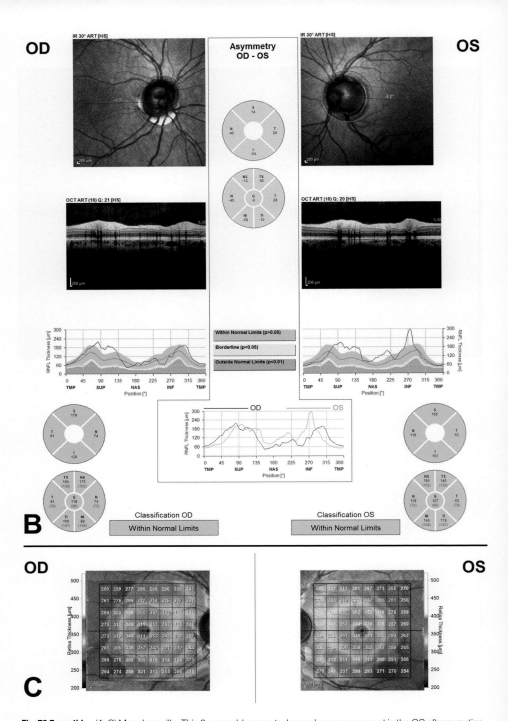

Fig. 70.7, cont'd (A-C) Megalopapilla. This 9-year-old presented as a glaucoma suspect in the OS after a routine eye examination showed asymmetry of optic nerve cupping (OS >OD), and elevated intraocular pressure (IOP) by noncontact tonometry (OD 19 mm Hg, OS 23 mm Hg). Past ocular history, medical history, and family history unremarkable. Examination revealed vision without correction 20/20 OU, intraocular pressure (IOP) OD 13 mm Hg, OS 15 mm Hg, central corneal thickness OD 605 um, OS 607 μm, large optic nerve head with inferior anomalous branching OD, even larger optic nerve head OS with absent inferior rim; cup-to-disc ratio 0.7 horizontal (h) × 0.85 vertical (v) OD, 0.9 h × 0.85 v OS (A). Heidelberg Spectralis SD-OCT showed normal retinal nerve fiber layer (RNFL) OD (average 118 μm OD, 127 μm OS) (B). Macular thickness was normal OU (C).

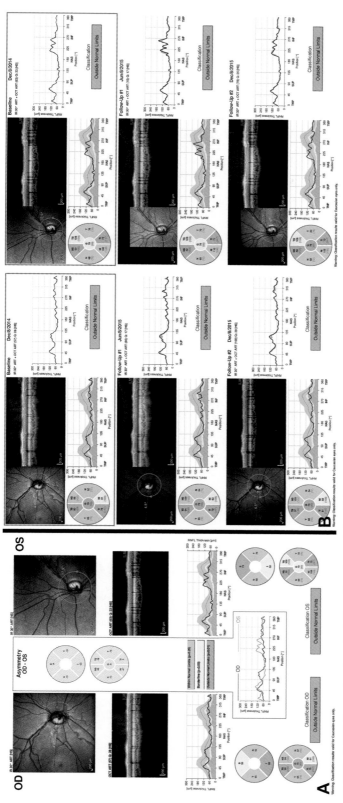

Fig. 70.8 (A,B) Optic nerve head cupping in the setting of prematurity with intraventricular hemorrhage. This 7-year old girl presented for evaluation of optic nerve head cupping. She was a twin born at 31 weeks' estimated gestational age, weighing 1230 g. While in the neonatal intensive care unit, she was diagnosed with a grade I intraventricular hemorrhage as well as stage 3 retinopathy of prematurity (ROP) requiring bilateral peripheral retinal laser photocoagulation. On initial examination, her vision was correctable to 20/20 OU with a mild myopic astigmatic correction, intraocular pressure (IOP) was 13 mm Hg in both eyes and optic nerve head cupping was estimated at 0.9 height (h) × 0.85 vertical (v) in both eyes. Heidelberg Spectralis SD-OCT showed thin, but relatively symmetric retinal nerve fiber layer (RNFL) OU (average 70 μm OD, 79 μm OS). (A) Observation over 1 year with serial IOP checks and repeat optical coherence tomography (OCT) imaging showed stable IOP and stable RNFL (B).

References

1. Beck AD, Chang TCP, Definition Freedman SF. Classification, Differential Diagnosis. In: Weinreb RN, Grajewski AL, Papadopoulos M, Grigg J, Freedman S, eds. *Childhood Glaucoma: Consensus Series 9. Amsterdam: Kugler.* 2013:3–10.
2. El-Dairi MA, Holgado S, Asrani S, Enyedi L, Freedman S. Correlation between Optical Coherence Tomography and glaucomatous optic nerve head damage in children. *Br J Ophthalmol.* 2009;93 (10):1325–1330.
3. Hess DB, Asrani SG, Bhide MG, Enyedi LB, Stinnett SS, Freedman SF. Macular and retinal nerve fiber layer analysis of normal and glaucomatous eyes in children using optical coherence tomography. *Am J Ophthalmol.* 2005;139(3):509–517.
4. Bussel II, Wollstein G, Schuman JS. OCT for glaucoma diagnosis, screening and detection of glaucoma progression. *Br J Ophthalmol.* 2014;98(suppl 2):ii15–ii19.
5. Ghasia FF, El-Dairi M, Freedman SF, Rajani A, Asrani S. Reproducibility of spectral-domain optical coherence tomography measurements in adult and pediatric glaucoma. *J Glaucoma.* 2015;24 (1):55–63.
6. Silverstein E, Freedman S, Zéhil GP, Jiramongkolchai K, El-Dairi M. The macula in pediatric glaucoma: quantifying the inner and outer layers via optical coherence tomography automatic segmentation. *J AAPOS.* 2016;20(4):332–336.
7. Reichel E, Ho J, Duker JS. *OCT Units: Which One is Right for Me? Rev Ophthalmol.* Available at https://www.reviewofophthalmology.com/article/oct-units-which-one-is-right-for-me; September 23, 2009.
8. Nassif N, Cense B, Park BH, et al. In vivo human retinal imaging by ultrahigh-speed spectral domain optical coherence tomography. *Opt lett.* 2004;29(5):480–482.
9. Menke MN, Dabov S, Knecht P, Sturm V. Reproducibility of retinal thickness measurements in healthy subjects using Spectralis optical coherence tomography. *Am J Ophthalmol.* 2009;147(3):467–472.
10. El-Dairi MA, Asrani SG, Enyedi LB, Freedman SF. Optical coherence tomography in the eyes of normal children. *Arch Ophthalmol.* 2009;127(1):50–58.
11. Yanni SE, Wang J, Cheng CS, et al. Normative reference ranges for the retinal nerve fiber layer, macula, and retinal layer thicknesses in children. *Am J Ophthalmol.* 2013;155(2):354–360 e351.
12. Bendschneider D, Tornow RP, Horn FK, et al. Retinal nerve fiber layer thickness in normals measured by spectral domain OCT. *J Glaucoma.* 2010;19(7):475–482.
13. Leung CK, Cheung CY, Weinreb RN, et al. Evaluation of retinal nerve fiber layer progression in glaucoma: a study on optical coherence tomography guided progression analysis. *Invest Ophthalmol Vis Sci.* 2010;51 (1):217–222.
14. Paunescu LA, Schuman JS, Price LL, et al. Reproducibility of nerve fiber thickness, macular thickness, and optic nerve head measurements using Stratus OCT. *Invest Ophthalmol Vis Sci.* 2004;45(6):1716–1724.
15. Chan CK, Miller NR. Peripapillary nerve fiber layer thickness measured by optical coherence tomography in patients with no light perception from long-standing nonglaucomatous optic neuropathies. *J Neuroophthalmol.* 2007;27(3):176–179.
16. Ye C, Yu M, Leung CK. Impact of segmentation errors and retinal blood vessels on retinal nerve fibre layer measurements using spectral-domain optical coherence tomography. *Acta Ophthalmol.* 2016;94(3): e211–e219.
17. Ely AL, El-Dairi MA, Freedman SF. Cupping reversal in pediatric glaucoma–evaluation of the retinal nerve fiber layer and visual field. *Am J Ophthalmol.* 2014;158(5):905–915.
18. Oct Lee H, Proudlock FA, Gottlob I. Pediatric Optical Coherence Tomography in Clinical Practice-Recent Progress. *Invest Ophthalmol Vis Sci.* 2016;57(9):69–79.
19. Rothman AL, Sevilla MB, Mangalesh S, et al. Thinner Retinal Nerve Fiber Layer in Very Preterm Versus Term Infants and Relationship to Brain Anatomy and Neurodevelopment. *Am J Ophthalmol.* 2015;160 (6):1296–1308.

Note: Page numbers followed by *f* indicate figures and *t* indicate tables.

Choroidal tuberculoma, 174
Choroidal vasculature
definition of, 63
development of, 63–64
Choroideremia
ancillary testing of, 127
brain connection of, 124
clinical features of
nonocular, 124
ocular, 125
OCT features of, 126, 126*f*
treatment of, 127
Circular/annular scans, for peripapillary RFNL
measurements, 23–24, 25*f*
Circumscribed choroidal hemangioma, 227–229
ancillary testing for, 227–229
brain connection and, 227
clinical features of, 227, 228*f*
OCT features of, 227, 229*f*
treatment for, 229
Clinic
image capture in, OCT, 18–27
OCTA image capture in, 18–27, 26*f*
optimizing systems and setup for OCT,
of children and infants in, 10–11, 10–11*f*
CME. *See* Cystoid macular edema
CNV membrane, and chorioretinal coloboma,
259–260, 259*f*
Coats disease, Coats plus syndrome and, 149–153
after treatment of, 152, 152*f*
ancillary testing of, 152, 153*f*
brain connection of, 149
clinical features of, 149–150, 150*f*
exudates and crystals of, 150
fibrotic nodule of, 151
intraretinal cystoid spaces of, 150
OCT features of, 150
retinal detachment of, 151
retinal layers and retinal thinning of, 151
treatment of, 153
vascular lesions of, 150, 151*f*
Coloboma, chorioretinal, 256–260
ancillary testing for, 258*f*, 260
brain connection and, 256–257
clinical features of, 257, 257–259*f*
CNV membrane and, 259–260, 259*f*
OCT features of, 257–258, 257–259*f*
retinal detachment and, 258*f*, 259
treatment for, 260
Combined hamartoma of the retina, 233–237
ancillary test for, 234
brain connection in, 233
clinical features of, 233, 234–236*f*
OCT features of, 234
treatment for, 235–237

Commotio retinae, 205–209
ancillary testing for, 208
clinical features of, 205, 206*f*
OCT features of, 206–208, 207–208*f*
treatment for, 209
Computed tomography (CT)
for ocular injury, 200
for papilledema, 303
Computed tomography venography (CTV), for
papilledema, 303
Congenital cerebral toxoplasmosis, 163
Congenital hypertrophy, of retinal pigment
epithelium, 247–250
ancillary testing for, 250, 250*f*
clinical features of, 247–248, 248*f*
OCT features of, 248–249, 249*f*
treatment for, 250
Congenital syphilis, 163
Congenital Zika syndrome, 163
Contrast magnetic resonance imaging (MRI), for
optic neuritis, 306
Conventional retinal photography, of coats disease, 152
Corneal curvature, of pediatric eye, 7
Corticosteroids, for Vogt-Koyanagi Harada
syndrome, 185
Crystals, of coats disease, 150
CSF diversion procedure, in papilledema, 303
CTV. *See* Computed tomography venography
Cube scan, 19–22, 20–22*f*
Cystoid hyporeflective spaces, 150
Cystoid macular edema (CME), 178–183
ancillary testing of, 182
brain connection of, 178
clinical features of, 178–180, 179–180*f*
OCT features of, 180–182, 181–183*f*
treatment of, 182–183
Cystoid spaces
intraretinal, 134
in optic atrophy, 293–294
Cytomegalovirus (CMV) retinitis, 166, 166*f*

D

DCP. *See* Deep capillary plexus
Declaration of Helsinki, 85
Deep capillary plexus (DCP), 42*t*
Deep vascular complex (DVC), 42*t*
DICOM. *See* Digital Imaging and Communications
in Medicine
Diffuse choroidal hemangioma, 223–226
ancillary testing for, 223
brain connection with, 223
clinical features of, 223, 224*f*
OCT features of, 223, 225*f*
treatment for, 224–225